Refractory Migraine

Refractory Migraine

Mechanisms and Management

Edited by

Elliott A. Schulman, MD, FACP
Department of Neurology
Jefferson School of Medicine
Lankenau Institute for Medical Research
Wynnewood, PA

Morris Levin, MD
Section of Neurology
Dartmouth-Hitchcock Medical Center
Lebanon, NH

Alvin E. Lake, III, PhD, BCIAC-SF
Division Director of Behavioral Medicine
Michigan Head-Pain & Neurological Institute
Ann Arbor, MI

Elizabeth Loder, MD, MPH
Division of Headache and Pain
Department of Neurology
Brigham and Women's/Faulkner Hospitals
Boston, MA

OXFORD
UNIVERSITY PRESS
2010

OXFORD
UNIVERSITY PRESS

Oxford University Press, Inc., publishes works that further
Oxford University's objective of excellence
in research, scholarship, and education.

Oxford New York
Auckland Cape Town Dar es Salaam Hong Kong Karachi
Kuala Lumpur Madrid Melbourne Mexico City Nairobi
New Delhi Shanghai Taipei Toronto

With offices in
Argentina Austria Brazil Chile Czech Republic France Greece
Guatemala Hungary Italy Japan Poland Portugal Singapore
South Korea Switzerland Thailand Turkey Ukraine Vietnam

Published by Oxford University Press, Inc.
198 Madison Avenue, New York, New York 10016
www.oup.com

Cover description: Käthe Kollwitz, Self-Portrait, Hand at the Forehead (Selbstbildnis mit der Hand an der Stirn), Kn 109 (Kl 106), Before mid-June, 1910 ?, Line etching and drypoint (a few etching spots appear like sandpaper), Käthe Kollwitz Museum Köln /©/ Artist Rights Society 2010.

Library of Congress Cataloging-in-Publication Data
Refractory migraine : mechanisms and management / edited by Elliot A. Schulman . . . [et al.].
p. ; cm.
Includes bibliographical references and index.
ISBN 978-0-19-539469-6 (alk. paper)
1. Migraine. I. Schulman, Elliot A.
[DNLM: 1. Migraine Disorders—therapy. 2. Migraine Disorders—diagnosis. WL 344 R332 2010]
RC392.R44 2010
616.8'4912—dc22 2009043872

9 8 7 6 5 4 3 2 1

Printed in the United States of America
on acid-free paper

To Bonnie, who encouraged me and who never had a doubt

– Elliott Schulman

To my wife Karen, who keeps putting up with my projects

– Mo Levin

To my wife Leslie Briggs, whose sense of humor, constant love and affection has kept me sane

– Al Lake

To my sister Karin, brother-in-law Mark, and delightful nephews Karl and Peter Otness

– Elizabeth Loder

Introduction

Headache experts have long recognized that a distinct subgroup of headache patients remains refractory to treatment. There is a long history of interest in the topic, but focused discussion is relatively recent. The area of refractory headache has gained visibility as a result of two recent physician surveys on the subject, a special section in the journal Headache devoted to refractory migraine (RM), and the formulation of a provisional definition for RM. However, refractory headache remains a frontier in headache management. The epidemiology and pathophysiology are poorly understood, the definition is still untested, and there is no consensus on "best practices" for treating these very needy patients. So, attempting a complete text on the subject may seem ambitious. Despite this, we have attempted to address the need for a systematic resource for RM by selecting authors who have particular expertise in key areas of the field.

The book is divided into three sections. The first section, "Definition, Epidemiology, Mechanisms and Diagnosis," addresses the history of the concept, definition, and classification of RM, as well as risk factors, epidemiology, postulated mechanisms, and approaches to accurate diagnosis. The second section, "Treatment," is devoted to management of these disorders. Pharmacological, physical, psychological, and alternative/complementary approaches are covered as well as treatment in the special populations of children, elderly, and lactating and pregnant women. The lack of firm evidence behind the recommended treatments is kept clearly in mind, with the hope that data will begin to emerge as RM is studied. Medication overuse, a highly significant problem in the refractory headache population, is addressed in this section along with inpatient treatment options. The third section, "Special Topics," includes a selection of information, suggestions, advice about issues of great import to refractory headache patients, but we think the concepts discussed in this section are applicable to all headache patients.

This book is designed to fill a growing need by the clinicians and researchers active in treating and investigating refractory headache for a comprehensive text. We hope that this book will serve to stimulate further discussion and research in the field, which will, in turn, lead to better understanding and treatment of this group of headache sufferers.

Acknowledgments

We are indebted to the many chapter authors who made this book possible. Their vision, hard work and support have made this first text devoted to Refractory Headache a meaningful one.

We would also like to thank all of our mentors who showed us the way. Their experience, insights and passion allowed headache to be seen as a legitimate medical problem.

We also express our thanks to Craig Panner at Oxford University Press and Jais K. Alphonse at Glyph International, for their unfailing encouragement and confidence in this book.

Finally, and most importantly, this book is dedicated to all our patients, past and future, whom we hope this book will serve.

Contents

Contributors

Avi Ashkenazi, MD
Doylestown Hospital
Doylestown, PA

Marcelo E. Bigal, MD, PhD
Department of Neurology
Global Director of Scientific Affairs
Division of Neuroscience
Merck Research Laboratories
Whitehouse Station, NJ

Stuart B. Black, MD
Chief of Neurology
Co-Director of the Neuroscience Center
Baylor University Medical Center at Dallas
Dallas, TX

Jonathan M. Borkum, PhD
Health Psych Maine
Waterville, ME

Roger K. Cady, MD
Founder and Consultant
Headache Care Center
Clinvest Research
Primary Care Network
Springfield, MO

Luzma Cardona, MD
Fellow, Headache Medicine
Graham Headache Center
Brigham and Women's/Faulkner Hospitals
Boston, MA

Kathleen Farmer, PsyD
Headache Care Center
Springfield, MO

Peter J. Goadsby, MBBS
Headache Group
Department of Neurology
University of California-San Francisco
San Francisco, CA

Steven Graff-Radford, DDS
Director, The Program for Headache and Orofacial Pain
Cedars-Sinai Medical Center
Los Angeles, CA

Phuu Pwint Han, DDS, PhD
Orofacial Pain and Oral Medicine Center
USC School of Dentistry
Los Angeles, CA

Richard Hargreaves, PhD
Department of Neuroscience
Merck Research Laboratories
West Point, PA

Andrew D. Hershey, MD, PhD, FAHS
Headache Center
Departments of Neurology and Pediatrics
Cincinnati Children's Hospital Medical Center
University of Cincinnati College of Medicine
Cincinnati, OH

Rigmor Jensen, MD, Dr. Med Sci
Professor Danish Headache Center
Department of Neurology, Glostrup Haspital
University of Copenhagen
Copenhagen, Denmark

Alvin E. Lake III, PhD, BCIAC-SF
Division Director of Behavioral Medicine
Michigan Head-Pain & Neurological Institute
Ann Arbor, MI

Morris Levin, MD
Department of Neurology
Dartmouth-Hitchcock Medical Center
Lebanon, NH

Richard B. Lipton, MD
Departments of Neurology, Epidemiology
And Population Health
Albert Einstein College of Medicine
The Montefiore Headache Center
Bronx, NY

Elizabeth Loder, MD, MPH
Division of Headache and Pain
Department of Neurology
Brigham and Women's/Faulkner Hospitals
Boston, MA

Ninan T. Mathew, MD, FRCP (C)
Houston Headache Clinic
Houston, TX

Alexander Mauskop, MD
Director, The New York Headache Center
New York, NY

Brian E. McGeeney, MD, MPH
Department of Neurology
Boston University School of Medicine
Boston, MA

Jes Olesen, MD, Dr Med Sci
Professor of Neurology
Danish Headache Center
Department of Neurology, Glostrup Hospital
University of Copenhagen
Copenhagen, Denmark

Donald B. Penzien, PhD
Head Pain Center
Department of Psychiatry and Human Behavior
University of Mississippi Medical Center
Jackson, MS

R. Allan Purdy, MD, FRCPC, FACP
Department of Medicine
Dalhousie Medical School
Halifax, NS Canada

Jeanetta C. Rains, PhD
Center for Sleep Evaluation
Elliot Hospital
Manchester, NH

Nabih M. Ramadan, MD, MBA, FAAN, FAHS
Chief Medical Officer,
Division of Development Disabilities,
NE Department of Health and Human Services
Beatrice, NE

Paul Rizzoli, MD
Director, Graham Headache Center
Brigham and Women's/Faulkner Hospitals
Boston, MA

Noah Rosen, MD
Director North Shore Headache Center
Harvey Cushing Institute of Neuroscience
Department of Neurology and Pysychiatry
North Shore LIJ Medical Center
Assistant Professor Albert Einstein University

John F. Rothrock, MD
Department of Neurology
University of Alabama College of Medicine
Director, Headache Treatment and Research Program
Editor-in-Chief, Headache
Birmingham, AL

Joel R. Saper, MD, FACP, FAAN
Director Michigan Head-Pain & Neurological Institute
Ann Arbor, MI
Clinical professor of Neurology
Michigan State University
Lansing, MI

Elliott A. Schulman, MD, FACP
Department of Neurology
Jefferson School of Medicine
Lankenau Institute for Medical Research
Wynnewood, PA

Todd A. Smitherman, PhD
Department of Psychology
University of Mississippi
University, MS

Christina Sun-Edelstein, MD
Department of Clinical Neurosciences
St. Vincent's Hospital
Melbourne, Australia

Deborah E. Tepper, MD
Center for Headache and Pain
Neurological Institute
Cleveland Clinic
Cleveland, OH

Stewart J. Tepper, MD
Center for Headache and Pain
Neurological Institute
Cleveland Clinic
Cleveland, OH

Thomas N. Ward, MD
Department of Neurology
Dartmouth Medical School
Dartmouth-Hitchcock Medical Center
Lebanon, NH

Refractory Migraine

Section I

Epidemiology, Definition, Mechanisms, and Diagnosis in Refractory Migraine

1

Historical Overview of Refractory Headache

Elliott A. Schulman, MD, FACP

Introduction

Episodic migraine headache is a common disorder, affecting approximately 35 million Americans at any given time. In the majority, pain is moderate or severe, with 53% reporting serious impairment or the need for bed rest.[1] Almost one third of migraineurs had missed at least one day of work or school in the previous year, and the productivity of individuals who worked with migraine often decreased by at least one half. Despite the increased public awareness of migraine, approximately half of migraineurs remain undiagnosed. Even among those who have been diagnosed with migraine, 57% treat with over-the-counter medicine.[2] Associated psychiatric comorbidity compounds their disability. The annual cost to American employers, due to impaired work function, is estimated to be 13 billion dollars.

Migraine subtypes have typically been distinguished based on the presence or absence of aura. Attack frequency, pain intensity, headache-related disability, and response to treatment have long been recognized to vary from patient to patient. Only attack frequency, however, has been incorporated into the *International Classification of Headache Disorders*, 2nd edition (ICHD-II).[4] Chronic migraine (CM) is defined by the presence of headache on at least 15 days per month, with at least 8 of those days linked to migraine.

The face of migraine treatment has changed over the past two decades. Since 1990, eight new antimigraine drugs, all triptans/triptan combinations, have become available, resulting in improved acute treatment.[5] They are effective, well-tolerated,[6] and safe.[7] Two preventive medications, divalproex sodium and topiramate, were approved as migraine treatments. They are both neuromodulators, and are often effective in decreasing migraine frequency, reducing disability, and in allaying concerns of experiencing additional migraines.

Treatment guidelines have summarized much of the emerging headache science into actionable approaches to optimize treatment. These approaches include accurately identifying headache types, eliminating triggers, addressing comorbid factors, and optimizing both pharmacological management and behavioral treatments, often resulting in effective headache control. Despite these advances, a group of patients remain "refractory" or "intractable" to standard approaches and continue to experience disabling headache despite optimal treatment.

Refractory migraine (RM) headache is often used interchangeably with intractable migraine. The *Oxford Dictionary* defines refractory as "not yielding to treatment." Intractable is defined as "hard to solve or deal with, stubborn." These terms are used interchangeably in the literature for the headache types we are addressing. We prefer to use the term "refractory" because it emphasizes lack of treatment response and it is used more frequently in the literature to describe this group of patients. Other terms used to describe this group include difficult, resistant, failed, and challenging.

Literature Review of Refractory Migraine

A literature search using PubMed was performed for articles containing the searchterms "refractory," "intractable," "difficult," "challenging," "nonresponsive," "resistant," and "fails/failed/failure," paired with either the word "headache" or "migraine" in the title. All searches were limited to the English language and humans. Any article that referred to a particular medication (e.g., "refractory to triptan X") or to any specific headache other migraine was excluded in Table 1.1. Of the 65 citations, 30 (46%) used the term "refractory," and 27 (42%) used the term "intractable." All terms in the search yielded articles except for the search

Table 1-1 Articles Categorized by Search Word Containing Migraine/Headache* ($n = 65$)

Search Term	Headache	Migraine
Refractory	13	17
Intractable	17	10
Difficult	2	0
Challenging	1	0
Resistant	0	2
Failure/fails/failed	2	0
Nonresponsive/nonresponsive	0	0

*Articles with more than one term were placed in the category that appeared first in the title.

Table 1-2 Articles Related to Refractory Headache Classified by Subject* (n = 65)

Type of Article	Headache*	Migraine*
Treatment-related (total)	14	20
Acute	7	9
Preventive	3	7
Procedure-based	2	1
Multidisciplinary	1	2
Psychological	1	0
Alternative	0	1
Case reports†	6	4
Epidemiology/registry	1	0
Diagnostic tools/diagnostic	1	0
Definitions	1	0
Commentaries/letters	5	5
Review	7	1

*Articles with more than one term were placed in the category that appeared first in the title.

†Case reports are defined as ≤4 cases.

term "nonresponsive." The 65 articles were characterized according to their content. Thirty-four (52%) were classified as treatment-related. Sixteen of these 34 articles (47%) addressed acute agents, and 10 (29%) discussed preventive agents. Ten of the 65 articles (15%) were case reports and 8 (12%) were reviews of the subject. Headache articles were also classified according to subject (Table 1.2).

Prior Approaches to Defining Refractory Migraine

Prior references to intractable migraine were included in the *International Classification of Diseases*, 9th edition (ICD-9).[8] New, more detailed descriptions of "intractable" headache have been revised in the ICD-9-CM. Additional types of migraine, including menstrual, persistent, and chronic migraine forms, have been added, although they remain undefined. The current classification is outlined in Table 1.3.

Integral Aspects of RM Definition

- Prophylactic medication
- Acute medication
- Adequate trial of medication
- Degree of disability
- Consider medication overuse
- Comorbid disorders addressed

Table 1-3 ICD-9-CM Migraine Classifications

Migraine with aura with intractability without status	346.01
Migraine without aura with intractability without status	346.11
Variants of migraine, not elsewhere classified with intractability without status	346.21
Hemiplegic migraine with intractability without status	346.31
Menstrual migraine with intractability without status	346.41
Persistent migraine aura without cerebral infarction with intractability without status	346.51
Persistent migraine aura with cerebral infarction with intractability without status	346.61
Chronic migraine with intractability without status	346.71
Other forms of migraine w/ intractability without status	346.81

In each migraine type listed, the specific intractable headache designation is also classified "with status."

Until recently, there was no well accepted definition for RM. Any characterization of RM has been tied to historical references in the literature. In the aforementioned PubMed search, only publications that specifically defined the term "refractory" or "intractable" were included. Articles that used the terms "drug resistant," "resistant to medication," or "usual therapies" as the definition for refractory or intractable were excluded. Of the identified, articles, 16 (76%) used the term "refractory" and 5 (24%) used the term "intractable." The earliest article that defines RM was a clinical trial that used diltiazem as a preventive medication in patients who had been "resistant" to nadalol.[9] Of the criteria considered as potential criteria for the definition, 16 (76%) addressed prevention, 7 (33%) addressed acute medication, and 4(19%) addressed medication overuse. Only 5% addressed either comorbidity or disability. The proposed definition by Goadsby et al.[10] was the most comprehensive.

Schulman and Traumuta[11] mailed a questionnaire to 300 members of AHS. They were asked if they agreed with the following definition for Refractory Headache (RH) including: headaches at least 15 days per month; unresponsive to multiple preventive medications, given at appropriate doses over a sufficiently reasonable time; and no analgesic rebound. Of the 40% who responded, 92% agreed with the definition. When they were asked for the etiology of RH, most named psychological factors, including abuse and stressful lifestyle. Other etiologies included secondary gain and malingering. Only 11% thought biochemical or organic factors were responsible.

Definitions for RM have been used in invasive treatment protocols. Patent foramen ovale (PFO) closure may lessen or eradicate headache. Clinical protocols were designed to test this concept. Actual and sham repairs of PFOs were included in the design. Because of the anticipated morbidity with this procedure, the challenge was to set a standard high enough for entry, without excluding patients who could benefit from such a procedure. The term "refractory" was used in three trials: MIST, ESCAPE, and PREMIUM.[12] Inclusion criteria in these studies required the failure of at least two preventive drugs, excluded patients with medication overuse, and required a degree of migraine disability. In another study, medically intractable headache patients were treated with occipital nerve stimulation.[13] These patients failed to respond to preventive medications from several classes, including combination pharmacotherapy, and all had a normal psychological profile. The U.S. Food and Drug Administration has considered a definition of RH to be used in a PFO closure trial. It proposes using the five groups of preventives outlined in the headache guidelines. Patients would have to fail treatment with either sodium valproate or topiramate, and one of three beta-blockers, including propranolol, nadolol, or timolol. If there were contraindications to these drugs, the definition of failure could be satisfied by failing drugs from classes of preventive agents whose effectiveness was based on consensus instead of scientific evidence.

Goadsby et al.[10] proposed a definition of intractable migraine and cluster headache, applicable to both trials and clinical practice. It required the failure of at least four preventive drugs applicable to the type of headache being treated. Success or failure of acute treatment was not addressed. Consideration was given to analgesic abuse, but degree of disability was not a criterion.

Why Define Refractory Migraine?

There are several reasons to define and characterize RM more accurately. Criteria are urgently needed to triage patients to appropriate levels of care and identify the best treatment modalities. RM definition will allow the design of studies to improve outcomes in patients with a poor prognosis.

Reasons Why a definition for RM Is Necessary

- Triage patients to appropriate levels of care.
- Identify "Best Practices."
- Serve as the criteria for inclusion in studies of novel pharmacological approaches.
- Better characterize the disorder.
- Identify risk factors for progression of migraine into the refractory type.
- Serve as a paradigm for treating physicians
- Improve the understanding of the pathophysiology of migraine

The definition will allow us to identify patients likely to improve and those likely to remain disabled, and to predict prognosis with a particular level of intervention. The criteria will also serve as a paradigm for physicians treating headache patients who have been labeled refractory. Finally, it may allow us to characterize better the pathophysiology of RM.

Improve Treatment of Migraine

The members of the Definition Committee (Committee) agreed that the primary impetus for the definition was to assist in obtaining the appropriate level of care for patients. Current guidelines for migraine treatment include a recommendation for stratified care. An algorithm and a headache staging system for treatment have been proposed. The five-item Migraine Disability Assessment

Questionnaire (MIDAS) assesses lost time due to headache over 3 months. This instrument correlates highly with physician judgments regarding patients' pain, disability, and need for medical care.[14] Patients are divided into four stages and treatment is individualized based in part on MIDAS stage.[15] Based on the MIDAS score, an algorithm for migraine management was proposed. This framework was based on the stratified care approach, with the emphasis on individualized management. It is unlikely that MIDAS grade alone will provide the information needed to define RM, although it is useful in stratifying care in primary care settings. A more comprehensive model was proposed by Saper[16] that uses the concept of headache staging. Headache type and frequency, drug usage, disability status, comorbid features, and utilization of medical resources are used to stage illness and select treatment. Factoring these variables into the model facilitates the triaging of patients to the proper level of care, which may include a multidisciplinary approach, utilizing behavioral medicine and psychological support. A formal definition for RM may result in a mandate to healthcare insurers. Patients who fulfill the RM criteria may be entitled to a higher level of care.

Identify "Best Practices"

Once the "Best Practices" of treatment are identified, all migraine patients may benefit. Approaches may be applicable to nonrefractory migraine patients as well. Goals of preventive therapy include reducing attack frequency, severity, and duration; improving function; and reducing disability.[17] Members of the AHS who responded to the first Refractory Headache Survey were asked "What do you believe works best for these patients?" The three treatments responders cited most frequently were (1) a multidisciplinary approach including psychological support, (2) being supportive and reassuring, and (3) educating patients about their disease. Polypharmacy and avoiding narcotics were also mentioned frequently.[18] Few good trials using multiple preventives in treatment-resistant patients have been performed. Saper[19] suggested that the treatment of RM include taking a more detailed history, employing creative use of medications and combinations, and inpatient treatment, if indicated. Current approaches to treatment, however, remain experience based.

Define Patient Criteria

More recently, there has been interest in polypharmacy[20,21] as a treatment option. Combining pharmacological and nonpharmacological treatments may yield better results than either alone. These will require novel trial design. Invasive treatments may require more stringent criteria than the RM definition alone. Making inclusion criteria too lax will subject inappropriate patients to substantial morbidity. Conversely, if criteria are too restrictive, patients who could truly benefit are excluded. Defining this group of patients could serve as the criteria for inclusion in studies of novel pharmacological approaches.

Better Characterize Migraine and Identify Current Patterns of Treatment and Unmet Medical Needs

The incidence and prevalence, sex and age distribution, and sociodemographic features of RM in population samples are unknown. In the first Refractory Headache Survey sent to AHS members, the estimated prevalence of RM in responders' practice ranged from "less than 5%" to "greater than 31%" (median 5–10%). Others have suggested that RM is "a relatively small minority" of the headache population.[22] In population-based studies, 4% to 5% of the general population have primary chronic daily headache.[23] This umbrella category, however, applies to many different headache types, including CM and chronic tension-type headache. Not all patients with CM will meet the criteria for RM. Because the proposed criteria for RM lack a frequency threshold, they may include patients diagnosed with episodic migraine.

Identify Risk Factors for Progression of Migraine

In some patients, migraine is a progressive disease. Modifiable risk factors for headache progression include obesity, caffeine, medication overuse, and sleep problems.[24] These factors should be identified and addressed. Migraineurs with major depression reported higher frequencies of physical and sexual abuse than those without depression.[25] Whether these factors are also important in contributing to RM is unclear. There are currently no biological markers that predict migraine progression. Because RM is a sufficiently unique entity, these biomarkers may be more readily identified. Identification of biological markers may stimulate research into disease-modifying agents for migraine.[26]

Serve as a Paradigm for Physicians

Healthcare professionals sometimes label migraine patients as refractory because they are challenging and difficult to manage, or make undue demands on their time or office staff. Often, patients have never been on a preventive regimen or have not had an appropriate trial of acute treatments. Secondary causes of headache should be excluded, and management of comorbid conditions should be optimized. This definition will set up criteria for treatment that can be applied in clinical practice.

Allow Better Characterization of the Pathophysiology of RM

Unique pathology been identified in some migraine patients. Whether these abnormalities are also seen in RM is uncertain. Identifying these patients will open new avenues of research in the areas of imaging, heredity, and central nervous system (CNS) function. Clarifying the pathophysiology of RM will undoubtedly lead to a better understanding of all headache mechanisms.

The Role of the American Headache Society in Refractory Headache

The AHS has held frequent workshops to address the pharmacological treatment of RH. Protocols for outpatient and inpatient treatment, addressing comorbid conditions, including mood disorders, and utilization of a multidisciplinary approach have also been discussed.

RHSIS was formed in 2000. Patients were characterized as "end of the line," "failure to respond." and failing "comprehensive therapy." Minutes of the meetings[27] state that defining RH is a primary goal. Other objectives included creating guidelines for treatment, including opioid use; addressing comorbid factors, particularly mood disorders; and increasing public awareness of the problem. Although various definitions were proposed, none ever achieved consensus (Larry Robbins, personal communication). RHSIS has met regularly since its inception. Continued focus has been on an acceptable definition and novel approaches to the entity.

The Committee (Schulman, Lake, Peterlin, Siegel, Markley, Goadsby, Lipton, and Levin) was charged with formulating a definition for RH in 2006. It was agreed that the definition would be operational in nature and have worldwide applicability. It would also address disability associated with the disorder. Most importantly, it would expedite appropriate care in RM patients. The proposed criteria[28] (Appendix 1.1) were formulated using the results of the Internet survey, a review of the literature, and collaborative discussions.

In 2006, the members of RHSIS formulated an Internet questionnaire addressing RH.[18] In addition to raising the visibility of RH, it would gauge interest in the entity and determine if there was a perceived need for a designation for RH. Respondents were asked for their opinions regarding appropriate criteria for RH, beliefs about pathophysiology, and whether RH should be added to the ICHD-II classification. The responses would also serve as a framework for future efforts of the section. Input on the content of the survey was obtained from AHS members with an interest in RH.

Of the 220 members who responded, 78.9% believed the definition should include an inadequate response to multiple abortive and preventive medications. Almost two-thirds of the respondents (63.6%) believed that an RH definition should be limited to headache occurring 15 days or more per month and 55.3% believed it should be associated with disability. When asked if RH should be added to the ICHD-II classification system, 57.5% believed it should be added, while 8.5% determined it should not, and 34% were unsure. More than four out of five respondents (83.6%) expressed interest in further education on RH, such as a focused RH course at the AHS Annual Meeting.

In a second survey, AHS members agreed that a definition for RM is needed (91%), that it should be added to the ICHD-II (86%), and that refractory forms of non-migraine headache disorders should be defined (87%). Responders believed a RM definition would be of greatest value in selecting patients for clinical drug trials.[29]

Appendix 1-1 Proposed Criteria for Definition of Refractory Migraine and Refractory Chronic Migraine

Primary diagnosis	A. ICHD-II Migraine or Chronic Migraine
	B. Headaches cause significant interference with function or quality of life despite modification of triggers, lifestyle factors, and adequate trials of acute and preventive medicines with established efficacy. 1. Failed adequate trials of preventive medicines, alone or in combination, from at least three (3) of four (4) drug classes: a. Beta-blockers b. Anticonvulsants c. Tricyclics d. Calcium channel blockers 2. Failed adequate trials of abortive medicines from the following classes, unless contraindicated: a. *Both* a triptan *and* DHE intranasal or injectable formulation b. *Either* nonsteroidal anti-inflammatory drugs (NSAIDs) *or* combination analgesics
Adequate trial	Period of time during which an appropriate dose of medicine is administered, typically at least two (2) months at optimal or maximum-tolerated dose, unless terminated early due to adverse effects.
Modifiers	1. With or without medication overuse, as defined by ICHD-II 2. With significant disability, as defined by MIDAS score ≥11

Proposed Definition of RM

The proposed criteria were formulated by consensus of the Committee (Appendix 1.1). Implicit in the headache criteria is an accurate diagnosis and that the patient has been compliant with the failed treatments. The following provides commentary and rationales on each element of the proposed definition.

A. Primary Diagnosis: ICHD-II migraine or chronic migraine.
The Committee agreed that limiting our definition to RM was an appropriate starting point and that incorporating additional primary headache disorders into the definition would add complexity. Formal guidelines are already in place for the treatment of migraine, although they will almost certainly require some modification in the RM patient. In addition, modifiers such as medication overuse headache (MOH) already exist.

B. Refractory: Headaches must cause significant interference with function or quality of life despite modification of triggers, lifestyle factors, and adequate trials of acute and preventive medicines with established efficacy.
Refractory headaches are associated with impairment in quality of life. Some individuals with relatively infrequent migraines may be refractory to treatment,

and a threshold for headache frequency was not included. Although all possible triggers may not be eliminated (e.g., weather change), those that are modifiable should be addressed and avoided. Management of certain lifestyle factors such as stress and mood disorders should be optimized. Because behavioral treatments are less accessible than pharmacological treatment and more variable in their application, we elected to define "refractory" as failure of the most commonly available pharmacological treatments. We decided to include both acute and preventive agents, as one alone would not constitute optimal treatment. Adequate trials of prophylactic agents were defined (see later). Acute agents should be tried in adequate doses, as early as possible, and in sufficient trials to establish efficacy.

B1. Failed adequate trials of preventive medicines, alone or in combination, from at least three of four drug classes: (1) beta-blockers; (2) anticonvulsants; (3) tricyclic antidepressants; (4) calcium channel blockers.
The specific classes were selected because they have shown clinical efficacy in evidence-based guidelines for migraine prevention.[30] The group struggled with determining the number of preventive medicine classes necessary before meeting the criteria for RM. Although a trial in each class is preferable, the optimal definition may depend on the consequences of receiving the label "refractory." For example, if this designation leads referral to a higher level of care (i.e., referral to headache center), then time needed to evaluate the effectiveness of each agent separately may inappropriately delay referral. The threshold for RM should be higher if the consequence is use of a high-risk invasive treatment.

B2. Failed adequate trials of abortive medicines from the following categories, unless contraindicated: (1) both a triptan and the intranasal or injectable formulation of dihydroergotamine (DHE); (2) either nonsteroidal anti-inflammatory drugs (NSAIDs) or combination analgesics.
A patient may not respond to a triptan and yet may respond to DHE, regardless of formulation. Trials on both a triptan and DHE, regardless of formulation, are a reasonable threshold. We agreed that NSAIDs or combination analgesics were effective agents in individuals. They are also more accessible in Third World countries where triptans are limited in choice or unavailable. Finally, some patients have a medical contraindication to triptans and DHE. This led to the caveat of including the qualifier "unless contraindicated," effectively lowering the threshold for meeting the criteria. If the patient has a contraindication to triptans and DHE, a trial on only NSAIDs or combination analgesics is necessary.

Adequate Trial: An adequate trial is defined as a period of time during which an appropriate dose of medicine is administered at optimal or maximum-tolerated dose, unless terminated early due to adverse effects.
Trials of a preventive 2 months in length were considered the shortest time before labeling a drug ineffective, especially with gradual upward titration.

Longer trials would be preferable, but this would prolong the time necessary to meet refractory criteria, and could delay patients receiving the appropriate level of care.

Modifiers: Modifiers include the following:

1. With or without medication overuse (MOH), as defined by ICHD-II.
Ideally, for migraine to be identified as refractory, patients should be withdrawn from medications with the potential for causing MOH. The group debated this point, but elected in this preliminary proposal to leave MOH as a modifier. Further, this modifier exists in the ICHD-II. In addition, the new criteria for chronic migraine no longer require that the headaches revert to a more episodic form after drug withdrawal in order to meet criteria for MOH.[31] Patients with chronic migraine and MOH now have two diagnoses. Some patients do undergo drug withdrawal, may remain abstinent from the offending medication for several months, and remain refractory. Also, because this definition was to have worldwide application, it may not be practical to avoid medication overuse in a less developed country. Using it as a modifier is a reasonable compromise.

2. With significant disability, as defined by MIDAS of 11 or higher.
There was a general agreement that disability must be addressed in the definition.

MIDAS was selected because it is widely used, well accepted as a valid and reliable measure of disability, and correlates highly with physicians' perceptions of the need for medical care.[14] The extent of disability may be a factor in deciding the appropriate level of care.

The optimal definition of RM is determined by the context of diagnosis and the consequences of assigning this label in that context. This definition has several shortcomings. Some of the aspects remain conceptual, despite the goal for the criteria to be operational. For example, "impairment in quality of life" is admittedly defined in broad terms. An alternative approach might be that the headaches significantly interfere with a patient's ability to work, attend school, or participate in family or social activities. A more formal definition might involve specific cut-scores on a specific health-related quality of life (HRQoL) measure. We suspect that the choice of measure and cut-score might be controversial. For this reason, MIDAS was used as a modifier to denote disability. Further, impairment in QOL and disability may correlate, but not necessarily.

What constitutes sufficient "improvement" from a preventive? A possible operational definition might be a sufficient improvement after preventive treatment so that adding a different or additional preventive would not be necessary. However, even the accepted criteria for a prophylactic agent are vague and need to be individualized. "Lack of response" to acute medicine is more descriptive than a definitive parameter. Is achieving a sustained pain-free state a reasonable endpoint? Although this is a high threshold, should we not expect this for our patients?

These criteria are meant as a starting point, and we view this as a work in progress. The operational criteria will depend on where the physician and patient live and approaches to take with individuals whose headaches are labeled as refractory. We acknowledge that there will undoubtedly be criticisms, which may lead to further modification and improvement of the proposed definition. Adequate field-testing will bring some of the deficiencies to light. It is our hope that these proposed criteria will stimulate further clinical and scientific attention to the nature of RM, its prevalence, and how best to treat those who suffer with it.

Summary

The study of migraine has yielded many benefits for headache patients. Little research, however, has been performed on RM headache, a term often used interchangeably with intractable migraine. This may be a consequence of a lack of a well accepted definition. Any characterization of RM has been tied to historical references in the literature. Results of a second survey of AHS members demonstrated agreement that a definition for RM is needed (91%), that it should be added to the ICHD-II (86%), and that refractory forms of non-migraine headache disorders should be defined (87%). An operational definition will allow us to characterize the condition more accurately, address unmet medical needs, and identify the most effective treatments. The RHSIS of the AHS has proposed a definition of RM wherein patients must meet the criteria for migraine or chronic migraine. Headaches need to cause significant interference with function or quality of life despite modification of triggers, lifestyle factors, and adequate trials of acute and preventive medicines with established efficacy. The definition requires that patients fail adequate trials of preventive medicines, alone or in combination, from at least three of four drug classes, including beta-blockers, anticonvulsants, tricyclics, and calcium channel blockers. Patients must also fail adequate trials of abortive medicines, including both a triptan and intranasal or injectable formulation DHE, and either NSAIDs or combination analgesics, unless contraindicated. An adequate trial is defined as a period of time during which an appropriate dose of medication is administered, typically at least 2 months at optimal or maximum-tolerated dose, unless terminated early due to adverse effects. The definition also employs modifiers for the presence or absence of medication overuse, and with or without significant disability. It is our hope that this definition will lead to further research in the area. Further understanding and characterization of RM will lead to improved treatment for all migraine patients.

References

1. Lipton RB, Bigal ME, Diamond M, et al. Migraine prevalence, disease burden, and the need for preventive therapy. *Neurology*. 2007;68(5):343–349.

2. Lipton RB, Diamond S, Reed M, Diamond ML, Stewart WF. Migraine diagnosis and treatment: results from the American Migraine Study II. *Headache.* 2001;41(7):638–645.
3. Hu XH, Markson LE, Lipton RB, Stewart WF, Berger ML. Burden of migraine in the United States: disability and economic costs. *Arch Intern Med.* 1999;159(8):813–818.
4. Headache Classification Subcommittee of the International Headache Society. The International classification of headache Disorders. *Cephalalgia.* 2004;24(suppl 1):8–152.
5. Goadsby PJ. The pharmacology of headache. *Prog Neurobiol.* 2000;62(5):509–525.
6. Ferrari MD, Roon KI, Lipton RB, Goadsby PJ. Oral triptans (serotonin 5–HT(1B/1D) agonists) in acute migraine treatment: a meta-analysis of 53 trials. *Lancet.* 2001;358(9294):1668–1675.
7. Dodick D, Lipton RB, Martin V, et al. Consensus statement: cardiovascular safety profile of triptans (5-HT agonists) in the acute treatment of migraine. *Headache.* 2004;44(5):414–425.
8. Hart A, Stegman M. ICD-9-CM. Ingenix. 2007.
9. Smith R, Schwartz A. Diltiazem prophylaxis in refractory migraine. *N Engl J Med.* 1984;310(20):1327–1328.
10. Goadsby P, Schoenen J, Ferrari M, Silberstein S, Dodick D. Towards a definition of intractable headache for use in clinical practice and trials. *Cephalalgia.* 2006;26(9):1168–1170.
11. Schulman EA, Traumuta G. Refractory Headache [abstract]. *Headache J Head Face Pain.* 1993;33(5):273–286.
12. Clinicaltrials.gov. www.clinicaltrials.gov/ct2/search (Accessed January 8, 2008). Bethesda, MD: National Library of Medicine.
13. Leone M, May A, Franzini A, et al. Deep brain stimulation for intractable chronic cluster headache: proposals for patient selection. *Cephalalgia.* 2004;24(11):934–937.
14. Lipton RB, Stewart WF, Sawyer J, Edmeads JG. Clinical utility of an instrument assessing migraine disability: the Migraine Disability Assessment (MIDAS) questionnaire. *Headache.* 2001;41(9):854–861.
15. Lipton RB, Silberstein SD. The role of headache-related disability in migraine management: implications for headache treatment guidelines. *Neurology.* 2001;56(6 suppl 1):S35–842.
16. Saper J, Lake III A, Lipton R. Staging headache cases: reconciling the complexity of a case with the required intensity of treatment. *Headache J Head Face Pain.* 2007;47(1):90–93.
17. Ramadan N, Silberstein S, Freitag F, Gilbert T, Frishberg B. Evidence-based guidelines for migraine headache in the primary care setting: pharmacological management for prevention of headache. www.aan.com/professionals/practice/guidelines. 2000 (Accessed January 10, 2008).
18. Schulman EA, Peterlin BL, Siegel SE, Lake III AE, Markley HG, Lipton RB. Refractory headache perceptions: results of an Internet survey of AHS members. American Headache Society. 2007.
19. Saper JR. Approach to the intractable headache case: identifying treatable barriers to improvement. *Continuum.* 2006;12(6):259–284.

20. Pascual J, Leira R, Láinez J. Combined therapy for migraine prevention? Clinical experience with a α-blocker plus sodium valproate in 52 resistant migraine patients. *Cephalalgia.* 2003;23(10):961–962.
21. Pascual J, Rivas M, Leira R. Testing the combination beta-blocker plus topiramate in refractory migraine. *Acta Neurol Scand.* 2007;115(2):81–83.
22. Lipton RB, Silberstein SD, Saper JR, Bigal ME, Goadsby PJ. Why headache treatment fails. *Neurology.* 2003;60(7):1064–1070.
23. Scher AI, Stewart WF, Liberman J, Lipton RB. Prevalence of frequent headache in a population sample. *Headache J Head Face Pain.* 1998;38(7):497–506.
24. Bigal ME, Lipton RB. Modifiable risk factors for migraine progression (or for chronic daily headaches)—clinical lessons. *Headache.* 2006;46(suppl 3):S144–146.
25. Tietjen GE, Brandes JL, Digre KB, et al. History of childhood maltreatment is associated with comorbid depression in women with migraine. *Neurology.* 2007;69(10):959–968.
26. Loder E, Biondi D. Disease modification in migraine: a concept that has come of age? *Headache J Head Face Pain.* 2003;43(2):135–143.
27 Minutes of Refractory Headache Special Interest Section: American Headache Society, 2000–2005.
28. Schulman EA, Lake AE, 3rd, Perlin BL, et al. Defining refractory migraine and chronic migraine [abstract]. *Headache JHead Face Pain.* 2007;47(5): 741–812.
29. Schulman EA, Peterlin BL, Lake AE, 3rd, et al. Defining refractory migraine: results of the RHSIS Survey of American Headache Society members. *Headache.* 2009;49(4):509–518.
30. Ramadan NM, Silberstein SD, Freitag FG. For the US Headache Consortium. Evidence-based guidelines for migraine headache in the primary care setting: pharmacological management for prevention of migraine. www.aan.com/professionals/practice/guidelines. 2000 (Accessed January 10, 2008).
31. Olesen J, Bousser M-G, Diener H-C, et al. New appendix criteria open for a broader concept of chronic migraine. *Cephalalgia.* 2006;26(6):742–746.

2

Refractory Migraine

Definition and Classification

Morris Levin, MD, and Elliott Schulman, MD

Introduction

The *Oxford English Dictionary* defines the word "refractory" as "not yielding to treatment." This seems an appropriate term for the many headache patients unresponsive to therapy who make up such a high percentage of visits to headache and pain specialty centers. But is "refractory" the best term? Defined as "resistant to treatment" by most references, the word does seem to describe a category often encountered. "Intractable" is another term that has been proposed, but it carries the implication that the condition may never be improved. The *International Classification of Diseases*, 9th edition (ICD-9) diagnostic coding system does include a modifier—"with intractable headache"—so this could be adopted to match coding system language. "Treatment-resistant" may be another option, but this might lead to the need to specify the treatment(s) used, and then numerous subtypes based on the specific therapeutic agent. "Severe" could be an equally meaningful term, but confusion could ensue regarding means of grading severity. The term "disabling" might lead to controversy about disability grading, with a large body of legal precedent to contend with. "Refractory" therefore seems a reasonable tag to apply to this group of patients—that is, those with headache conditions that, for whatever reason, do not improve despite concerted efforts with several appropriate treatment trials.

There are a number of reasons, discussed in Chapter 1, to define and characterize refractory headache (RH) disorders better, including refractory migraine (RM). To summarize, diagnostic criteria will allow this group of patients to be studied regarding natural history, pathophysiology, management, and prognosis, and properly triaged to appropriate levels and centers for care.

Advantages to Defining Refractory Migraine and Other Refractory Headaches

- To better characterize the disorder and its natural history
- To allow further studies of mechanism
- To identify risk factors for progression
- To allow for consistent treatment trials
- To identify "best practices"
- To promote triage of patients to appropriate centers for care

In this chapter, we propose a definition for RM as well as its underlying rationale. We also address the important task of classifying RHs, especially RM, in the array of primary and secondary headache disorders.

Schulman and Traumuta[1] proposed a definition for RH as follows: (1) headaches occurring on at least 15 days per month; (2) lack of response to multiple preventive medications, given at appropriate doses over a sufficiently reasonable time; and (3) no analgesic rebound. Three hundred members of the American Headache Society (AHS) were mailed a questionnaire asking if they agreed with these criteria, and of the 40% who responded, 92% agreed with the definition. The proposed definition of RH by Goadsby et al.[2] was designed as a tool to select patients for enrollment in treatment trials aimed at intractable headaches. Their criteria were stricter, including the failure of at least four preventive drugs applicable to the type of headache being treated. Success or failure of acute treatment was not addressed. Consideration was given to analgesic abuse, but degree of disability was not a criterion. The Food and Drug Administration considered a definition of RM to be used in a patent foramen ovale (PFO) closure trial.[3] It proposes using the five groups of preventives outlined in the headache guidelines. Patients would have to fail either sodium valproate or topiramate, and one of the beta-blockers, including propranolol, nadolol, or timolol. If there were contraindications to either a neuromodulator and/or beta-blockers, the definition of failure could be satisfied by failing drugs from classes of preventive that based their effectiveness on consensus, rather than scientific evidence.

Working Definition of RM and Refractory Chronic Migraine

For several years, the American Headache Society's Refractory Headaches Special Interest Section (RHSIS) has been attempting to define and classify RH using several approaches. Discussion among this group and with others has yielded fruitful consensus opinion about the components of useful definitions of RM and refractory chronic migraine (RCM). In addition, two surveys have been sent by the AHS to its membership in an attempt to broaden the consensus. The first survey revealed significant agreement among responders that RH should occur 15 or more days per month and be associated with disability. Most respondents believed the definition of RH should include an inadequate response to multiple abortive and preventative medications. In the second survey there was broad agreement that RM should be defined and added to the *International Classification of Headache Disorders*, 2nd edition (ICHD-II), and that refractory forms of non-migraine headache disorders should be defined as well.[4,5]

Based on these surveys, the RHISIS endeavored to formulate a definition that was (1) easily employed in clinical practice, (2) useful for research purposes, (3) able to have worldwide applicability, and (4) also addressed disability. Tools in crafting the criteria also included reviews of previous definitions of intractable or refractory headache, both in the literature and used as inclusion criteria in treatment studies. There was consensus that the definition should address appropriate use and lack of effectiveness of both acute and preventive medications with attention to medication overuse. The definition arrived at by consensus of the RHSIS is provided in Table 2.1 and is discussed in the text that follows. Although not included in the proposed criteria, it is implicit that the headache diagnosis is accurate (i.e., refractoriness not due to misdiagnosis) and that the patient has been compliant with the failed treatments (i.e., not apparent refractoriness due to improper treatment).

Table 2-1 Proposed criteria for definition of Refractory Migraine (RM) and Refractory Chronic Migraine (RCM)

A. Headaches meet the ICHD-II Migraine or Chronic Migraine criteria.
B. Headaches cause significant interference with function or quality of life despite modification of triggers, lifestyle factors, and adequate trials of acute and preventive medicines with established efficacy.
   1. Failed adequate trials of preventive medicines, alone or in combination, from at least 3 out of the following drug classes:
      a. Beta-blockers
      b. Anticonvulsants
      c. Tricyclics
      d. Calcium channel blockers
D. Failed adequate trials* of abortive medicines from the following classes, unless contraindicated:
      a. Both a triptan and dihydroergotamine (DHE) intranasal or injectable formulation
      b. Either nonsteroidal anti-inflammatory drugs (NSAIDs) or combination analgesics

Source: Schulman et al. (2008).

*Adequate trial: Period of time during which an appropriate dose of medicine is administered, typically at least 2 months at optimal or maximum-tolerated dose, unless terminated early due to adverse effects.

Modifiers: +MO, –MO: with or without medication overuse, as defined by ICHD-II.

+D, –D: with or without significant disability, as defined by MIDAS, >11.

Table 2-2 A Practical "Screening" Version of the Definition of Refractory Migraine

- Diagnosis of migraine
- Significant impact on quality of life, despite lifestyle changes
- Failure of three out of four recommended classes of preventive medication
- Failure of all appropriate acute medications.

The practical "screening" version of the definition of RM is provided in Table 2.2.

Criterion A, requiring that the headaches meet ICHD-II)[6] criteria for migraine or chronic migraine (CM), was crafted to ensure that at least as a starting point, a discrete group of patients would be defined, without overlap into other primary headache categories such as cluster headache. The definition of CM favored by the authors is that found in the most current Appendix of the ICHD–II, which allows for some headaches not to meet strict migraine criteria.[7]

Criterion B, specifying refractoriness, includes a clause requiring basic lifestyle adjustment before determining refractoriness. The committee debated whether an adequate trial of behavioral treatment should be included in the definition. Although a number of meta-analytic studies have shown that biofeedback, relaxation, and cognitive–behavior therapy are efficacious for migraine[8] behavioral treatments are less accessible than pharmacological treatment and more variable in their application. Thus, this requirement was not included. There is no threshold for headache frequency, as some individuals with relatively infrequent migraines may be refractory to treatment.

The "refractoriness" segment of the definition includes lack of effectiveness of both acute and preventive agents, as one alone would not constitute optimal treatment. Prophylactic agent classes were chosen based on evidence-based guidelines for migraine prevention,[9] and include (1) beta-blockers; (2) anticonvulsants; (3) tricyclic antidepressants; and (4) calcium channel blockers. Choosing as a requirement the failure with three of the four proven prophylactic drug classes was somewhat arbitrary but based on consensus, results of the second AHS survey described earlier, and the imperative to achieve a reasonable level of specificity, which requiring failure with only two classes would probably not have accomplished. While a trial in each of the four classes might be preferable, it was felt that this would lead to a sacrifice in sensitivity, which in turn could exclude patients who would appropriately benefit from inclusion into a refractory category. For example, if this designation leads referral to a higher level of care (i.e., referral to headache center), then time needed to evaluate the effectiveness of each agent separately may inappropriately delay referral.

The requirement of failure to respond to acute medication is stringent: (1) both a triptan and dihydroergotamine (DHE) in either the intranasal or injectable formulation and (2) either nonsteroidal anti-inflammatory drugs (NSAIDs) or combination analgesics. It was concluded that a nonrefractory patient may fail to respond to a triptan and yet may respond to DHE. NSAIDs and combination analgesics were included because they are effective agents in some individuals. They are also more accessible throughout the world. Because there are patients who cannot tolerate triptans and/or DHE, the qualifier "unless contraindicated" was added to this requirement, effectively lowering the threshold for meeting the criteria.

An adequate trial of prophylactic medication is required. This is defined as treatment over a period of time generally required to assess effectiveness, and in an appropriate dose. This is typically at least 2 months at optimal or maximum-tolerated dose, unless terminated early due to adverse effects. Although longer trials would be preferable, lengthening this requirement was viewed as too restrictive.

Modifiers were added to this definition to include the often important concomitant issues of medication overuse headache (MOH) and disability. Modifier 1, "With or without medication overuse (MOH), as defined by ICHD-II," allows for patients to carry the diagnosis of RM as well as MOH. Ideally, for migraine to be truly refractory, attempts to withdraw overused medication should be made. But this often proves very difficult or impossible, highlighting the need for specialized or intensive treatment. There are, of course, some patients who assert that their headaches do respond to acute interventions that they have to take frequently, presumably leading to MOH. These patients would not meet RM or RCM criteria (lack of response to acute medications). However, clinical experience teaches that this is generally not a stable situation, and that these patients' conditions will worsen and improve only after acute medications are reduced. To complicate things even more, some patients with MOH will not improve after the removal of acute medications. The use of "Probable" and multiple diagnoses might be the best approach with many of these patients.

Modifier 2, "With significant disability, as defined by Migraine Disability Assessment Score (MIDAS) of 11 or higher," is designed to characterize further the population of RM based on this measure of life impact. The MIDAS was selected because it is widely used, well accepted as a valid and reliable measure of disability, and correlated highly with physicians' perceptions of the need for medical care.[10]

Defining Non-migraine RHs

Clearly, there are several categories of primary and secondary headaches that include significant numbers of patients refractory to treatment.

Without much effort one can visualize many, including cluster headaches, chronic paroxysmal hemicranias, SUNCT (short unilateral neurlalgiform headaches with conjunctival injection and tearing), new daily persistent headache (NDPH), hemicrania continua, exertional headaches, posttraumatic headaches, idiopathic intracranial hypertension, and neuralgias. How to define these groups will depend on their individual features. For example, refractory hemicrania

Primary Refractory Headache Types

- Migraine
- Chronic tension-type headache
- Chronic migraine
- Cluster headache
- Paroxysmal hemicrania
- SUNCT
- Hemicrania continua
- New daily persistent headache
- Exertional headaches

Secondary Refractory Headache Types

- Post-traumatic
- Medication overuse headache
- Intracranial hypertension
- Intracranial hypotension
- Neuralgias

continua might be an appropriate term for patients who either do not respond to indomethacin or cannot tolerate it; refractory idiopathic intracranial hypertension (IIH; pseudotumor cerebri) might be defined as failure of surgical treatment. It makes sense to define and characterize these groups in order to pursue studies of pathophysiology, treatment, and prognosis. Some of these considerations are discussed in Chapter 21.

Difficulties in Defining RHs

There are a number of shortcomings in the proposed RM definition. First, some of the criteria remain conceptual, despite our attempt to be specific. For example, "impairment in quality of life" is admittedly vague. A more formal definition might involve specific cut-scores on a particular health-related quality of life (HRQoL) measure. But which tool to choose? The disability modifier could be a yes or no qualitative measure, that is, evidence that the headaches interfere with a patient's ability to work, attend school, or participate in family or social activities. This of course overlaps into the disability modifier that does have a specific numerical threshold—MIDAS >11—albeit an arbitrary one. Second, it will be debatable as to what actually constitutes "failure" to respond to preventive or acute therapy. Is it the patient's perception? Is it lack of headache frequency or pain severity reduction to some percentage less than the initial level? Finally, is not refractoriness a contextual concept, depending on the environment in which physician and patient exist, and mutual expectations?

Despite these limitations, it seems reasonable to propose these criteria as a starting point, with the final definition seen as a goal not to be reached until further data point toward revisions in this definition.

Classification of RM: Historical Perspective

The first recorded classification of headache disorders was formulated by Arateus of Cappadocia, who lived in Alexandria in the 1st century AD.[11] His headache classification divided disorders into (1) Cephalea (frequent, severe, long-lasting headaches), (2) Cephalalgia (infrequent milder headaches), and (3) Heterocrania ("half head" headaches). The British pioneer of neurology, Thomas Willis (1621–1675), described headaches as "within or without the skull"; "universal or particular"; "short, continuous or intermittent"; "wandering or uncertain"; "before, behind or the side"; and "occasional or habitual."[12] The National Institutes of Health formed an Ad Hoc Committee in 1962 to classify headaches who devised a glossary-format list of 15 headache types, ostensibly based on etiology.[13] The first evidence-based classification was produced by the International Headache Society in 1988 as the International Classification of Headache Disorders (ICHD).[14] This classification divided headache disorders into primary headaches, secondary headaches, and neuralgias and related disorders, and contained specific criteria for each diagnosis. The ICHD was revised and published as the *International Classification of Headache Disorders*, 2nd edition (ICHD-II) in 2004.[6] It is 160 pages long and contains roughly 200 diagnostic entities (depending on how one counts subtypes). It contains four sections: Primary Headaches, Secondary Headaches, Neuralgias and facial pain, and the Appendix. The ICHD-II's Appendix serves several functions: (1)"to present research criteria for a number of novel entities that have not been sufficiently validated by research studies," (2) to provide "alternative sets of diagnostic criteria to those in the main body of the classification....because clinical experience and a certain amount of published evidence suggest that this may be a good idea," and (3) to include previous diagnoses as "a first step in eliminating disorders included as diagnostic entities in the first edition because of tradition but for which sufficient evidence has still not been published."

The ICHD-II is comprehensive, fairly specific regarding exact features of each type, hierarchical (i.e., with built-in subtypes and sub-subtypes), and clearly organized. However, by virtue of its size, complexity, and relative arbitrariness in some areas (despite sincere efforts to base definitions on evidence), it has serious limitations as a practical tool for clinicians. The most significant challenge faced by the Classification Committee of the International Headache Society in producing the ICHD and, later, the ICHD-II, is that for the primary headaches there are no known biological markers. Thus, diagnostic criteria for migraine, tension type headache, cluster headache, and so forth must be based on subjective criteria. This has led to significant overlap among definitions.

Table 2-3 Appendix Criteria for A1.5.1 Chronic Migraine

A. Headache (tension-type and/or migraine) on 15 days per month for at least 3 months
B. Occurring in a patient who has had at least five attacks fulfilling criteria for 1.1 Migraine without Aura
C. On 8 days per month for at least 3 months headache has fulfilled C1 and/or C2 below, that is, has fulfilled criteria for pain and associated symptoms of migraine without aura
  1. Has at least two of a–d:
     a. Unilateral location
     b. Pulsating quality
     c. Moderate or severe pain intensity
     d. Aggravation by or causing avoidance of routine physical activity (e.g., walking or climbing stairs)
     And at least one of a or b:
     a. Nausea and/or vomiting
     b. Photophobia and phonophobia
  2. Treated and relieved by triptan(s) or ergot before the expected development of C1 above
D. No medication overuse and not attributed to another causative disorder

Source: Headache Classification Committee (2006).

For example, there are many patients whose headaches seem to satisfy more than one diagnosis.

Already there have been several revisions of the ICHD–II; therefore, the ICHD-II is referred to now as the ICHD-II, revised (ICHD-IIR). One revision in particular illuminates an expedited approach to amending or changing the ICHD when it becomes necessary—the addition of an appendix classification for Chronic Migraine. It was felt by a number of practitioners that the Chronic Migraine definition in ICHD-II did not represent the majority of patients with this condition because it required that all of the headaches that patients experienced fulfill ICHD criteria for migraine. The American Headache Society proposed a looser definition that was accepted by the IHS Classification Committee as an Appendix definition awaiting further evidence for inclusion in the classification proper (Table 2.3).[7]

Currently, the ICHD-II does delineate a category for any type of refractory headache. If one accepts the rationale for defining RM, it seems essential for it to be included in the classification schema of headache disorders. There are a number of options for doing this that are discussed below. Interestingly, as mentioned above, diagnostic coding for refractoriness has already been put into place in the *International Classification of Diseases*, 9th edition (ICD-9) system via modifiers for "intractable" (e.g., migraine with intractable headache—346.11).

Challenges in RM Classification

Like other primary headaches, there are no biological markers for RM. Thus, any diagnostic criteria will have to be descriptive, as is generally true for other primary headaches. Another major challenge has to do with the concept of refractoriness itself. A key question is whether refractoriness in headache disorders represents less treatable versions of particular headache types, or whether all refractory headaches share common pathophysiology and thus represent a discrete category in itself. Another problem is the possibility that the group of patients defined by, for example, RM, may include several disparate subgroups with different pathological mechanisms. Finally, a patient's "refractoriness" may change over time. Can a patient lose a diagnosis of refractory migraine? Can a patient have refractory headache which evolves to a nonrefractory headache type? The framers of the ICHD certainly accept diagnosis as a potentially dynamic process, as the Introduction states it is "possible for a patient to have one diagnosis at one time and another diagnosis a few years later." But should a history of former refractoriness imply something about the patient's underlying genotype or pathophysiology, thus directing classification?

Current ICHD-IIR Categories that Include Various Types of RH

There are currently no categories in the ICHD II which classify refractory headaches. Even Chronic Migraine, which has a high frequency of migraines as part of its definition, may not be refractory if the proposed definition is applied (although presumably most of these patients have failed to respond to previous treatment trials). Chronic Tension-Type Headache is similar. Chronic Cluster Headache and Chronic Paroxysmal Hemicrania suggest a refractoriness based on failure to remit as hoped for, but do not require that all effective therapies have failed. New Daily Persistent Headache (NDPH) carries the implication of daily frequency, again despite presumed therapy (although refractoriness is not actually part of the explicit inclusion criteria for NDPH). None of these diagnostic definitions includes any of the several parameters that could describe refractoriness in explicit diagnostic criteria, so even though the implication of refractoriness seems logical, it is actually not specified for any disorder in the ICHD.

Classification Options for RHs

There are several classification options for RH including the following: (1) A new ICHD diagnostic chapter or section entitled "Refractory Headaches," with subdivisions based on headache type; (2) diagnostic subsections for each headache type that can "be" refractory; (3) creation of a modifier (e.g., "R") that could be appended to any headache diagnosis; and (4) creation of a new axis ("Axis 2"), in addition the original ICHD axis, to describe factors like refractoriness as well as perhaps other factors such as disability, contributing conditions, and so forth.[15]

Option 1: A New ICHD Chapter for the RHs

The current ICHD-IIR primary headache section (Part 1) consists of four chapters: (1) Migraine; (2) Tension-Type Headache; (3) Cluster Headache and Other Trigeminal Autonomic Cephalalgias (TACs); and (4) Other Primary Headaches. A fifth chapter entitled "Refractory Primary Headaches" could be added that could be subdivided into various refractory headaches as follows:

5.1 Refractory Migraine
5.2 Refractory TTH
5.3 Refractory TACs
5.4 Other Refractory Primary Headaches

Unfortunately, this would constitute a large new chapter. The sheer size of the ICHD-II is already daunting enough to discourage many practitioners from using it. More importantly, this approach might send the unproven message that different types of refractory headaches are more alike than nonrefractory and refractory headaches of the same type (e.g., migraine and refractory migraine).

Option 2: A Subset of Each Headache Type that Can Be Refractory

Currently, the ICHD's Migraine chapter contains six subtypes. Adding a final category of "Refractory Migraine" would extend the migraine chapter as follows:

Chapter 1: Migraine

1.1 Migraine without Aura
1.2 Migraine with Aura
1.3 Childhood Periodic Syndromes that Are Commonly Precursors of Migraine
1.4 Retinal Migraine
1.5 Complications of Migraine
1.6 Probable Migraine
1.7 Refractory Migraine

Similarly, other chapters in the ICHD-IIR could have an additional subsection, so that another example, using the Cluster Headache and Other Trigeminal Autonomic Cephalalgias chapter, would look like the following:

3.1 Cluster Headache
3.2 Paroxysmal Hemicrania
3.3 Short-Lasting Unilateral Neuralgiform Headaches with Conjunctival Injection and Tearing
3.4 Probable Trigeminal Autonomic Cephalalgia
3.5 Refractory TAC

This approach of adding subsections for each headache type that can "be" refractory seems logical, but it again would lead to a large amount of new text and diagnoses. Does the inclusion of all of these really matter or is it important for just a few? If the latter, perhaps just including refractory subdiagnoses for migraine with aura, migraine without aura, chronic migraine, cluster headache, and paroxysmal hemicranias might suffice.

There are actually several ways this could be done depending on which hierarchical level is addressed. One way to add a refractory category for migraine might be to list it as follows:

Chapter 1: Migraine

- 1.1 Migraine without Aura
- 1.2 Migraine with Aura
- 1.3 Childhood Periodic Syndromes that Are Commonly Precursors of Migraine
- 1.4 Retinal Migraine
- 1.5 Complications of Migraine
- 1.6 Probable Migraine
- 1.7 Refractory Migraine
  - 1.7.1 Refractory Migraine without Aura
  - 1.7.2 Refractory Migraine with Aura
  - 1.7.3 Refractory Chronic Migraine
  - 1.7.4 Refractory Probable Migraine

Or, alternatively the Refractory Migraine diagnosis could be inserted at the second digit level; e.g.:

Chapter 1: Migraine

- 1.1 Migraine without Aura
  - 1.1.1 Refractory Migraine without Aura
- 1.2 Migraine with Aura
  - 1.1.1 Refractory Migraine with Aura

And for Chronic Migraine:

- 1.5.1 Chronic Migraine
  - 1.5.1.1 Refractory Chronic Migraine

For the sake of illustration, specific classification criteria are proposed in Tables 2.4 and 2.5 for Refractory Migraine and Refractory Chronic Migraine using this approach to classification.

Option 3: A Modifier for Refractoriness—"R"

The psychiatry classification schema, *Diagnostic and Statistical Manual of Mental Disorders, 4th edition—text revision* (DSM IV-TR), includes "severity specifiers" such as mild, moderate, and severe, to help further characterize the illness. For example, Major Depressive Episode—mild refers to the patient who meets diagnostic criteria for Major Depressive Disorder, but with few symptoms (e.g., delusions or hallucinations) and only mild impairment in function and social activities and relationships.[16] To apply this to the migraine

Table 2-4 Proposed Criteria for Refractory Migraine without Aura A1.1.1

A. Headache fulfills criteria A, B, C, and D for 1.1 Migraine without Aura.
B. Significant reduction in quality of life is reported.
C. The patient has failed adequate trials of three classes of preventive medication.
D. The patient has failed three classes of acute medication.
E. Not attributed to another disorder (i.e., secondary causes of headache excluded, including medication overuse headache [MOH]).

Table 2-5 Proposed Criteria for Refractory Migraine without Aura A1.1.1

A. Headache fulfills criteria A, B, C, and D for 1.1 Migraine without Aura.
B. Significant reduction in quality of life is reported.
C. The patient has failed adequate trials of three classes of preventive medication.
D. The patient has failed three classes of acute medication.
E. Not attributed to another disorder (i.e., secondary causes of headache excluded, including medication overuse headache [MOH]).

chapter, one could specify refractory migraine as: 1.1R—Migraine without Aura, R (refractory), with the definition for the "R" suffix to include the features of the refractory migraine definition (poor quality of life, failure of several medications in preventive and acute categories).

Carrying this further, the ICHD could someday employ other modifiers such as *Mild, Moderate, Severe, Progressive, Resolving,* or *Associated with Medication Overuse.* In fact, some modifiers already exist in the ICHD. For example: 5.2.2 Posttraumatic headache resulting from *mild* head injury and 5.2.1 Posttraumatic headache resulting from *moderate or severe* head injury. Because our definition for RM proposes modifiers for disability and the presence of medication overuse headache, these could be encompassed by this option as well.

This option might have fewer ramifications on the rest of the ICHD. However, it does tend to add one more layer to each patient's diagnosis, and practitioners already balk at using more than one digit in using ICHD for diagnostic purposes. In addition, however, this "R (refractory) modifier" approach would lend itself most easily to meeting diagnostic coding and reimbursement needs because it is so similar to the ICD-9 modifiers for "intractable" (see earlier—e.g. "migraine with intractable headache—346.11" could be equivalent to a "1.2,R" diagnosis). Simply expanding the use of the ICD modifiers would then closely match a refractory headache clinical diagnostic system

Option 4: A New Axis

The DSM IV-TR classification schema currently contains the well-known five-axis "Multiaxial Assessment" protocol:

Axis 1—Clinical Psychological Disease
Axis 2—Personality Disorders and Mental Retardation
Axis 3—Medical Disorders

Table 2-6 Options for Classifying Refractory Headaches Including Refractory Migraine

1. New category in ICHD IIR—"Refractory Headaches"
2. Subcategories in each appropriate chapter for refractory subtypes—e.g., Refractory Migraine with aura, Refractory Post-traumatic Headaches, etc.
3. Modifier "R" for refractoriness that can be appended to any diagnosis.
4. New axis describing the presence or lack of refractoriness

Axis 4—Psychosocial and Environmental Problems
Axis 5—Global Assessment of Functioning

Similarly, the ICHD could be transformed into a multiaxis system to include, for example, an Axis 2 concerning Refractoriness. Thus, a diagnosis could look like:

Axis 1—1.1 Migraine without Aura
Axis 2—Refractory Headache

Other features of the headache disorder, such as disability, severity of pain, and so forth, could also be included in this axis. This approach would have similarities to the multi-axis headache staging system of Saper et al.,[17] which classifies patients into categories that predict use of resources. Adding an Axis 2 to the ICHD to refer to refractoriness, disability, and so forth makes sense if one wishes to add information to a patient's formal diagnosis. However, this would dramatically change the format of the ICHD, and if not rejected out of hand immediately by the IHS classification committee, it would likely lead to prolonged controversy, as well as a delay in acceptance and use by practitioners of yet another new tool. Options for classifying RH including RM are summarized in Table 2.6.

Of the options described, the authors would support either option 2—adding diagnostic definitions within categories of headaches, or option 3—adding a modifier for refractoriness ("R") that could simply be appended to any diagnosis. Both have the advantage of simplicity, although there are pros and cons to each

Here is a specific case example: A woman who describes frequent throbbing nauseating hemicranial headaches, lasting several hours in duration, associated with phonophobia and photophobia, but without focal neurological deficits, has been unresponsive to many prophylactic and abortive agents. Her quality of life has been severely reduced. A thorough neurological examination, laboratory testing, and brain magnetic resonance imaging (MRI) have been entirely normal. The following are possible diagnoses:

Option 2 diagnosis: 1.1.1 Refractory Migraine without Aura
Option 3 diagnosis: 1.1R Migraine without Aura, Refractory

Medication Overuse headache

It is now well accepted that overuse of acute medications often leads to refractory migraine. Many authors have demonstrated that frequent use of virtually

Table 2-7 Appendix Criteria for A8.2 Medication Overuse Headache

A. Headache present on >15 days/month.
B. Regular overuse (>10 days/month or >15 days/month, depending on the medication) for >3 months of one or more acute/symptomatic treatment drugs as defined under subforms of 8.2.
C. Headache has developed or markedly worsened during medication overuse.

Source: Headache Classification Committee (2006).

Note: This revised list of criteria for medication overuse headache (MOH) eliminates the requirement for improvement once the medication is withdrawn).

any abortive or analgesic agent can "transform" intermittent migraine to a chronic daily headache pattern (>15 days per month).[18–20] And, as for treatment resistance, Matthew et al. showed that frequent use of analgesics made migraines resistant to prophylactic medications.[21] Differentiating medication overuse migraine (MOH) from chronic migraine *not* related to MOH can be challenging, particularly as headache morphology is not particularly helpful.[22] The ICHD-II recommended assigning "probable MOH" to those patients using acute medications frequently and experiencing migraine or migrainous headaches greater than 15 days per month, and considered this a clear diagnosis only if headaches resolved or reverted to intermittent occurrence after the offending medication was removed. Of note, new criteria for MOH have been added to the Appendix of the ICHD II (see Table 2.7), specifically abolishing the need for MOH to resolve after medications are removed, and it is likely that this new set of criteria will be employed by most researchers and clinicians in the future.[7]

Because many patients generally fulfilling "refractory headache" criteria will have MOH, a classification schema for RM should somehow deal with this subset. This is the purpose for the modifiers seen at the end of the RM definition (see Table 2.1). For example, using option 2 above, Refractory Migraine without Aura, could be further subdivided into Refractory Migraine without Aura, with MOH, and Refractory Migraine without Aura, without MOH.

To maintain the format and spirit of the ICHD-II's current handling of MOH, it might actually be best to consider MOH to be a secondary cause of refractory headache, with the existence of subtypes: (1) Refractory MOH (or using option 3—MOH-R) and 2) Nonrefractory MOH (if there are any cases). It must be said, however, there will always be patients with apparently refractory migraine in whom the role of medication overuse may be difficult or impossible to assess. MOH is discussed in more detail in Chapter 9.

Conclusions

There are a number of important reasons to define and classify RM. Obstacles include the lack of clear consensus concerning the specific details of what constitutes refractoriness, and the possibility that the group defined may include disparate subgroups. A proposed definition is provided that carries the weight of an iterative collaborative process. Requirements include: (1) a diagnosis of migraine; (2) significant impact on quality of life, despite lifestyle changes and avoidance of triggers; (3) failure of three out of four accepted classes of preventive medication; and (4) ineffectiveness of all appropriate acute medications.

The current classification system produced by the International Headache Society—the International Classification of Headache Disorders, 2nd edition, revised (ICHD-IIR)—does not provide any usable classification for this important group of patients. Challenges to amending the ICHD to include a RM definition include the lack of biological or other pathognomonic markers, and the similarity of several features of RM and those of other already existent headache classification definitions. Still, there are several workable options, which are in some ways similar but involve different levels of the hierarchy in the ICHD IIR. In the case of refractory migraine, the best options for classification are either to add diagnostic definitions within categories of migraine, for example, "Migraine without Aura, Refractory," or to add a modifier for refractoriness such as "R" that could simply be appended to the primary diagnosis, thus: "Migraine without aura, R."

Because definitions and classifications of diagnostic entities are valid only if they serve clinical needs, the proposed definition of RM should be "field tested" using one or more populations of headache patients that include patients felt to be refractory. If such a diagnostic definition can be validated, it will help to determine the best directions for future research into and treatment of this important group of patients. Once validated, the definition of RM should be proposed for inclusion into the Appendix of the ICHD-II, using one of the approaches outlined in this chapter. This could then be subjected to further scrutiny and testing worldwide, leading to better understanding of mechanisms, natural history, and best treatment options.

References

1. Schulman EA, Traumuta G. Refractory headache. *Headache.* 1993;33:273–286.
2. Goadsby PJ, Schoenen J, Ferrari MD, Silberstein SD, Dodick D. Towards a definition of intractable headache for use in clinical practice and trials. *Cephalalgia.* 2006;26:1168–1170.
3. Clinicaltrials.gov. National Library of Medicine: Bethesda, MD. Available at: www.clinicaltrials.gov/ct2/search (Accessed May 11, 2010).
4. Schulman EA, Peterlin BL, Siegel SE, Lake AE, Markley H, Lipton RB. Refractory headache perceptions: Results of an Internet Survey of AHS Members. Chicago: American Headache Society, 2007.
5. Schulman EA, Peterlin BL, Lake AE III, Lipton RB, Hanlon A, Siegel S, Levin M, Goadsby PJ, Markley HG. Defining Refractory Migraine: Results of the RHSIS Survey of American Headache Society Members. Headache. 2009,4:509–518.
6. Schulman, EA, Lake AE, Goadsby, PJ, et al. Defining refractory migraine (RM) and refractory chronic migraine (RCM): Proposed criteria for the Refractory Headache Special Interests Section of the American Headache Society. *Headache.* 2008; 48:778–782.
7. Headache Classification Subcommittee of the International Headache Society. *The International Classification of Headache Disorders*, 2nd ed. *Cephalalgia.* 2004; 24(suppl 1):9–160.

8. Headache Classification Committee, Olesen J, Bousser M-G, Diener H-C, et al. New appendix criteria open for a broader concept of chronic migraine. *Cephalalgia.* 2006,26:742–747.
9. Campbell JK, Penzien DB, Wall EM. For the US Headache Consortium (American Academy of Family Physicians, American Academy of Neurology, American Headache Society, American College of Emergency Physicians, American College of Physicians—American College of Internal Medicine, American Osteopathic Association, National Headache Foundation). Evidence-based guidelines for migraine headache: Behavioral and physical treatment. www.aan.com 2000 (Accessed May 11, 2010).
10. Ramadan NM, Silberstein SD, Freitag FG. For the US Headache Consortium (American Academy of Family Physicians, American Academy of Neurology, American Headache Society, American College of Emergency Physicians, American College of Physicians– American College of Internal Medicine, American Osteopathic Association, National Headache Foundation). Evidence-based guidelines for migraine headache in the primary care setting: pharmacological management for prevention of migraine. www.aan.com 2000 (Accessed May 11, 2010).
11. Lipton RB, Stewart WF, Sawyer J, Edmeads JG. Clinical utility of an instrument assessing migraine disability: the migraine disability assessment (MIDAS) questionnaire. *Headache.* 2001;41:854–861.
12. Isler H. Headache classification prior to the Ad Hoc criteria. *Cephalalgia.* 1993; 12(suppl 2):9–10.
13. Pearce JMS. Historical aspects of migraine. *J Neurol Neurosurg Psychiatry.* 1986;49:1097–1103.
14. Ad Hoc Committee on Classification of Headache of the National Institutes of Health. Classification of Headache. *JAMA.* 1962;179:717–718.
15. International Headache Society Classification Committee. Classification and diagnostic criteria for headache disorders, cranial neuralgias and facial pain. *Cephalalgia.* 1988;8(suppl 7):1–96.
16. Levin M. Refractory Headache: Classification and Nomenclature. *Headache.* 2008;48:783–790.
17. American Psychiatric Association. *Diagnostic and Statistical Manual of Mental Disorders, Fourth Edition, Text Revision* (DSM-IV-TR®). Arlington, VA: American Psychiatric Publishing, 2000.
18. Saper J, Lake AE, Lipton RB. Staging headache cases: reconciling the complexity of a case with the required intensity of treatment. *Headache.* 2007:47:90–93.
19. Limmroth V, Katsarava Z, Fritsche G, Przywara S, Diener HC. Features of medication overuse headache following overuse of different acute headache drugs. *Neurology.* 2002;59(7):1011–1014.
20. Rapoport AM. Analgesic rebound headache. *Headache.* 1988;28:662–665.
21. Zeeberg P, Olesen J, Jensen R. Probable medication-overuse headache: the effect of a 2-month drug-free period. *Neurology.* 2006;66:1894–1898.
22. Mathew NT, Kkurman R, Perez F. Drug induced refractory headache-clinical features and management. *Headache.* 1990;30:634–638.
23. Silbertstein SD, Olesen J, Bousser M-G, et al. *The International Classification of Headache Disorders,* 2nd ed. (ICHD-II)—revision of criteria for 8.2 Medication-Overuse Headache. *Cephalalgia.* 2005;25:460–465.

3

Epidemiology of Refractory Migraine

Richard B. Lipton, MD, and Marcelo E. Bigal, MD, PhD

Introduction

A large number of epidemiological studies have measured the prevalence, distribution, burden, and patterns of treatment for a range of primary headache disorders, as defined by the *International Classification of Headache Disorders*, 1st and 2nd editions (ICHD-I and ICHD-II).[1–4] These studies show that migraine affects 10% to 15% of the general population while tension-type headache affects about 40% of the population.[5–8] Chronic daily headache, defined as headache 15 or more days per month, occurs in about 4% of the general population.[9,10]

These epidemiological studies have also shown that headache-related disability and impairment in health-related quality of life (HRQoL) are concentrated in specific segments of the headache population.[11,12] For example, the impact of migraine on the individual headache sufferer exceeds the individual impact of tension type headache. Among migraineurs, there is also a spectrum of disability.[11,12] Some individuals with migraine are refractory to guideline based treatment and continue to experience disability and disruption in HRQoL despite optimal treatment.

Defining the epidemiology of this group, referred to herein as refractory migraine (RM), is important because of its disproportionate contribution to the overall burden of illness. Considering the epidemiology of refractory migraine is timely, as operational diagnostic criteria have only recently become available. These criteria were developed by a subcommittee of the Refractory Headache Special Interest Section of the American Headache Society (the Committee).[14] They have not been tested in a deliberate and rigorous epidemiological studies but should have a substantial impact on headache research. In this chapter, we present an approach to assessing the epidemiology of RM and R-CM based on the five key components of the proposed definitions. Herein, we summarize what is known about the epidemiology of each component, focusing on data from North America.

Epidemiological Research on RM

For purposes of epidemiological research, the definition of RM has five key components. First, RM and R-CM can be diagnosed only in individuals meeting the ICHD-II criteria for migraine or chronic migraine.[3] Second, these individuals must experience significant interference with function or disruption in HRQoL due to headaches. Interference must be present despite treatment efforts in three areas: modification of triggers and lifestyle factors, adequate trials of acute medication, and adequate trials of preventive medicines. These three domains of treatment comprise the third, fourth, and fifth components of RM and R-CM definitions.

For applications to epidemiologic research, each component of the definition must be operationalized. In addition, two "modifiers" of RM and R-CM have been proposed. One distinguishes RM and R-CM with and without medication overuse. The other distinguishes RM and R-CM with and without disability based on a Migraine Disability Assessment (MIDAS) scale score of 11 or greater. In the sections that follow, we consider each of these five components of the RM or R-CM definition as well as the modifiers from an epidemiological perspective.

Epidemiology of Migraine and Chronic Migraine

The epidemiology of both episodic and chronic migraine has been well studied.[3,4] The 1-year period prevalence of migraine typically ranges from 15% to 20% in women and from 4% to 7% range in men.[1,2,6–8,15] Three large-scale studies in nationally representative samples of the U.S. population were conducted in 1989 (American Migraine Study 1 [AMS-1]),[16] 1999 (American Migraine Study 2 [AMS-2]),[6] and in 2004 (American Migraine Prevalence and Prevention Study [AMPP]).[8] These studies generated remarkably similar results regarding the basic epidemiology of migraine over a 15-year period, suggesting that migraine prevalence has been stable in the United States. (Fig. 3.1).

For chronic migraine, population studies have been more limited. Most have used the Silberstein–Lipton criteria[17] rather than the chronic migraine

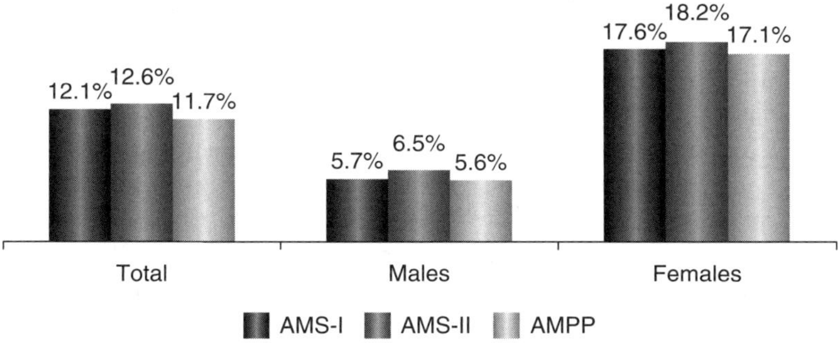

Figure 3-1 Prevalence of migraine in the American Migraine Study (AMS)-1, AMS-2, and AMPP for total sample and by gender.

criteria proposed in ICHD-II[3] and in its revision.[18] Chronic migraine occurs in about 2% of the adult population and is more common in women than in men.[9,10] The prevalence of episodic migraine varies with age with an inverted U-shaped function; the prevalence of chronic migraine is more stable with age. The differences among the various case definitions for chronic/transformed migraine, the epidemiology of chronic daily headache, and the risk factors for new-onset chronic daily headache have been recently reviewed.[19]

Interference with Function or HRQoL

Significant interference with function or HRQoL requires an operational definition for epidemiological research. We consider three approaches: asking a directed question or questions, using HRQoL measures, or using measures of disability. Any definition of significant interference must be applied over a specified period of time while particular treatments are being used. The definitions of RM and R-CM require significant interference or reduced HRQoL despite optimal treatment. Therefore, this aspect of the definition must be repeatedly applied as treatment changes.[20]

One approach might be to ask the patient a yes–no question such as, "Do your headaches substantially interfere with your ability to function?" or "Do your headaches substantially reduce your quality of life?" These sorts of yes–no questions may generate false-positive responses if the headaches ever interfere with function, even to a small degree. They may generate false-negative responses in a patient having a good week. Instead, we prefer questions with graded response options based on frequency, severity, or both. For example, one could ask, "Over the last 3 months, how often have your headaches significantly interfered with your ability to function?" or "Over the last 3 months, how often have your headaches significantly interfered with your quality of life?" Categorical response options could include never, rarely, some of the time, much of the time, most of the time, all of the time. With this kind of question, responses of never and rarely are usually considered negative responses to reduce false-positives. This approach has the great advantage of simplicity but has not been validated.[2] As each patient applies his or her idea of what constitutes significant interference in ability to function and reduced quality of life,[21] reliability may be difficult to achieve.

One alternative is to use instruments specifically designed to measure functional ability or HRQoL. Functional impairment in migraine may occur both during (ictal burden) and between (interictal burden) attacks.[22,23] Using the MIDAS questionnaire, functional ability is assessed in three domains during attacks over a 3-month recall period: work and school, household work, and chores as well as family, social and leisure activity.[24] As the MIDAS questionnaire is used as a modifier to define RM and R-CM with and without disability, we discuss it further in the section on modifiers.

HRQoL instruments generally measure the impact of illness across a range of domains such as physical health, mental health, social functioning, role-functioning, and general well-being.[25–29] Generic and disease-specific HRQoL instruments have been used to evaluate migraine sufferers.[25] Generic instruments, such as the Short Form-36 from the Medical Outcomes Study, are designed to measure the impact of a range of illnesses on HRQoL.[25] Disease-specific HRQoL questionnaires are designed to address the quality-of-life impact of a specific illness. For purposes of defining RM, comparing illness is not an issue. Therefore, disease specific HRQoL measures may be preferable.

Several population-based studies in the United States and Europe have evaluated HRQoL among migraine sufferers and a control population, often using generic HRQoL measures.[30–32] These studies often include a contemporaneous non-migraine control population. Scores in the migraine population were significantly lower (indicating worse HRQoL) than those in the control population.

Some studies described the relationships among HRQoL, migraine frequency, disability, and depression. As migraine frequency and disability increased, HRQoL decreased. Migraine has an impact on HRQoL independent of the influence of comorbidities such as depression.[32] The use of these instruments in well defined populations may help define RM and R-CM. For diagnostic purposes, an empirical cut score is needed. Individuals scoring below a particular cut score would be said to have significant interference for purposes of applying the proposed RM case definition.

Adequate Trial of Trigger and Lifestyle Management

There is not a consensus on the key components of an adequate trial of trigger and lifestyle modification. The U.S. Headache Consortium Guideline summarizes the evidence that supports particular interventions.[33] In our view, an adequate trial in this domain should, at minimum, include: (1) education on the nature of migraine and the factors that trigger it; (2) use of a diary to identify headache patterns and trigger factors; and (3) advice on diet, sleep, exercise, stress management, and trigger avoidance. Many refractory patients would likely benefit from intervention with a psychologist with expertise in cognitive–behavioral therapy, biofeedback, as well as trigger and lifestyle modification. The frequency of use of these interventions in the general migraine population is not well known. These aspects of treatment will have to be better specified before they can be studied in epidemiological surveys.

Adequate Trial of Acute Pharmacotherapy

The definitions of RM[14] and R-CM[14] require that the patient fail adequate trials of acute treatment. These trials include a triptan and dihydroergotamine (DHE) as well as at least one nonsteroidal anti-inflammatory drug (NSAID) or a combination analgesic. These criteria are explicit and reasonable. Nonetheless, clinicians might disagree on what constitutes an adequate trial of a treatment. More problematic for epidemiological research is that this sort of information is difficult to obtain by questionnaire or phone survey. Study participants can usually report their current medications accurately but may have difficulty in reporting prior treatments, particularly from the remote past.

Nonetheless, studies have examined the patterns of acute treatment for migraine in the United States and around the world. Rather than reviewing the literature, we highlight data from the American Migraine Prevalence and Prevention Study (AMPP).[8,34] In the AMPP, migraine-specific acute treatments were used by 31.6% of respondents with CM and 24.8% with episodic migraine.

Triptan use was common, but the use of any ergot, including DHE, was rare. As a consequence, few migraine sufferers would meet this criterion for RM or R-CM. Over-the-counter (OTC) medications were used by 83% of respondents with CM and 89% of those with episodic migraine. In the CM group, NSAIDs were used by 63% of the sample, with ibuprofen (45% of NSAID use), naproxen (26%), and aspirin (24%) being the most common. It seems likely that the prevalence of RM and RCM in the United States is low, based in no small measure on the very low rates of use for ergot alkaloids. The definition of RM and R-CM may encourage treatment trials with DHE. It would be useful to know how often DHE provides relief in otherwise refractory patients.

Though we are not in a position to assess rates of treatment success or failure, about 48% of the individuals with CM were satisfied with their acute therapies; 23% were dissatisfied and the remaining were neutral (AMPP data on file).

Adequate Trial of Preventive Pharmacotherapy

The definitions of RM and RCM require adequate trials with three or four classes of preventive drugs. The crucial classes include beta-blockers, anticonvulsants, tricyclic antidepressants, and calcium channel blockers. In the AMPP study, medications specifically taken to prevent headaches had ever been used by a minority of CM sufferers (40.0%). Just 33.3% were currently using preventive medications for CM. For episodic migraine, only 12.4% are current users of preventive medications.[34]

Table 3.1 displays the medications used by individuals in the U.S. population with episodic migraine and CM, specifically to prevent their headaches. For each type of preventive medication, use was higher for the CM sufferers than the episodic migraine sufferers. For CM, 32.7% had used topiramate whereas gabapentin and divalproex each had been used by approximately 20% of individuals. Antidepressants, antihypertensive medications,

Table 3-1 Preventive Therapies Used by Individuals with Chronic Migraine in the U.S. Population in 2006

	Chronic Migraine (%)	Episodic Migraine (%)
Antiepileptic Drugs		
Divalproex	19.7	9.7
Topiramate	32.7	19.2
Gabapentin	21.6	11.4
Other	7.1	5.5
Antidepressant Medications		
Amitriptyline	32.7	17.3
Nortriptyline	9.1	4.6
Duloxetine	7.2	2.1
Venlafaxine	7.2	4.9
Paroxetine	8.2	5.8
Sertraline	12.0	6.7
Fluoxetine	10.6	5.5
Antihypertensive Medications		
Propranolol	21.6	19.9
Nadolol	3.4	2.7
Metoprolol	7.2	4.6
Atenolol	7.2	5.4
Verapamil	9.1	5.2
Diltiazem	0.5	0.2
Nutraceuticals		
Feverfew	10.1	11.8
Magnesium	10.6	9.6
Vitamin B_2	9.6	9.9
Butterbur	1.4	1.2

and calcium channel blockers all showed significant use. Nutraceuticals were frequently used including magnesium (10.6%), feverfew (10.1%), and riboflavin (9.6%).

The definition of RM or R-CM requires impaired HRQoL or function despite adequate trials of the required treatments. This definition has not been applied to existing data sets to the best of our knowledge. However, among individuals with CM overall satisfaction with treatment was high. For example, more than 70% of subjects with CM, treated with topiramate or amitriptyline were satisfied or very satisfied with treatment. Satisfaction was slightly lower for propranolol or verapamil.

Modifiers

The diagnosis of RM or R-CM may be qualified with the modifier "disabling" if the MIDAS score is 11 or greater. The MIDAS questionnaire measures lost days in three domains (work and school; chores and household work; as well as family, social, and leisure activity) over a 3-month recall interval. A score of 11 means that the patient had substantial limitations, usually in more than one domain. A score of 11 could arise from 11 separate attacks each preventing function for a single domain for a single day. It could also arise from multiday attacks or attacks that limited activities in more than one functional area for a day. The cut-score of 11 was developed based on diary validation and clinical utility studies, though it is admittedly somewhat arbitrary.[24] In population studies, about 22% of migraine sufferers and 41% of CM migraine sufferers have MIDAS scores greater than 11.

Table 3.2 provides a more detailed assessment of the frequency of significant interference as measured by MIDAS, for both EM and CM in the population. We report the proportion of individuals losing at least one day of work or school; household work; or family, social, and leisure activity over 3 months as one measure of significant interference. We also report reduced productivity days at work or school and household work or chores. The table reveals

Table 3-2 "Significant" Interference over the Last 3 Months: AMPP 2005 Survey

	Proportion of Cases in the Population (%)	
	Episodic Migraine ($n = 494$)	Chronic Migraine ($n = 520$)
Missed work or school (≥1 day)	17.1	23*
Reduced productivity (≥5 days)	12.3	33.8*
Missed household work (≥1 day)	68.5	56.9*
Reduced productivity (≥5 days)	24.3	57.4*
Missed family, social and leisure activity (≥1 day)	40.3	64.7*

that activity limitations are more common in CM than EM but that both disorders have substantial disability.

The ICHD-IIR provides an operational definition for the diagnosis of medication overuse headache.[35,36] Excessive use of symptomatic medication is a risk factor for migraine chronification and perhaps for refractoriness to treatment.[37–40] Excessive symptomatic medication (ESM) use is common in the population.[41] It has been estimated that nearly 4.4% of men and almost 7% of the women in Switzerland use analgesics at least twice a week, and more than 2% use it daily.[42] In the United States, frequent use of analgesics is also common. According to the Slone survey, headache is the second most common reason for taking medication in the U.S. adult population.[39] Other conditions associated with frequent analgesic use include pain not secondary to arthritis (third most frequent) and medications to relieve arthritis and joint pain (sixth most frequent).[43]

Medication overuse is associated with R-CM. In headache clinics, more than 80% of patients with CDH use acute medications on more days than not;[39,44,45] in the population, the prevalence of CM with medication overuse (use of acute medications on more than 10 or 15 days per month, depending on the medication class) is approximately 1.5%.[9,10]

Future Directions

The proposed definitions for RM and R-CM should be assessed in field studies to determine if they can be reliably applied. That is, experienced clinicians seeing the same patients should agree on the diagnosis of RM or R-CM. Once reliability is established, validity studies are needed. These studies might assess diagnostic groups with external validators including diary-based assessments.

When the diagnostic criteria are finalized, better defining the epidemiology of RM and R-CM will require specifically designed studies. There are well developed approaches for identifying ICHD-II migraine and chronic migraine in the population. An operational definition for impairment of function or reduced HRQoL is required. Better approaches for defining adequate trials of nonpharmacologic, acute, and preventive treatment are also needed.

References

1. Stovner LJ, Hagen K, Jensen R, et al. The global burden of headache: a documentation of headache prevalence and disability worldwide. *Cephalalgia.* 2007;27(3):193–210.
2. Lipton RB, Bigal ME. Ten lessons on the epidemiology of migraine. *Headache.* 2007;47(suppl 1):S2–9.

3. Headache Classification Committee of the International Headache Society. Classification and diagnostic criteria for headache disorders, cranial neuralgias and facial pain. *Cephalalgia.* 1988;8(suppl 7):1–96.
4. Headache Classification Subcommittee of the International Headache Society. *The International Classification of Headache Disorders*, 2nd ed. *Cephalgia.* 2004;24(suppl 1):1–15.
5. Schwartz BS, Stewart, WF, Simon D, Lipton RB. The epidemiology of tension type headache *JAMA.* 2004;279:381–383.
6. Lipton RB, Stewart WF, Diamond S, et al. Prevalence and burden of migraine in the United States: data from the American Migraine Study II. *Headache.* 2001;41:646–657.
7. Steiner TJ, Scher AI, Stewart WF, et al. The prevalence and disability burden of adult migraine in England and their relationships to age, gender and ethnicity. *Cephalalgia.* 2003;23:519–527.
8. Lipton RB, Bigal ME, Diamond M, Freitag F, Reed ML, Stewart WF; AMPP Advisory Group. Migraine prevalence, disease burden, and the need for preventive therapy. *Neurology.* 2007;68(5):343–349.
9. Scher AI, Stewart WF, Liberman J, Lipton RB. Prevalence of frequent headache in a population sample. *Headache.* 1998;38:497–506.
10. Castillo J, Muñoz P, Guitera V, Pascual J. Epidemiology of chronic daily headache in the general population. *Headache.* 1999;39:190–196.
11. Stewart WF, Ricci JA, Chee E, et al. Lost productive time and cost due to common pain conditions in the US workforce. *JAMA.* 2003;290: 2443–2454.
12. Hu XH, Markson LE, Lipton RB, et al. Burden of migraine in the United States: disability and economic costs. *Arch Intern Med.* 1999;159:813–818.
13. Lipton RB, Silberstein SD, Saper JR, Bigal ME, Goadsby PJ. Why headache treatment fails. *Neurology.* 2003;60(7):1064–1070.
14. Schulman EA, Lake III AE, Goadsby PJ, Peterlin BL, Siegel SE, Markley HG, Lipton RB. Defining refractory migraine and refractory chronic migraine: proposed criteria from the Refractory Headache Special Interest Section of the American Headache Society. *Headache.* 2008;48(6):778–782.
15. Scher AI, Stewart WF, Lipton RB. Migraine and headache: a meta-analytic approach. In: Crombie IK, Croft PR, Linton SJ, eds. *Epidemiology of Pain.* Seattle: IASP Press, 1999:159–170.
16. Stewart WF, Lipton RB, Celentano DD, Reed ML. Prevalence of migraine headache in the United States. Relation to age, income, race, and other sociodemographic factors. *JAMA.* 1992;267:64–69.
17. Silberstein SD, Lipton RB, Sliwinski M. Classification of daily and near-daily headaches: field trial of revised IHS criteria. *Neurology.* 1996;47:871–875.
18. Headache Classification Committee. New appendix criteria open for a broader concept of chronic migraine. *Cephalalgia.* 2006;26:742–746.
19. Bigal ME, Lipton RB. When migraine progresses: transformed or chronic migraine. *Expert Rev Neurother.* 2006;6(3):297–306
20. Lipton RB, Bigal ME, Stewart WF. Clinical trials of acute treatments for migraine including multiple attack studies of pain, disability, and health-related quality of life. *Neurology.* 2005;65(12 suppl 4):S50–58.

21. Cady R, Farmer K, Beach ME, Tarrasch J. Nurse-based education: an office-based comparative model for education of migraine patients. *Headache.* 2007; [Epub ahead of print]
22. Leonardi M, Steiner TJ, Scher AT, Lipton RB. The global burden of migraine: measuring disability in headache disorders with WHO's Classification of Functioning, Disability and Health (ICF). *J Headache Pain.* 2005;6(6):429–440.
23. Hamelsky SW, Lipton RB, Stewart WF. An assessment of the burden of migraine using the willingness to pay model. *Cephalalgia.* 2005;25(2):87–100.
24. Stewart WF, Lipton RB, Dowson AJ, Sawyer J. Development and testing of the Migraine Disability Assessment (MIDAS) Questionnaire to assess headache-related disability. *Neurology.* 2001;56(6 suppl 1):S20–28.
25. Solomon GD. Evolution of the measurement of quality of life in migraine. *Neurology.* 1997;48(suppl 3): 10–15.
26. Solomon GD, Skobieranda FG, Gragg LA. Quality of life and well being of headache patient: measurement by the Medical Outcomes Study. *JAMA.* 1989;262:907–913.
27. Hurst B, Macclesfield U. Assessing outcomes of treatment for migraine headache using generic and specific measurements. Neurology 1998;50 (suppl 4):180–181.
28. Jhingran P, Osterhaus JT, Miller DW, et al. Development and validation of the Migraine-Specific Quality of Life Questionnaire *Headache.* 1998;38:295–302.
29. Santanello NC, Hartmaier SL, Epstein RS, Silberstein SD. Validation of a new quality of life questionnaire for acute migraine headache. *Headache.* 1995;35:330–337.
30. Gobel H, Petersen-Braun M, Soyka D. The epidemiology of headache in Germany: a nationwide survey of a representative sample on the basis of the headache classification of the International Headache Society. *Cephalalgia.* 1994;14:97–106.
31. Terwindt GM, Ferrari MD, Tijhuis M, Groenen SM, Picavet HS, Launer LJ. The impact of migraine on quality of life in the general population: the GEM study. *Neurology.* 2000;55(5):624–629.
32. Lipton RB, Liberman JN, Kolodner KB, et al. Migraine headache disability and quality of life: a population-based case-control study. *Headache.* 1999;39:365.
33. Campbell JK, Penzien D, Wall EM. Evidence-based guidelines for migraine: Behavioral and physical treatments. Available at: http://www.aan.com/professionals/practice/pdfs/gl0089.pdf
34. Diamond S, Bigal ME, Silberstein S, Loder E, Reed M, Lipton RB. Patterns of diagnosis and acute and preventive treatment for migraine in the United States: results from the American Migraine Prevalence and Prevention study. *Headache.* 2007;47(3):355–363.
35. Silberstein SD, Olesen J, Bousser MG, et al; International Headache Society. The *International Classification of Headache Disorders*, 2nd ed. (ICHD-II)–revision of criteria for 8.2 Medication-overuse headache. *Cephalalgia.* 2005; 25(6):460–465.
36. Olesen J, Bousser MG, Diener HC, et al. New appendix criteria open for a broader concept of chronic migraine. *Cephalalgia.* 2006;26(6):742–746.

37. Katsarava Z, Schneeweiss S, Kurth T, et al. Incidence and predictors for chronicity of headache in patients with episodic migraine. *Neurology.* 2004;62:788–790.
38. Bigal ME, Lipton RB. Modifiable risk factors for migraine progression (or for chronic daily headaches)—clinical lessons. *Headache.* 2006;46(suppl 3): S144–146.
39. Mathew NT. Drug-induced headache. *Neurol Clin.* 1990;8:903–912.
40. Krymchantowski AV, Moreira PF. Out-patient detoxification in chronic migraine: comparison of strategies. *Cephalalgia.* 2003;23:982–993.
41. Compton WM, Volkow ND. Major increases in opioid analgesic abuse in the United States: concerns and strategies. *Drug Alcohol Depend.* 2006;81(2):103–107.
42. Compton WM, Stein JB, Robertson EB, Pintello D, Pringle B, Volkow ND. Charting a course for health services research at the National Institute on Drug Abuse. *J Subst Abuse Treat.* 2005;29(3):167–172.
43. Kaufman DW, Kelly JP, Rosenberg L, Anderson TE, Mitchell AA. Recent patterns of medication use in the ambulatory adult population of the United States: the Slone survey. *JAMA.* 2002;287(3):337–344.
44. Bigal ME, Rapoport AM, Sheftell FD, et al. Transformed migraine and medication overuse in a tertiary headache centre—clinical characteristics and treatment outcomes. *Cephalalgia.* 2004;24:483–490.
45. Rapoport A, Stang P, Gutterman DL, et al. Analgesic rebound headache in clinical practice: data from a physician survey. *Headache.* 1996;36:14–19.

4

Medically Refractory Primary Headache*[1]

Some Mechanistic Considerations[1]

Peter J. Goadsby MD, PhD, DSc, and Richard Hargreaves PhD

Introduction

Migraine is a brain disorder with a complex pathophysiology that until recently has been relatively poorly understood.[2] It is common,[3] disabling,[4] and economically costly.[5] In this chapter we address some possible mechanisms underlying medically refractory primary headache, and to do so we have arbitrarily adopted some definitions to frame our discussions in an area that has not been formally addressed in the past. First, we recognize the definitions of the International Headache Society for migraine[6] and for chronic migraine.[7] However, for this exercise the rigid use of the 15-day cutoff is probably not suitable, and we try to address whether frequency of headache is an issue for tractability for treatment. Second, the definition of refractory to treatment is here taken to mean pharmacologic medical treatment. Precise definitions for this, such as the number of failed preventives, have been suggested,[8,9] but for our purpose this is less important than the general principle that some patients with clinically indistinguishable phenotypes seem refractory to medical management. Third, we have assumed that refractoriness is not due to diagnostic errors or inappropriate use of normally effective medicines,[10] the most common reasons for apparent intractability. Lastly, we set aside a natural history argument: that many patients would improve or

*This chapter is based on an earlier published review

become responsive to therapy if given time. This may be true for some individuals but is not helpful as a blanket explanation.

Is There a Genetic Basis for Medically Intractable Migraine?

Migraine appears to be a condition that has a substantial inherited component. It is clear from clinical practice that many patients have first-degree relatives who also suffer from migraine,[11,12] and numerous published studies have reported a positive family history.[13] The genetic underpinning of primary headaches remains somewhat speculative. In migraine with aura, epidemiological studies have identified the methyltetrahydrofolate reductase gene mutation C677T as over-represented, but its potential role in the disorder is currently unexplained.[14] Most discussions on the genetics of primary headache have their base in findings from studies of rare migraine variants with deep genetic penetrance in a few families that have profound and well described phenotypes. The specific genetic cause of familial hemiplegic migraine has been identified in a number of cases. Mutations involving the $Ca_v2.1$ (P/Q) type voltage-gated calcium channel *CACNA1A* gene are causative in familial hemiplegic migraine-I (FHM-I).[15] Mutations in the *ATP1A2* gene[16,17] encoding the catalytic α_2-subunit of the glial Na^+, K^+-ATPase cause FHM-II. This mutation results in a smaller electrochemical gradient for Na^+ that has the effect of reducing the activity of glutamate transporters, leading to a synaptic buildup of the excitatory neurotransmitter glutamate. Two missense mutations (Q1489K and L1649Q) in *SCN1A* encoding the pore-forming α-subunit of the voltage-gated sodium channel Nav1.1 have been linked to what is now known as FHM-III. *SCN1A* mutations have previously been associated with childhood epilepsies of varying severity. A third mutation (l236V) has recently also been identified in an FHM family in which the majority of mutation carriers also have epilepsy. Electrophysiological studies[18] have shown that the sodium channel mutations associated with FHM have divergent effects on channel function. Relative to "wild-type" Nav1.1 channels, Q1489K shows increased persistent current but faster entry to slow inactivated as well as delayed recovery characteristics that is essentially a loss of function that is compounded by a greater loss of channel availability during repetitive stimulation. L236V, however, showed gain of function features such as accelerated recovery and increased persistent current and delayed entry into slow inactivation. Interestingly, the mutations that are associated with loss of function are linked to typical FHM, but L263V occurred in a family having both FHM and a high incidence of epilepsy. These findings indicate the complex relationship between migraine and epilepsy and suggest that the disorders may have a common molecular basis. Although devastating, FHM is not more troublesome to treat than any other form of migraine, often responding to the calcium channel/dopamine blocker flunarizine.[19]

The physiological consequences of the FHM mutations are only now being explored in genetically engineered animal models expressing mutant forms of the channels. Certainly, there is a reduced threshold to initiation of cortical spreading depression (CSD) in the rat;[20] however, because most antimigraine preventives have actions to reduce susceptibility to CSD,[21] a CSD-based mechanism for intractability is unlikely. Changes in neurotransmitter expression, specifically calcitonin gene-related peptide (CGRP) in trigeminal ganglion of animals with an FHM-I mutation, have also been reported.[22] Perhaps there is a paradigm here for starting to understand how genetic change may alter treatment responses, especially as CGRP antagonists[23] are now being developed as potential antimigraine therapies.[24–26] Future studies on the potential role of these channels in migraine-associated brain dysfunction should address conditional expression of these mutant channels in specific brain regions and neuronal subpopulations that have relevance to migraine pathogenesis

Population-based family studies in migraine probands who had either disabling or very painful migraine showed higher levels of family aggregation of migraine.[27] Interestingly, in the more recent study, the early age at onset of migraine in the proband was also associated with increased family aggregation and increased severity.[28] Because migraine is a complex multifactorial genetic disorder,[29]it could be speculated that probands with more severe pain, more disability, or an earlier age at onset may have a greater genetic load and perhaps greater risk of being refractory but this has yet to be proven. Treatment-refractory migraine is certainly a subset of all migraine, suggesting that there must be an intersecting problem of migraine genetics plus something else that confers refractoriness.

Is There a Structural Explanation?

One possible explanation for treatment-refractory migraine would be structural changes in the brain. Raskin[30] initially reported, and Veloso confirmed,[31] that stimulation of the periaqueductal gray region can produce migraine in otherwise non–headache-prone people. Similarly, Welch and colleagues[32] noted excess iron in the periaqueductal gray (PAG) of patients with episodic and chronic migraine. Indeed chronic migraine can develop after a hemorrhage into a cavernoma in the region of the PAG,[33] or with a lesion of the pons.[34,35] Functional brain imaging with positron emission tomography (PET) similarly points to the brain stem by the demonstration of activation of the dorsal midbrain, including the PAG, and the dorsal pons, near the locus coeruleus, in studies during migraine without aura.[36] Dorsolateral pontine activation is seen with PET in spontaneous episodic[37–38] and chronic migraine,[40] and with nitroglycerin-triggered attacks.[41,42] However, in patients with chronic migraine successfully treated with occipital nerve stimulation, who had been previously refractory to medical treatment, these brain areas, interestingly, remained active.[40] It has been speculated, with support from preclinical studies[43–46] that extracranial disease at the back of the head or upper neck may make headaches refractory through sensitizing neurons in the trigeminocervical complex that receive convergent input from both the trigeminal and occipital nerves. Persistent input from extracranial sources nerves enhances the sensitivity to input from intracranial pain producing structures, thereby potentially exacerbating headache. Anecdotal reports have suggested that addressing these extracranial structural problems may, for some people, be the key to effective treatment.

Is One Plausible Explanation for Medically Refractory Migraine Structural Changes in the Brain Stem?

If this were the explanation, one might expect to see it on brain imaging. Careful comparisons of migraine and non-migraine brains using voxel-based morphometry initially failed to demonstrate changes.[47] Subtle changes in the visual processing network have now been shown in migraine with and without aura.[48] However, there is no suggestion these change with time or are related strictly to attack load or any other measure of disease burden,[49] so they may be an anatomical trait.

Do Structural Changes on MRI Account for Refractory Migraine?

Migraine with aura has been associated with a number of "vascular" pathologies. There is a relationship between migraine with aura and patent foramen ovale (PFO),[50] yet simple closure of PFO in migraine is not curative.[51] Migraine with aura is seen in **c**erebral **a**utosomal **d**ominant **a**rteriopathy with **s**ubcortical **i**nfarcts and **l**eukoencephalopathy (CADASIL)[52] and in the Trex1 mutations,[53] and there are white matter abnormalities seen on brain magnetic resonance imaging (MRI) in migraine with aura.[54] Moreover, migraine with aura is associated with increased stroke risk in young females.[49] One view has been to see these as mechanistic associations, that vascular or cerebrovascular disease is somehow pathogenetic in migraine. An alternative view would be to see migraine with aura, broadly, sometimes being part of a cerebral–neurovascular syndrome of coexistent manifestations of sometimes codependent pathologies. In this construct aura gene(s) convey or are associated with structural vascular change, much as is seen in cerebral–cardiac associations such as those of Friedrich's ataxia. Such a view suggests that the vascular components may complicate migraine, for example, PFO may trigger migraine attacks, but that the vascular changes are not causal. This construct would also suggest that such changes are not predictive of refractoriness in migraine, and so far they seem not to be so.

Is There a Systems Functional Explanation?

Central nervous system (CNS) plasticity changes are an attractive way to conceptualize medically intractable migraine. Clearly changes in brain function, without overt lesions, can be seen on PET studies of chronic migraine. There is persistence of pontine activation without any change on MRI.[40] One common theme in medically intractable migraine is the coexistence of medication overuse.[55]

Medication overuse headache is to be found in about one percent of Western populations, so it is very common as a problem.[56] Medication overuse headache can be seen in patients using analgesics for other reasons, such as in rheumatology[57] or gastrointestinal indications,[58] or indeed in patients with cluster headache.[59] There are two common themes here. First, not all patients overusing analgesics will develop medication overuse headache, indeed perhaps only about one-third do so. Second, almost all patients who develop the problem in these settings have a personal or family history, or both, of migraine or disabling headache.[60] Some patients do extremely well when medication overuse is controlled, although many do not.[61] Further, it has generally been held that medication overuse plays a substantial role in medical intractability such that medication withdrawal is recommended as part of the management of frequent migraine. However, it is clear from randomized placebo-controlled trials that this is not necessarily always correct, as topiramate is effective in a proportion of patients with chronic migraine and medication overuse.[62,63]

There is certainly a trait in migraine that can be demonstrated interparoxysmally using electrophysiological methods. Visual,[64] auditory,[65] and event-related[66] potentials are each exaggerated between attacks, suggesting a lack of habituation, which normalise during attacks,[67] and can be altered by standard migraine preventives.[68] Remarkably, patients without migraine but with a family history can also be shown to have impaired habituation of the nociception-specific blink reflex, behaving like migraineurs rather than controls.[69] A marker of unknown importance is a change in orbitofrontal cortex. [^{18}F] Flurodeoxyglucose PET activity that has been observed in patients with medication overuse headache.[70]

Taken together, there is considerable emerging evidence for CNS dysfunction in migraine; however, none specifically has been implicated in medical intractability. The tools are available and electrophysiological[71] and functional imaging[72] studies in cohorts of relatively tractable and intractable patients may in the future yield insights into potential brain systems and circuits that influence tractability.

Is There a Pharmacologic Explanation?

A seemingly obvious possibility for medically intractable migraine would be a pharmacological explanation. This must exclude a simple pharmacokinetic argument that posits lack of exposure to medication, as one can always augment absorption with antiemetics and prokinetics, or indeed turn to non-oral routes. Few migraineurs do not respond to sumatriptan 6 mg subcutaneously,[73] and in clinical practice they are neither phenotypically obvious, nor necessarily those that do not respond to preventive medicines.

Is there then any rational pharmacological explanation for medically refractory primary headache? Receptor polymorphisms for the serotonin receptors that mediate the actions of triptans,[74] such as the 5-HT$_{1B}$ receptor,[75,76] are unrelated to clinical responses to sumatriptan. 5-HT$_{1F}$ receptor genetics[77] also seem unrelated to anti-migraine activity. But perhaps other genes that mark a good response will, when absent, lead to refractoriness (e.g., it has been suggested that particular dopamine receptor 2 forms may be important for rizatriptan effectiveness[78]); but this is unproven by rigorous clinical trial. Perhaps understanding how genes such as those in dopamine pathways that have been associated with increased severity[79] or protection from migraine[80] intersect with those increasing risk of migraine will hold the key to understanding the basis of refractoriness. Now that the genetics of rare profound family migraine variants are becoming better understood, it is hoped that the observations made can be used to focus future studies into the molecular genetics of primary headaches and medically intractable migraine and provide the basis for new therapeutic advances.

From the preventive migraine literature there is little as yet to be gleaned. Chronic migraine has barely been studied, with the notable exception of its responsiveness to topiramate.[62,63,81] Although these studies suggest that patients previously considered difficult to treat are tractable, they were not designed to give insights into nonresponsive subjects.

Summary

Basic science studies of potential mechanisms in migraine have shown a high potential for sensitizing changes within trigeminal sensory pathways[82] that could influence headache severity and associated sensory symptoms. Cutaneous allodynia has been proposed as a clinical marker of central sensitization and its presence appears associated with frequency, severity, and disability of migraine in more than 60% of migraineurs,[83,84] although it does not influence therapeutic responses at least to triptans.[85–87] It therefore seems remarkable that the treatment of migraine is not more intractable and that most patients seen in practice remain, to some degree, responsive to therapy. However, despite increased understanding of the mechanisms involved in idiopathic primary headache and its therapy, the condition of refractory migraine remains somewhat of an enigma. There are many exciting new technological advances that may enable us to understand refractory migraine better and place it within or outside current theories of migraine pathogenesis. Neuroimaging studies may point to the CNS structures, transmitter systems, and circuits involved in refractory migraine. Pharmacogenetics may hold a crucial key to identify ion channel, receptor-based, or biochemical differences that could provide a rational basis for strategies to improve clinical care. Refractory migraine is a worthy challenge for the science and treatment of headache that demands increased research.

References

1. Goadsby PJ, Hargreaves R. Refractory migraine and chronic migraine: pathophysiological mechanisms. *Headache.* 2008;48:799–804.
2. Goadsby PJ, Oshinsky M. The pathophysiology of migraine. In: Silberstein SD, Lipton RB, Dodick D, eds. *Wolff's Headache and Other Head Pain,* 8th ed. New York: Oxford, 2008:105–119.
3. Lipton RB, Stewart WF, Diamond S, Diamond ML, Reed M. Prevalence and burden of migraine in the United States: data from the American Migraine Study II. *Headache.* 2001;41:646–657.
4. Menken M, Munsat TL, Toole JF. The global burden of disease study - implications for neurology. *Arch Neurol.* 2000;57:418–420.
5. Stewart WF, Ricci JA, Chee E, Morganstein D, Lipton R. Lost productive time and cost due to common pain conditions in the US workforce. *JAMA.* 2003;290:2443–2454.
6. Headache Classification Committee of The International Headache Society. The International Classification of Headache Disorders, 2nd ed. *Cephalalgia.* 2004;24(suppl 1):1–160.
7. Olesen J, Bousser MG, Diener HC, Dodick D, First M, Goadsby P, et al. New appendix criteria open for a broader concept of chronic migraine. *Cephalalgia.* 2006;26:742–746.
8. Goadsby PJ, Schoenen J, Ferrari MD, Silberstein SD, Dodick D. Towards a definition of intractable headache for use in clinical practice and trials. *Cephalalgia.* 2006;26:1168–1170.
9. Schulman EA, Lake AE, 3rd, Goadsby PJ, Peterlin BL, Siegel SE, Markley HG, et al. Defining refractory migraine and refractory chronic migraine: proposed criteria from the refractory headache special interest section of the American Headache Society. *Headache.* 2008;48:778–782.
10. Lipton RB, SIlberstein SD, Saper J, Bigal ME, Goadsby PJ. Why headache treatment fails? *Neurology.* 2003;60:1064–1070.
11. Silberstein SD, Lipton RB, Goadsby PJ. *Headache in Clinical Practice,* 2nd ed. London: Martin Dunitz, 2002.
12. Lance JW, Goadsby PJ. *Mechanism and Management of Headache,* 7th ed. New York: Elsevier, 2005.
13. Russell MB. Genetic epidemiology of migraine and cluster headache. *Cephalalgia.* 1997;17:683–701.
14. Scher AI, Terwindt GM, Verschuren WM, et al. Migraine and MTHFR C677T genotype in a population-based sample. *Ann Neurol.* 2006;59:372–375.
15. Ophoff RA, Terwindt GM, Vergouwe MN, et al. Familial hemiplegic migraine and episodic ataxia type-2 are caused by mutations in the Ca^{2+} channel gene CACNL1A4. *Cell.* 1996;87:543–552.
16. Marconi R, De Fusco M, Aridon P, et al. Familial hemiplegic migraine type 2 is linked to 0.9Mb region on chromosome 1q23. *Ann Neurol.* 2003; 53:376–381.

17. De Fusco M, Marconi R, Silvestri L, et al. Haploinsufficiency of ATP1A2 encoding the Na$^+$/K$^+$ pump 2 subunit associated with familial hemiplegic migraine type 2. *Nat. Genet.* 2003; 33: 192–196.
18. Kahlig KM, Rhodes TH, Pusch M, et al. Divergent sodium channel defects in familial hemiplegic migraine. *Proc Natl Acad Sci USA.* 2008; 105: 9799–9804
19. Mohammed BP, Goadsby PJ, Prabhakar P. To report the use of flunarizine in children with headache in a tertiary centre. *Cephalalgia.* 2009; 29 (Suppl 1):143.
20. van den Maagdenberg AMJM, Pietrobon D, Pizzorusso T, et al. A Cacna1a knock-in migraine mouse model with increased susceptibility to cortical spreading depression. *Neuron.* 2004;41:701–710.
21. Ayata C, Jin H, Kudo C, Dalkara T, Moskowitz MA. Suppression of cortical spreading depression in migraine prophylaxis. *Ann Neurol.* 2006;59:652–661.
22. Mathew R, Chami L, Bergerot A, van den Maagdenberg AMJM, Ferrari MD, Goadsby PJ. Reduced expression of calcitonin gene related peptide (CGRP) in mice with the familial hemiplegic migraine (FHM) 1 mutation. *Cephalalgia.* 2007;27:1190.
23. Doods H, Arndt K, Rudolf K, Just S. CGRP antagonists: unravelling the role of CGRP in migraine. *Trends Pharmacol Sci.* 2007;28:580–587.
24. Olesen J, Diener H-C, Husstedt I-W, et al. Calcitonin gene-related peptide (CGRP) receptor antagonist BIBN4096BS is effective in the treatment of migraine attacks. *N Engl J Med.* 2004;350:1104–1110.
25. Ho T, Mannix L, Fan X, et al. Randomized controlled trial of an oral CGRP antagonist, MK-0974, in acute treatment of migraine. *Neurology.* 2008;70:1004–1012.
26. Ho TW, Ferrari MD, Dodick DW, et al. Efficacy and tolerability of MK-0974 (telcagepant), a new oral antagonist of calcitonin gene-related peptide receptor, compared with zolmitriptan for acute migraine: a randomised, placebo-controlled, parallel-treatment trial. *Lancet.* 2008;372:2115–2123.
27. Stewart WF, Staffa J, Lipton RB, Ottman R. Familial risk of migraine: a population-based study. *Ann Neurol.* 1997;41:166–172.
28. Stewart WF, Bigal ME, Kolodner K, Dowson A, Liberman JN, Lipton RB. Familial risk of migraine: variation by proband age at onset and headache severity. *Neurology.* 2006;66:344–348.
29. Ferrari MD, van den Maagdenberg AMJM, Frants RR, Goadsby PJ. Migraine as a cerebral ionopathy with impaired central sensory processing. In: Waxman SG, ed. *Molecular Neurology.* London: Elsevier Academic Press, 2007:439–461.
30. Raskin NH, Hosobuchi Y, Lamb S. Headache may arise from perturbation of brain. *Headache.* 1987;27:416–420.
31. Veloso F, Kumar K, Toth C. Headache secondary to deep brain implantation. *Headache.* 1998;38:507–515.
32. Welch KM, Nagesh V, Aurora S, Gelman N. Periaqueductal grey matter dysfunction in migraine: cause or the burden of illness? *Headache.* 2001;41:629–637.
33. Goadsby PJ. Neurovascular headache and a midbrain vascular malformation-evidence for a role of the brainstem in chronic migraine. *Cephalalgia.* 2002;22:107–111.

34. Afridi S, Goadsby PJ. New onset migraine with a brainstem cavernous angioma. *J Neurol Neurosurg Psychiatry.* 2003;74:680–682.
35. Obermann M, Gizewski ER, Limmroth V, Diener H-C, Katsarava Z. Symptomatic migraine and pontine vascular malformation: evidence for a key role of the brainstem in the pathophysiology of chronic migraine. *Cephalalgia.* 2006;26:763–766.
36. Weiller C, May A, Limmroth V, et al. Brain stem activation in spontaneous human migraine attacks. *Nat Med.* 1995;1:658–660.
37. Afridi S, Giffin NJ, Kaube H, et al. A PET study in spontaneous migraine. *Arch Neurol.* 2005;62:1270–1275.
38. Denuelle M, Fabre N, Payoux P, Chollet F, Geraud G. Brainstem and hypothalamic activation in spontaneous migraine attacks. *Cephalalgia.* 2004;24:775–814.
39. Denuelle M, Fabre N, Payoux P, Chollet F, Geraud G. Hypothalamic activation in spontaneous migraine attacks. *Headache.* 2007;47:1418–1426.
40. Matharu MS, Bartsch T, Ward N, Frackowiak RSJ, Weiner RL, Goadsby PJ. Central neuromodulation in chronic migraine patients with suboccipital stimulators: a PET study. *Brain.* 2004;127:220–230.
41. Bahra A, Matharu MS, Buchel C, Frackowiak RSJ, Goadsby PJ. Brainstem activation specific to migraine headache. *Lancet.* 2001;357:1016–1017.
42. Afridi S, Matharu MS, Lee L, et al. A PET study exploring the laterality of brainstem activation in migraine using glyceryl trinitrate. *Brain.* 2005;128:932–939.
43. Bartsch T, Goadsby PJ. Stimulation of the greater occipital nerve induces increased central excitability of dural afferent input. *Brain.* 2002;125:1496–1509.
44. Bartsch T, Goadsby PJ. Increased responses in trigeminocervical nociceptive neurones to cervical input after stimulation of the dura mater. *Brain.* 2003;126:1801–1813.
45. Bartsch T, Goadsby PJ. Anatomy and physiology of pain referral in primary and cervicogenic headache disorders. *Headache Curr.* 2005;2:42–48.
46. Le Doare K, Akerman S, Holland PR, et al. Occipital afferent activation of second order neurons in the trigeminocervical complex in rat. *Neurosci Lett.* 2006;403:73–77.
47. Matharu MS, Good CD, May A, Bahra A, Goadsby PJ. No change in the structure of the brain in migraine: a voxel-based morphometric study. *Eur J Neurol.* 2003;10:53–58.
48. Granziera C, DaSilva AFM, Snyder J, Tuch DS, Hadjikhani N. Anatomical alterations of the visual motion processing network in migraine with and without aura. *PLoS Med.* 2006;3:e402.
49. Kurth T. Migraine and ischaemic vascular events. *Cephalalgia.* 2007;27:965–975.
50. Diener HC, Kurth T, Dodick D. Patent foramen ovale and migraine. *Curr Pain Headache Rep.* 2007;11:236–240.
51. Dowson A, Mullen MJ, Peatfield R, et al. Migraine Intervention with STARFlex Technology (MIST) Trial. A Prospective, Multicenter, Double-Blind, Sham-Controlled Trial to Evaluate the Effectiveness of Patent Foramen Ovale Closure with STARFlex Septal Repair Implant to Resolve Refractory Migraine Headache. *Circulation.* 2008;117:1397–1404.

52. Joutel A, Corpechot C, Ducros A, et al. Notch3 mutations in CADASIL, a hereditary adult-onset condition causing stroke and dementia. *Nature.* 1996;383:707–710.
53. Richards A, van den Maagdenberg AM, Jen JC, et al. C-terminal truncations in human 3'-5' DNA exonuclease TREX1 cause autosomal dominant retinal vasculopathy with cerebral leukodystrophy. *Nat Genet.* 2007;39:1068–1070.
54. Kruit MC, van Buchem MA, Hofman PA, et al. Migraine as a risk factor for subclinical brain lesions. *JAMA.* 2004;291:427–434.
55. Silberstein SD, Olesen J, Bousser MG, Diener HC, Dodick D, First M, et al. *The International Classification of Headache Disorders,* 2nd ed (ICHD-II)–revision of criteria for 8.2 Medication-overuse headache. *Cephalalgia.* 2005;25:460–465.
56. Scher AI, Lipton RB, Stewart W. Risk factors for chronic daily headache. *Curr Pain Headache Rep.* 2002;6:486–491.
57. Bahra A, Walsh M, Menon S, Goadsby PJ. Does chronic daily headache arise de novo in association with regular analgesic use? *Headache.* 2003;43:179–190.
58. Wilkinson SM, Becker WJ, Heine JA. Opiate use to control bowel motility may induce chronic daily headache in patients with migraine. *Headache.* 2001;41:303–309.
59. Paemeleire K, Bahra A, Evers S, Matharu MS, Goadsby PJ. Medication-overuse headache in cluster headache patients. *Neurology.* 2006;67:109–113.
60. Goadsby PJ. Is medication-overuse headache a distinct biological entity? *Nat Clin Pract Neurol.* 2006;2:401.
61. Zeeberg P, Olesen J, Jensen R. Discontinuation of medication overuse in headache patients: recovery of therapeutic responsiveness. *Cephalalgia.* 2006;26:1192–1198.
62. Diener H-C, Bussone G, van Oene JC, Lahaye M, Schwalen S, Goadsby PJ. Topiramate reduces headache days in chronic migraine: a randomized, double-blind, placebo-controlled study. *Cephalalgia.* 2007;27:814–823.
63. Silberstein SD, Lipton RB, Dodick DW, et al. Efficacy and safety of topiramate for the treatment of chronic migraine: a randomized, double-blind, placebo-controlled trial. *Headache.* 2007;47:170–80.
64. Schoenen J, Wang W, Albert A, Delwaide PJ. Potentiation instead of habituation characterizes visual evoked potentials in migraine patients between attacks. *Eur J Neurol.* 1995;2:115–122.
65. Wang W, Timsit-Berthier M, Schoenen J. Intensity dependence of the auditory cortical evoked potentials is pronounced in migraine: an indication of cortical potentiation and low serotonergic transmission? *Neurology.* 1996;46:1404–1409.
66. Wang W, Schoenen J. Interictal potentiation of passive "oddball" auditory event-related potentials in migraine. *Cephalalgia.* 1998;18:261–265.
67. Afra J, Sandor P, Schoenen J. Habituation of visual and intensity dependence of cortical auditory evoked potentials tend to normalise just before and during migraine attacks. *Cephalalgia.* 2000;20:347.
68. Sandor PS, Afra J, Ambrosini A, Schoenen J. Prophylactic treatment of migraine with beta-blockers and riboflavin: differential effects on the

intensity dependence of auditory evoked cortical potentials. *Headache.* 2000;40:30–35.
69. Di Clemente L, Coppola G, Magis D, et al. Interictal habituation deficit of the nociceptive blink reflex: an endophenotypic marker for presymptomatic migraine? *Brain.* 2007;130:765–770.
70. Fumal A, Laureys S, Di Clemente L, et al. Orbitofrontal cortex involvement in chronic analgesic-overuse headache evolving from episodic migraine. *Brain.* 2006;129:543–550.
71. Magis D, Ambrosini A, Bendtsen L, Ertas M, Kaube H, Schoenen J. Evaluation and proposal for optimalization of neurophysiological tests in migraine: part 1—electrophysiological tests. *Cephalalgia.* 2007;27:1323–1338.
72. Magis D, Bendtsen L, Goadsby PJ, et al. Evaluation and proposal for optimization of neurophysiological tests in migraine: Part 2—neuroimaging and the nitroglycerin test. *Cephalalgia.* 2007;27:1339–1359.
73. Ferrari MD, The Subcutaneous Sumatriptan International Study Group. Treatment of migraine attacks with sumatriptan. *N Engl J Med.* 1991;325:316–321.
74. Goadsby PJ. The pharmacology of headache. *Prog Neurobiol.* 2000;62:509–525.
75. MaassenVanDenBrink A, Vergouwe MN, Ophoff RA, Saxena PR, Ferrari MD, Frants RR. 5-HT_{1B} receptor polymorphism and clinical response to sumatriptan. *Headache.* 1998;38:288–291.
76. Velati D, Viana M, Cresta S, et al. 5-Hydroxytryptamine(1B) receptor and triptan response in migraine, lack of association with common polymorphisms. *Eur J Pharmacol.* 2007;580:43–47.
77. VanDenBrink AM, Vergouwe MN, Ophoff RA, et al. Chromosomal localization of the 5-HT_{1F} receptor gene: no evidence for involvement in response to sumatriptan in migraine patients. *Am J Med Genet.* 1998;77:415–420.
78. Asuni C, Cherchi A, Congiu D, Piccardi MP, Del Zompo M, Stochino ME. Association study between clinical response to rizatriptan and some candidate genes. *J Headache Pain.* 2007;8:185–189.
79. Park J, Lee KS, Kim JS, Kim YI, Shin HE. Genetic contribution of catechol-*O*-methyltransferase polymorphism in patients with migraine without aura. *J Clin Neurol.* 2007;3:24–33.
80. Akerman S, Goadsby PJ. Dopamine and migraine: biology and clinical implications. *Cephalalgia.* 2007;27:1308–1314.
81. Silvestrini M, Bartolini M, Coccia M, Baruffaldi R, Taffi R, Provinciali L. Topiramate in the treatment of chronic migraine. *Cephalalgia.* 2003;23:820–824.
82. Burstein R, Jakubowski M. Analgesic triptan action in an animal model of intracranial pain: a race against the development of central sensitisation. *Ann. Neurol.* 2004;55:27–36.
83. Lipton RB, Bigal ME, Ashina S, et al. Cutaneous allodynia in the migraine population. *Ann Neurol.* 2008;63:148–158.
84. Bigal ME, Ashina S, Burstein R, et al. Prevalence and characteristics of allodynia in headache sufferers: a population study. *Neurology.* 2008;70:1525–1533.
85. Cady R, Martin V, Mauskop A, et al. Symptoms of cutaneous sensitivity pre-treatment and post-treatment: results from the rizatriptan TAME studies. *Cephalalgia.* 2007;27:1055–1060.

86. Goadsby PJ, Zanchin G, Geraud G, et al. Early versus non-early intervention in acute migraine— "Act when Mild- AwM." A double-blind placebo-controlled trial of almotriptan. *Cephalalgia.* 2008;28:383–391.
87. Diaz-Insa S, Goadsby PJ, Zanchin G, et al. Early treatment with almotriptan allows a good outcome even in allodynic migraine patients: an Act when Mild (AwM) substudy. *Cephalalgia.* 2009;29:119.

5

History Taking and Examination of Patients with Refractory Headache

Thomas N. Ward, MD

Introduction

Whereas this book is focused on the topic of refractory migraine, this chapter concentrates on the process of making an accurate diagnosis in patients with the *symptom* of headache. According to the *International Classification of Headache Disorders*, 2nd edition (ICHD-II), there are more than 200 causes of headache.[1] The clinician's task is to ascertain what specific headache diagnosis/diagnoses the patient has, which will allow for proper treatment and prognosis. Diagnostic tests are chosen based on the initial clinical impression and are discussed at length in Chapter 6.

One useful diagnostic strategy is to remember that headaches may be *primary* (sui generis) such as migraine, or *secondary* (due to some underlying cause which might even be threatening and which, if treated, might cure the patient). In evaluating the patient with headache, the goal is to gather enough information to allow for classification of the headache type(s).

Specific headache diagnosis is made primarily from a careful history. Examination of the patient may add useful clues but often is normal in headache patients. Tests, if necessary, are then chosen based on the clinician's diagnostic impression, and to confirm or refute the various possibilities. Excluding secondary causes of headache is essential.

The various exigencies of clinical practice mandate management strategies that require optimal use of the appointment time allotted. Much has been made of the fact that clinicians interrupt patients early on during the interview and this sometimes leads to conflict and the feeling from some patients that they have not been "heard." On the other hand, a disorganized patient or one who rambles on aimlessly without direction can also waste a significant portion of the clinic visit. I shall now present my view of how to proceed, allowing the clinician to obtain the necessary data, but that also engages the patients and affords them their right to give their headache history.

History Taking

Ideally, the interview is best conducted in person with a sufficient amount of time allotted to gather the history, examine the patient and review the records, as well as time at the end for education, and initiating the therapeutic plan. Conducting the interview in person allows rapport to be established and is an important part of the therapeutic alliance. Some clinicians, in the interest of efficiency and time management, send patients questionnaires to fill out before their appointment. If this is done, it is important to ensure that the document(s) will contain enough information to assist in making a proper assessment of the patient and that there is time to review it with the patient for accuracy. There are many examples of such forms, which can be modified by clinicians to suit their particular needs.[2] The downside to using such forms is that the patient will have less time with the clinician. Motivated patients may do a better job of filling out the form and others may not make an adequate effort to provide sufficient information to benefit fully. In any event, someone must review the forms with the patient to ensure accuracy and clarify any discrepancies.

I begin the interview by asking the patient his or her age and if he or she is right- or left-handed. I then ask the patient to tell me about his or her headaches. The initial interaction may provide important information about the patient. Patients with borderline traits may disparage previous clinicians and/or elevate you by inappropriate flattery. Noting this can help set the stage for discussions about reasonable expectations and boundaries at the conclusion of the visit.

Most patients start by telling me how they are currently, and I gently interrupt them and redirect them by asking them at what age they first had headaches that were a problem for them. Various headache types have typical ages at onset, and this is an important diagnostic clue (see Box 5.1). In females, I ask when they had their menarche and if that was related to their headaches (onset, worsening, or change). Then I inquire as to *why* they remember those headaches. Were they associated with vomiting, or otherwise disabling so they missed school or other important events, or was the pain just severe and memorable in its own right? Was there some possibly inciting event such as the introduction of birth control pills, a new medical condition, a stressful life event, or a head/neck injury? Was the pattern infrequent, or frequent, or

Box 5-1 Typical Ages at Onset for Headaches

1. Migraine: Unusual before 4 years old, unusual to begin after 40 years old
2. Cluster headache: Usually second to fourth decades but onset as young as 2 years old has been suspected (based on behavioral observation) and also can begin in old age.
3. Tension-type headache: Childhood to old age
4. Hypnic headache: Usually >50 years old
5. Giant cell (temporal) arteritis: Usually >50 years old
6. Trigeminal neuralgia: Usually >40 years old. For patients <50 years old be particularly wary of secondary causes such as multiple sclerosis.

possibly constant from onset (in which case New Daily Persistent Headache is a possibility)?[1]

It is important to try to get patients to describe in detail the clinical features of their prior headaches to allow for a retrospective diagnosis, as well as asking about any previous clinicians they may have seen, and what diagnoses, tests, and treatments occurred. As much detail as possible should be sought, and requesting outside records and interviewing family members, especially parents, can be extremely useful. Many migraine patients have sinus symptoms due to a reflex involving the superior salivatory nucleus and others have neck discomfort.[3,4] The result is they may carry a false label of "sinus headache" or "tension headache" when in fact they have migraine. The original headache may have changed over time to a daily headache from a pattern of intermittent migraine, based on the concept of transformed migraine.[5] Or, a hemicranial headache that clearly was hemicrania continua may have become bilateral in the setting of medication overuse.[1,6]

Next, I ask the patient to tell me, then or now, if there been any triggers for the headaches. Triggers are most relevant for migraine, but are also known to occur with other headache conditions such as during bouts of cluster headache. Triggers do not necessarily cause headache every time, but perhaps more often than not, and within a few hours at most of exposure. I also ask about any ameliorating factors and what treatments in the past have worked, as they may also provide diagnostic clues. Patients should be asked if they have had a prodrome, possibly a hypothalamic manifestation of an impending headache, which may include food cravings, yawning, irritability, fatigue, or elation and that may occur hours to a few days before an attack. A history of an aura should be sought. This is a reversible neurological phenomenon, usually visual, which is thought to occur in 10% to 20% of migraineurs. An aura, however, may occur in association with other types of headache or may occur in isolation. When they occur in patients in later life, older than 40 years old, with or without history of migraine, transient ischemic attacks must be considered ("late-life migraine accompaniments").[1,7]

As migraineurs often have abnormalities of the autonomic nervous system, I ask if they have a history of motion sickness, fainting, or cold extremities (Raynaud's phenomenon is comorbid with migraine).[8] In my experience, it is common for a migraine patient to have at least one of these three conditions.

Then, after having obtained this background for perspective, and only *then*, do I ask the patient "How are you now, by which I mean over the past several months, and regarding the headache issue that has bought you here now?" The patient realizes he or she has had not only an opportunity to reflect on and convey his or her life's headache history, but now can approach the problem at hand. I ask patients, in a typical month currently, do they have any headache-free days? I carefully ask patients how many *types* of headaches they have. Specifically I ask if they have *one* type of headache that may vary, or perhaps *two* types "big ones (even big ones with vomiting) and little ones". I learned this particular question from Dr. Egilius L.H. Spierings, who informed me his mentor, Dr. John Graham of the Faulkner Headache Clinic, used this question[9] (personal communication). Rarely does a patient have more than one or two types of headache. I need to know if the headaches are daily and if so, are they constant or is there any headache-free time? I also need to know the duration of the headache attacks (untreated) if they are discrete.

Next, we delve into the characteristics of the headache pain. *Where* is it located? For example, hemicrania (always on one side, or can it alternate?), holocranial, elsewhere? *What* does it feel like—sharp, pressure, pounding, other; some patients may have multiple pain characteristics? Is the pain *mild/moderate/severe*? How long does it take to escalate to its maximum severity level? How *long* does it last? How *often* do attacks occur, and *when* do the attacks occur? I also need to know if there are associated features. I ask about nausea, vomiting, anorexia, light and/or sound sensitivity, even osmophobia. I inquire if there are any unusual types of pain such as the scalp/hair being painful, inability to wear jewelry/eyeglasses, or other manifestations of cutaneous allodynia (a sign of central sensitization) either during or outside of headache attacks as this has diagnostic and potentially treatment implications.[10] Patients are asked about their behavior during attacks; are they agitated and perhaps pace about during attacks (as in cluster headache), or do they lie down or sit quietly in a dark quiet place as migraineurs generally do? Has this headache changed? Is it worsening (i.e., more frequent, more severe or with a new feature such as nocturnal awakening or vomiting)? Of note, some things that worry headache sufferers are reassuring to the seasoned headache clinician. For example, a migraineur whose headaches are usually on one side who experiences a headache once on the other side may be concerned about a change in headache presentation while the clinician is reassured that occurrence on the opposite side argues against a migraine mimic such as an arteriovenous malformation or other underlying structural lesion. Or as noted earlier, medication overuse may change a headache, such

Box 5-2 Red Flags in Headache Evaluation

1. Sudden ("thunderclap") onset
2. *Any* abnormality on the neurological examination, including mental status
3. Age >50 years or <5 years
4. New-onset headache in patients with cancer or HIV infection
5. Abnormal vital signs, especially fever, Cushing's reflex, or paroxysmal elevations of blood pressure or blood pressure at the levels of malignant hypertension
6. *First/worst* (severe) headache
7. Seizures associated with headache
8. Onset during exertion
9. Worsening under observation

as making hemicrania continua become bilateral, or making migraine "transform" by an increase in headache frequency.[11] However, a change in headache pattern otherwise is a "red flag" and suggests the need for further investigation (Box 5.2).[12]

It is important to ask about treatments and diagnostic testing done in relation to the current problem. *As much detail as possible should be obtained.* Were medications trials given at sufficient dosage for adequate amounts of time (usually at least 2–3 months)? If the patient failed to tolerate or respond to a preventative agent(s), was he or she in analgesic rebound, which is felt to render preventative drugs ineffective? *I make specific and detailed inquiry into exactly how patients treat their current headaches.* This includes any nonprescription remedies and herbal/alternative treatments. Patients often do not consider these "medications" but some can cause analgesic rebound (medication overuse headache) and some may interact with prescription remedies. The timing of usage during an attack, the amounts ingested, and the frequency of use are essential pieces of information. I also often record a total weekly and/or monthly amount of any medications that might be causing analgesic rebound. I ascertain what tests were obtained, what the results were, and who else was consulted. It is best to obtain copies of test results and to review any diagnostic imaging personally by obtaining the images in addition to the reports.

The remainder of the history consists of detailing current and past general medical conditions (e.g., hypertension, thyroid disease, HIV, cancer), history of surgeries/procedures and of any physical trauma (whiplash, concussion), medications (doses, frequency of intake including any herbal/alternative/nonprescription remedies including especially over-the-counter/off-the-shelf analgesics), and medication allergies/intolerances. If the patient has a history of concussion and/or whiplash I specifically inquire as to the date(s), circumstances, and whether or not he or she made a full recovery from that particular event. Many patients with neck injuries are left with residual neck symptoms that may be relevant to their overall clinical presentation.

Psychiatric history should include any diagnoses applied by mental health workers and can also be made retrospectively based on patient-supplied symptomatology. I ask about energy, mood, and especially about sleep. Do they snore and is there "excessive daytime somnolence" (falling asleep during the daytime inappropriately, suggesting possible sleep apnea)? Is there significant trouble falling asleep and/or mid-cycle awakening? I ask if the patient has nightmares and also if he or she has any history of "abuse" (physical, emotional, or sexual). If the answer is positive I ask if it is ongoing or in the past. If there is a positive history, I also ask if the patient has been treated or is in ongoing therapy. If the abuse is ongoing, I make an intervention (referral to psychiatric services, shelter, and law enforcement as appropriate).

Family history is important to record, especially in cases of migraine. Some family members may have been given this diagnosis, but many migraineurs feel they have "sick headache" or "sinus headache" (see earlier). Asking if there is any recollection of family members lying down with a headache is helpful. Family histories are notoriously unreliable. I often give patients who seem to be migraineurs, but who tell me they have no relatives with migraine, a little detective work to do at their next family gathering. By asking the same questions I asked them, many return telling me of relatives who indeed manifested attacks clearly suggestive of migraine. I ask patients about their social history. Do they smoke? If they drink alcohol, how much and how often do they imbibe (does alcohol set off their headaches as may occur with some migraineurs and cluster patients during bouts)? I ask about their employment if they work outside the home. If so, have they missed work (absenteeism) or are they at work struggling due to the headaches (presenteeism)? Are their jobs in jeopardy because of the headaches? I also ask about their living situation; are they alone, separated, recently divorced? What is the impact of their pain problem on their friends, relatives? Further information may be gathered when appropriate to assess the level of disability/impact caused by the headaches. The *Migraine Disability Assessment score* (MIDAS) is one instrument that clinicians may use. It is a validated and reliable assessment of the prior 3 months.[13] In addition, some clinicians use published scales to try to quantify the levels of anxiety and/or depression the patient may be experiencing such as the Beck Depression Inventory.

By this point, most patients feel they have participated in the history and may even feel a bit fatigued. I then ask of each and every new headache patient "is there anything else you think I should know about your headache problem or anything you feel I neglected to ask?" Most patients appreciate this question and it does give them the opportunity to clarify any important points or to bring up anything else important to them. Most feel that the above questions covered their history quite adequately.

I then give the patient a brief break of several minutes and actually leave the room while the patient prepares for the physical examination. Generally removing shoes and socks is sufficient although sometimes a gown is necessary.

The real reason for leaving the room is to give them a brief respite and allow them and anyone else in the room (often their significant other), to collect their thoughts. Often, when I return, they will have thought of something else important to reveal to me or want to clarify/modify some piece of history. Perhaps 50% of the time I am rewarded with another historical fact that helps me make the diagnosis. Years ago, this surprised me, but with experience I came to realize most patients want the clinician to succeed and will do their best to help you if you give them a chance.

The Physical Examination

The physical examination needs to be appropriate for headache patients and the setting (acute, subacute, or chronic presentation). Each piece of information should potentially help diagnose the patient's headache type. Vital signs are important. *Fever*, appropriately measured (which usually means rectally in the acute/subacute encounter) is not a sign of primary headache. Pulse and blood pressure are also important (consider thyroid disease, anemia or infection if tachycardic, mass lesion if blood pressure is rising and pulse is slowing (Cushing's reflex). Essential hypertension is not generally associated with headaches, but malignant hypertension is.[14]

If the assessment is of an acutely/subacutely ill patient, we look especially for signs of trauma. Is there a Battle sign or raccoon eyes (both signs of basilar skull fracture)? If so, I look for otorrhea or fluid behind the tympanic membrane. Once cervical spine films have been rapidly done and known to be negative if there has been trauma, I look for nuchal rigidity (meningismus). Remember that this sign of meningeal irritation may be lost in deep coma. The skin should be examined looking for rashes (meningococcal meningitis, Rocky Mountain spotted fever, Lyme disease, and lupus).

The general examination of the headache patient may include listening to the heart (irregular rhythm?) and over the orbits, mastoid processes, and carotid and vertebral arteries (a bruit could suggest an arteriovenous malformation or a vascular dissection).

In the clinic, I usually next do something relatively nonthreatening with the patient to help him her feel at ease for the remainder of the examination. I examine the temporomandibular joints. Placing my index and middle fingers over the joints, I have the patient open and close the mouth, looking for the distance he or she can open the mouth in the midline, if there is limitation of opening/closing, if there is crepitus, and *most importantly* if there is pain with opening and closing. I then percuss the sinuses and palpate the biceps insertions. I determine the range of motion of the neck and if there is any pain/limitation of movement. I palpate the posterior paraspinous cervical musculature and ascertain if the greater occipital nerves are tender. I test pin sensation in the C2 and C3 dermatomes.[15] Details of the neurological examination are available in many fine standard texts.[16]

Next I check to see if the pupils are symmetrical and equally reactive to light. I examine the ocular fundi, looking for evidence of papilledema and to see if there are spontaneous venous pulsations. Papilledema is a sign of increased intracranial pressure but it should be noted some patients, presumably due to anatomical defects in the optic nerve sheaths, may never develop this sign despite having raised intracranial pressure.[17] (The presence of spontaneous venous pulsations suggests normal intracranial pressure). I check visual acuity (with the glasses on) and look for evidence of field defects and constriction of visual fields.

The remainder of the cranial nerve (CN) examination is easy and can be accomplished rapidly. CN I (olfaction) should be tested with a nonirritant substance such as coffee grounds (irritating substances test trigeminal nerve function instead). Loss of smell can be due to many conditions ranging from the mundane (smoking, upper respiratory infection), to trauma (shearing of olfactory filaments in the cribriform plate), and to olfactory groove tumors or tumors of the base of the skull. Extraocular movements should be tested including upgaze and looking for the presence of nystagmus (it is best to record what you observe and not to resort to jargon so there is less possibility of miscommunication). I test facial sensation with a tiny wisp of cotton with the patent's eyes closed. One looks for a facial droop ("peripheral" or "central" VIIth) and tests hearing (screening for hearing by finger rub or watch tick is usually sufficient). One then tests the gag reflex/palatal elevation (CN IX, X) and head turning/shoulder shrug (CN XI). Lastly, hypoglossal (CN XII) function is assessed by checking tongue protrusion/movement and assessing for atrophy/fasciculations.

Motor examination is performed looking for symmetry/asymmetry of strength, remembering that a pronator drift may be the subtlest sign of pyramidal tract weakness. Tone is also assessed. Sensory examination should include screening for light touch, double-simultaneous light touch, temperature, vibration, proprioception, and graphesthesia and/or stereognosis (assuming the primary modalities are intact). I include, as noted earlier, pin testing in at least the C2 and C3 dermatomes, looking for evidence of upper cervical root entrapment, especially in cases of posttraumatic headache/neck pain. Testing (light touch) about the face is crucial, especially looking for the presence of trigger zones, a clue to trigeminal and other neuralgias. Lastly, for the sensory examination, a Romberg test is performed. Hover about the patient when this is done, ready to catch him or her should the test be positive (the patient does fall!). The test is positive only if the patient does not fall with eyes open but does topple once he or she closes the eyes. Again, describe what you see (swaying, falling).

I next perform a cerebellar examination, looking for both abnormalities of appendicular and axial/midline function. I assess rapid repetitive alternating movements (finger tapping, patting the thigh with the hand), finger-to-nose, heel-to-shin, and tandem walking, which suffice for a quick screen. I then watch the patient walk in his or her bare feet, including sudden turns to either side. The neurological examination concludes with deep tendon reflexes and assessment of the plantar response (is there a Babinski sign?).

Once the history and examination have been concluded, a differential diagnosis may be created. The clinician is entitled to a "favorite" diagnosis but it is important to keep an open mind. Some patients will fit nicely into one or more categories of the ICHD-II. Some will not and will be "probable" diagnoses (they miss the classification category by one diagnostic feature). I counsel caution in these cases and the clinician should then be especially wary of secondary cases of headache. When the diagnosis is not clear it is crucial to default to the most conservative position and investigate further whether by tests, further history gathering, or observation. There are numerous diagnostic pitfalls, especially in patients with refractory headache, that can confound therapy (Box 5.3).[18]

An important feature of the initial encounter is the conclusion when diagnosis is discussed with the patient, therapeutic goals are set, and treatment plans are made. Some headache can be "cured." Usually, however, the more likely scenario is that the headaches will be "managed." We set reasonable expectations as to what we, as clinicians, can provide for services and availability. Patients need education about what to expect as far as a reasonable time course for improvement, medication effects, and long term prognosis. Education is essential. I recommend that clinicians find some headache references for patients that they feel comfortable with and that they can endorse. In our headache clinic, we try to be "evidence-based" whenever possible and educate patients about unproven therapies and potentially dangerous or counterproductive treatments. These resources can be reviewed by the

Box 5-3 Diagnostic Pitfalls in Headache

1. Incorrect diagnosis
2. Failure to consider the presence of more than one headache diagnosis/etiology
3. Missing sinus disease/base of skull pathology (e.g., contact points, sphenoid sinusitis, nasopharyngeal carcinoma)
4. Missing cervical/cranio–cervical junction contributions (e.g., upper cervical root entrapment, cervical dystonia/torticollis, Chiari malformation, syrinx)
5. Missing medication overuse headache (analgesic rebound)
6. Failure to consider the emergence of a second headache superimposed on an initial headache type
7. Missing intracranial hypertension (can occur without papilledema) or intracranial hypotension
8. Mistaking a treatment response for a diagnosis (e.g., the headache due to subarachnoid hemorrhage may respond to a triptan drug or dihydroergotamine).
9. Misdiagnosing a secondary headache (e.g., arteriovenous malformation) as a primary headache (e.g., migraine with aura)

patients and their families, and are reassuring and also save time. Patients in my clinic are given a written plan with contact phone numbers for the clinician's office and the clinic nurse, in case they are having problems. I write out the treatment plan and any additional tests as well as consultations that will be necessary. I also write out my differential diagnosis.

Taking care of refractory headache patients is challenging but can also be very rewarding. I always remember the "aphorism that a second examination is the most helpful diagnostic test in a difficult neurologic case."[16] I would point out that that includes keeping an open mind and taking any further information, history or physical findings, into account. Having a therapeutic partnership with patients can lead to improved outcomes.

References

1. Classification Committee of the International Headache Society: *International Classification of Headache Disorders II. Cephalalgia.* 2004;24(suppl 1):1–160 (also available at www.i-h-s.org with most recent updates).
2. Silberstein SD, Lipton RB, Goadsby PJ. *Headache in Clinical Practice*, 2nd ed. London: Martin Dunitz; 2002:15.
3. Barbanti P, Fabbrini G, Pesare M, Vanacore N, Cerbo R. Unilateral cranial autonomic symptoms in migraine. *Cephalagia.* 2002;22(4):256–259.
4. Ward TN, Levin M. Diagnosis and pathophysiology of migraine. *Expert Rec Neurother.* 2004;4(3):383–390.
5. Mathew NT, Stubits E, Nigam MR. Transformation of episodic migraine into daily headache: analysis of factors. *Headache.* 1982;27:66–68.
6. Young WB, Silberstein SD. Hemicrania continua and symptomatic medication overuse. *Headache.* 1993;33:485–487.
7. Fisher CM. Late-life migraine accompaniments as a cause of unexplained transient ischemic attacks. *Can J Neurol Sci.* 1980;7(1):9–17.
8. Kuritzky A, Ziegler DK, Hassanein R. Vertigo, motion sickness, and migraine. *Headache.* 1981;21:227–231.
9. Spierings ELH. Migraine, Big and small (letter). *Headache.* 2001;41(9):918–919.
10. Ashkenazi A, Sholtzow M, Shaw JW, Burstein R, Young WB. Identifying cutaneous allodynia in chronic migraine using a practical clinical method. *Cephalalgia.* 2007;27(2):111–117.
11. Mathew NT, Kurman R, Perez F. Drug-induced refractory headache—clinical features and management. *Headache.* 1990;30:634–638.
12. Ward TN, Levin M, Phillips JM. Evaluation and Management of Headache in the Emergency Department. *Med Clin North Am.* 2001;85(4):971–985.
13. Stewart WF, Lipton RB, Kolodner K. Migraine Disability Assessment (MIDAS) score: relation to headache frequency, pain intensity, and headache symptoms. *Headache.* 2003;433:258–265.
14. Ward TN. Headache in cerebrovascular disease. In: Samuels MA, Freske S, eds.*Office Practice of Neurology.* New York: Churchill Livingstone; 1996:1141–1144.
15. Pikus HJ, Phillips JM. Characteristics of patients successfully treated for cervicogenic headache by surgical decompression of the second cervical root. *Headache.* 1995;35(10):621–629.

16. Ropper AH, Brown RH (eds): *Adams and Victor's Principles of Neurology*, 8th ed. New York: McGraw-Hill; 2005.
17. Mathew NT, Ravinshankar K, Sanin LC. Coexistence of migraine and idiopathic intracranial hypertension without papilledema. *Neurology.* 1996;46:1226–1230.
18. Lipton RB, Silberstein SD, Saper JR, Bigal ME, Goadsby PJ. Why headache treatment fails. *Neurology.* 2003;60:1064–1070.

6

Differential Diagnosis and Investigation of Refractory Headache

R. Allan Purdy, MD, FRCPC, FACP

Introduction

In every neurological disorder, there is always a differential diagnosis and for headache, especially refractory headache (RH), the same is true for refractory migraine (RM). Actually, although not evidence based to the knowledge of this author, it would be highly unlikely that any patient with RH would ever come to the attention of a headache specialist without having had considerable thought, time, and effort put into looking at alternative diagnoses or extensive investigations having been done. At least this would be the common experience and one should serve the patients well. However, headache diagnosis is not precision science at the best of times, and thus there is ample leeway for going down the wrong path in any individual patient or error. Thus, it is absolutely necessary that prudence and diligence reign in this area of diagnostic uncertainty, and if this chapter could deliver one message it would be, "If in doubt, check it out!" With this in mind, we now look at the differential diagnosis of RH and appropriate investigations to be done. Other chapters of this volume deal with history and physical assessments of patient with RH and classification is covered in prior chapters.

Remember that primary and secondary headaches are brain disorders and diseases, and when patients have RH it is probably because they have been not been properly diagnosed or treated or both, or are simply just very difficult to treat and manage. Clinicians can become overwhelmed very quickly in managing patients with RH, and thus a team approach with multiple professionals and treatment options probably offers the best chance for managing RH patients.

Differential Diagnosis of RH

To begin with the operational criteria for RM have now been defined[1–3] nevertheless the nosology of this entity remains confusing.[4] Any variance from these criteria requires a differential diagnosis. In particular, note that the criteria are operative only if the headaches cannot be attributed to another disorder, a criterion that is similar for the primary headache disorders classification as well.[5] Also recall that RH is usually an end-stage diagnosis after all other therapies have failed, and thus the differential diagnosis includes any primary headache disorder that did not respond to therapy and a myriad of secondary disorders that can cause chronic daily headache (CDH) or RH, or both.

It is best to begin from primary principles in dealing with the diagnostic considerations in patients with RH. In fact, it might be better to have the patient seen anew by another consultant, as a completely unbiased or fresh opinion may be exactly what is needed to clarify the history, and to a lesser extent the physical examination, of a RH case. Only when diagnosticians are willing to keep an open mind and think anew or differently about the patient and their complaints, is it possible to find new causes or suggest new ways of investigation or a repetition of prior investigations—these suggestions express opinion and are not evidence based but do follow the thinking of classical neurological diagnosis.

Primary Headache Disorders Presenting as RH or RM

One can start with the recognized common primary headache disorders that can lead to or present as RH or RM and go from there. In this way, the causes are most easily sought, and once these are examined carefully and found wanting then and only then does one go on to revisit other diagnostic considerations, including secondary headache disorder that can present as RH or even rarer or uncommon causes of RH. Secondary headache disorders presenting with characteristics of primary headache disorders usually declare themselves at some point by showing features not consistent with the original primary phenotype, and this is the clue to making the diagnosis.

The primary RH types include several well-recognized disorders as outlined in Chapter 2 and some that are less well recognized or diagnosed. The purpose here is to highlight some diagnostic thoughts about these types of headache that may prove useful in dealing with patients with RH, as the criteria for several types of RH headaches are outlined in Chapter 1 in this volume, and other disorders are dealt with in detail in other chapters.

Migraine is usually not a problem in the differential diagnosis of RH, as in many cases it serves as the underlying prototypic primary headache disorder that has transformed into CDH with or without medication overuse headache (MOH), along the way to becoming RM or chronic migraine (CM). It is thus not surprising that elements of migraine persist and exist in many RH patients.

Chronic tension-type headache, on the other hand, has to be separated out from CDH, MOH, and RH. Using *International Classification of Headache Disorders* (IHCD) criteria[5] that again should not prove problematic, unless it is comorbid with other medical or affective disorders that can also can occur in patients with CM. Also CM can also be parsed out from the background noise of comorbid disorders and MOH quite easily can be differentiated by headache physicians as on its own CM should be sufficiently well delineated, as outlined in Chapter 2, to cause no problems in differential diagnosis. The trigeminal autonomic cephalalgis (TACs) do represent a problem, in that it can be difficult to separate out secondary from the primary subtypes, with the possibility that some can go on to become TACs which represent RH in their own right—these entities have been fully delineated in their primary form in the ICHD classification and many excellent review articles.[6,7] The characteristics of each TAC is outlined in Chapter 21 but it is important to recognize that the TACs are sufficiently rare in the experience of most physicians, including those with a special interest in headache medicine, that any time a TAC is encountered clinically then secondary causes need to be considered and appropriately investigated. For example, brain neoplasms are increasingly found to be associated with TAC and TAC-like headache.[8–10]

Certainly, any cluster headache (CH) that has any atypical features, such as female predisposition, short duration or frequent attacks, or lack of association with agitation or restlessness should not be ignored particularly if the patient has any fixed neurological signs or does not respond to the usual therapies for cluster headache. Thus, paroxysmal hemicrania, Short-lasting Unilateral Neuralgiform headache with Conjunctival injection and Tearing (SUNCT), and hemicrania continua (HC) need to be accurately diagnosed clinically and investigated if necessary and treated. In fact, with respect to HC, the diagnosis is probably missed[11] frequently and without an adequate trial of indomethacin[12] or a failure to respond to indomethacin, it is likely another cause for the headache or diagnosis will arise. Importantly, it should be noted that the clinical features of TACs are starting to intermingle with other primary headache disorders such as migraine and vice versa,[13] and thus the definitive nosology for these entities is becoming less clear over time. It may prove best from the diagnostic point of view that all of these disorders should be considered secondary until proven otherwise, as all of them can ultimately present as RH.

New daily persistent headache (NDPH)[14] remains an enigmatic and difficult differential diagnostic consideration in CDH and now in RH. Although some forms are thought to be self-limiting, most clinicians identify the nonremitting and untreatable form to be part of the spectrum of CDH—operational diagnostic criteria exist outlined in Chapter 2 but are of little help in making a definitive diagnosis. The single most important criteria to make the diagnosis might be the patient's memory of the onset of headache at a specific time on specific day, without any other cause to be found or ever found. In some ways, NDPH is the classical RH, as it may never remit or respond to any therapy. On the other hand, exertional headaches are well recognized by clinicians, when the history is sufficiently well done, to be a distinct category of common and generally treatable disorders.[15] They have also been associated with some significant and serious secondary etiologies such as Chiari I malformation and subarachnoid hemorrhage (SAH), but generally upon a new clinical presentation exertional headaches are taken seriously and properly investigated or confused with RH or RM.

Secondary Headache Disorders Presenting as RH

In this section the secondary headache disorders presenting as RH, as outlined in Chapter 2, are discussed. Post-traumatic headache (PTH) is of course one cause of RH, given its long duration and chronicity in some patients.[16] It should not be difficult to make the diagnosis in patients who meet the criteria for chronic post-traumatic headache, and also to recognize if the pattern of headache mimics one of the primary headache disorders such as migraine or tension-type headache. Close attention to the relationship to the trauma is of course important, as is the necessity of finding by way of history or collateral information from prior records as to the presence of preexisting headache disorders. It is clear that a small percentage of patients persist with chronic post-traumatic headache that appears resistant to all forms of reasonable treatment including some of the usual treatments of the primary chronic headache disorders. In this group of patients is always important to ensure that no new cause of chronic headache has arisen so, once again, an open mind to a larger differential diagnosis is prudent and warranted.

Medication overuse headache (MOH)[17] is dealt with in some detail in Chapters 1 and 9 of this volume and always becomes a compounding variable in assessing anyone with potential RH or RM. This usually does not become a problem if common causes of MOH are excluded and managed and other medications become ineffective, raising the question of evolving RH. Some feel that medication misuse with rebound headache is likely the single most common secondary disorder that causes intractability.[18]

In patients with RH, it is important to continue to explore their use of any medication and any alternative therapies that contain active ingredients that could cause headache. Also, a careful review of medications taken for other medical and comorbid conditions is vital as many of these can actually cause headache. The percentage of patients that actually get ongoing headaches from their medicinal agents is usually low, in the single digits;

nevertheless, all treatments need to be carefully scrutinized to ensure they are not important in the generation and ongoing RH.

Some common medications causing headache include:[18]

- Monoamine oxidase inhibitors
- Calcium-channel blockers
- Nonsteroidal anti-inflammatory agents
- Caffeine
- Citrates
- Ranitidine
- Estrogen compounds
- Vasopressor agents

Idiopathic intracranial hypotension (IIH) can be a difficult diagnosis in some patients and not infrequently the actual diagnosis and ultimate resolution of the causation can be delayed for months or years.[19] Straightforward cases of positional headache relieved by recumbency in patients with post-lumbar puncture headache for instance will most likely be easily recognized and treated without much problem, however a chronic cerebrospinal fluid (CSF) leak arising in the upper spinal cord area may easily escape diagnosis, particularly if the patient evolves from a positional headache into a chronic daily headache or one in which the positional components are absent or paradoxical in nature.[19] At that point, it is necessary to go back and carefully review the history and early imaging to ensure that a cause for a presumable spontaneous intracranial hypotension was not missed. Of great importance are patients presenting with what appears to be a Chiari I malformation and upon gadolinium enhancement by magnetic resonance imaging (MRI) are found to have pachymeningeal enhancement and the other characteristics of the "sagging brain" so often seen in this disorder.[20] Low-pressure headache is a real problem area in neurological diagnosis in headache medicine, and if a patient with CDH or what appears to be RH is seen to have any of the MRI findings suggesting intracranial hypotension, then it is necessary, despite the history, to pursue further tests to find the putative leak, including CSF pressure measurement, radionuclide cisternography, and computed tomography (CT) myelogram.[19]

Intracranial hypertension without mass lesion[21] can lead to chronic headache with or without papilledema if idiopathic in nature, and this can be difficult to diagnose if the imaging is negative or shows some minimal ventricular change, and the papilledema is not striking or if a secondary cause is present without papilledema.[22] Also, these patients need accurate measurement of CSF pressure and neuro-ophthalmological assessments to make the diagnosis and exclude other etiologies. Most space-occupying lesions such as tumors are usually not a problem in RH as they can be identified with imaging in most cases early on in their presentation; however, every clinician knows of cases of early glioma or glioblastoma presenting with a primary type headache[23] leading to RH, when subsequent neuroimaging showing the white matter lesion and tumor at a later date.

Cranial neuralgias can present as RH or facial pain, but at least on clinical diagnostic criteria[5] they are relatively easy to sort out from other causes of RH. This is because they display true neuralgic pain with typical pain qualities that are distinct, and clearly different from other causes of facial pain, including the not so uncommon "atypical facial pain," which usually has non-neuralgic features. When the diagnosis of facial pain is unknown, it is probably better to name it facial pain of undetermined etiology. The clue to facial pain differential diagnosis is to remember the clinical anatomy of the fifth cranial nerve at the bedside and also to know the radiological course of that nerve and associated neural and other structures are in the head. Thus any neurological findings whatsoever will raise clinical suspicion of secondary causation, as would any unusual neuroradiological findings along the intracranial and extracranial pathways for this important nerve in the head. Cases of a Meckel's cave meningioma or multiple sclerosis can present with chronic facial pain unresponsive to any medical therapy and thus becoming RH. Also, dental and otolaryngological conditions can mimic these disorders as well and need to be excluded.

Chronic fungal infections such as coccidiomycosis; bacterial infections such as Lyme disease and tuberculosis; and parasitic infections such as neurocysticercosis should be considered as potential causes of chronic and/or refractory headache in susceptible populations.[23] Sphenoid sinusitis can present as daily headache and present with few nasal symptoms. These rare etiologies will be seen in practice on occasion and if you live in an area where some of these infections are endemic, then a high index of suspicion is warranted. Chronic meningitis, meningeal carcinomatosis, and neurosarcoidosis can present as chronic and RH, and thus may require further investigation, such as lumbar puncture, because neuroimaging, especially when contrast is not employed, may be unrevealing.

Some Further Thoughts on Serious and Secondary Headaches

"Red flags" are useful in looking at patients with RH and should always be reviewed when seeing any patient, in large part because RH and serious new causes of headache are not mutually exclusive. Thus, it bears repeating that any patient with RH who has any of the following red flags needs evaluation for serious causes of headache:[23]

- Any headache beginning suddenly with peak intensity within minutes
- Any new or different headache for the patient
- Progressive headache, facial or neck pain
- Headache associated with fever or other systemic symptoms
- Headache with neurological signs, especially if new

- Head pain precipitated by Valsalva's maneuver such as coughing or sneezing or bending down
- Onset of headache in an adult older than 50 years of age

It is vital to consider a longer differential diagnosis beyond the usual causes of CDH and RH. A list of serious etiologies is best to consider in the approach to each patient:[23]

- Space-occupying lesion—tumor, abscess, hematoma
- Infection—meningitis or encephalitis
- Stroke, including infarction, subarachnoid or intracerebral hemorrhage, and cerebral venous sinus thrombosis
- Systemic disorders—thyroid disease, hypertension, inflammatory disorders
- Arteritis including temporal and CNS vasculitis
- Traumatic injuries to the head and neck
- Cervical spine causes of headache
- Ophthalmological and otolaryngological causes of headache
- Dental or maxillofacial cause of headache and facial pain

The detailed clinical and differential diagnosis of secondary headaches that sometimes lead to CDH or intractable headache, some with an acute or subacute onset have been dealt with in great detail in recent publications.[18,24] Some comments, however, are worth reemphasizing from these reviews.

- Sphenoid sinusitis may produce intractable headache.
- Postpartum headache can be secondary to venous sinus thrombosis and papilledema maybe missing.
- Intracranial hypertension can present without papilledema and cause chronic headache.
- Postural headache upon standing suggests a CSF leak, which can occur spontaneously, after prior lumbar puncture or epidural block.
- Headache with coughing, or sneezing suggests a Chiari I malformation, a problem at the cervical medullary junction or increased intracranial pressure.
- Headache associated with fever suggests an infectious causation.
- Dermatological lesions may suggest that Lyme disease, herpes zoster, sarcoidosis, collagen vascular disease, or other systemic illness plays a role in the chronic headache.
- In patients with HIV unusual opportunistic infections, including toxoplasmosis and cryptococcal meningitis, can occur
- A history of recent dental work or oral infections raises the question of intracranial infection, including brain abscess.
- Cancer of the head or neck can produce chronic head and face pain that can be hard to diagnose.

Diagnostic Testing in RH

Radiological Assessment

Frishberg[25] outlined the usual reasons for imaging patients with headache disorders as follows: "...patients with new-onset headaches, headaches with a progressive course, headaches with a significant change in pattern, headaches that never alternate sides, and headaches associated with any neurological findings or seizures have a substantially higher likelihood of a secondary cause such as tumor, arteriovenous malformation, or other structural lesion." In these situations, imaging must be considered as part of the workup.

Neuroimaging is very important in the initial and ongoing evaluation of patients with RH. Ultimately, gadolinium-enhanced MRI would be the best test for patients with RH, although it could miss some cases of RH such as cerebral venous thrombosis. This test is more sensitive than enhanced or unenhanced CT scans, especially when looking at the structures in the posterior fossa, craniocervical junction, leptomeninges, and dura.

Plain CT should be good screening test for the majority RH patients, with enhanced CT probably yielding more with minimal risk in most patients and CT scans also may include bone windows and sinus views if needed. Nevertheless, an unenhanced CT scan in a patient with RH and a normal neurological examination may be negative or appear normal in many disorders including the following:[23,24]

- Temporal arteritis
- Infiltrating glioma
- Ethmoidal or sphenoidal sinusitis
- Central nervous system vasculitis
- Some posterior fossa or craniocervical lesions
- Some aneurysms and vascular malformations
- Venous sinus or cortical vein thrombosis
- Meningitis (including viral, bacterial, or carcinomatous) and encephalitis
- IIH without papilledema
- Bilateral isodense subdural hematomas
- CSF hypovolemia secondary to CSF leak (intracranial hypotension)

Finally, it should be noted that CT scan maybe helpful in avoiding the finding of non-specific white matter changes, now commonly seen on MR imaging.[26]

Laboratory Assessment of RH

Numerous diagnostic tests are available to assist in assessing causes of CDH and RH. Clinical evaluation needs to guide the selection of any specific diagnostic test(s).[23,24] A complete blood count and differential may show anemia suggesting a hematological or systemic disease, and the presence of a left-shift and elevated white blood cell count would suggest a bacterial infection. An elevated erythrocyte sedimentation rate (ESR) and/or C-reactive protein suggests arteritis, especially temporal arteritis in the elderly patient, or other form of vasculitis or systemic disorder. If giant cell arteritis is suspected, then a temporal artery biopsy is indicated. Systemic disorders may be suggested by abnormal liver and renal function. In metastatic cancer, calcium is frequently elevated, and a low serum sodium may suggest syndrome of inappropriate antidiuretic hormone (SIADH), which can be associated with systemic disease and intracranial diseases, including primary and secondary tumors, and chronic subdural hematoma.

Drug screening is useful if the headaches are associated with the use or overuse of medications. Blood gases in patients with headache and pulmonary disease may reveal reduced oxygen saturation and elevated carbon dioxide, leading to chronic headache and RH. In patients suspected of obstructive sleep apnea, overnight pulse oximetry may demonstrate oxygen desaturations during sleep directing the investigation to sleep studies and overnight polysomnogram. Thyroxin and thyroid-stimulating hormone tests are helpful if there is any suspicion of thyroid dysfunction that can cause or be contributing to RH. Where Lyme disease is endemic, do a screening enzyme-linked immunosorbent for *Borrelia burgdorferi* antibodies. Primary and secondary headaches occur in patients with human immunodeficiency virus (HIV) infection and acquired immune deficiency syndrome (AIDS). Therefore, do an HIV titer and possibly a VDRL test (for venereal disease). Testing for hypercoagulability is indicated if the patient is suspected of having intracranial venous thrombosis. Rare mitochondrial encephalopathies, including MELAS (mitochondrial encephalomyopathy, lactic acidosis, and stroke-like episodes) can present with chronic and RH headache, and may require special investigations, such as muscle biopsy.

Lumbar Puncture and Other Tests in RH

Lumbar puncture and CSF examinations are done in those patients suspected of having intracranial hypertension, hypotension, or chronic meningitis due to infections or cancer. Elevated or low intracranial pressure disorders may be missed if CSF opening pressure is not studied. or not performed correctly.[24]

EEG in patients with CDH or RH can occasionally be useful when a metabolic derangement is causing both an encephalopathy and the chronic headache syndrome. Nevertheless, the report of the Quality Standards Subcommittee of the American Academy of Neurology in 1994 recommended: "EEG is not useful in the routine evaluation of patients with headache" (guideline).[27] This does not exclude the use of EEG to evaluate headache patients with associated symptoms, suggesting a seizure disorder, such as an atypical migrainous aura, or episodic loss of consciousness. Assuming that head imaging capabilities are readily available, EEG is not recommended to exclude a structural cause of headache (option).

The Minnesota Multiphasic Personality Inventory (MMPI) can detect comorbid psychological problems in patients with CDH.[28] However, the presence of comorbid psychological disorders does rule out the presence of serious causes of RH so psychological testing is ancillary in RH cases.

Conclusions

The differential diagnosis and investigation of patients with RH can be challenging; however, patients with RH are usually significantly disabled, and require detailed medical and neurological evaluations using a methodical and systematic approach. By the time most patients develop RH they have been examined and investigated many times, however, their cases demand that the cardinal principle of clinical neurology be utilized in each and every case, which means going back to basics, repeating the history and physical and pursing appropriate investigations or seeking other opinions. Laboratory testing and neuroimaging are important in the diagnostic evaluation of patients with RH.

References

1. Levin, M. Refractory headache: classification and nomenclature. *Headache.* 2008;48:783–790.
2. Schulman EA, Peterlin BL, Lake AE, 3rd, et al. Defining refractory migraine: results of the RHSIS Survey of American Headache Society members. *Headache.* 2009;49(4):509–518.
3. Goadsby PJ, Schoenen J, Ferrari MD, Silberstein SD, Dodick D. Towards a definition of intractable headache for use in clinical practice and trials. *Cephalalgia.* 2006;26:1168–1170.
4. Goadsby PJ, Hargreaves R. Refractory migraine and chronic migraine: pathophysiological mechanisms. *Headache.* 2008;48(6):799–804.
5. Headache Classification Subcommittee of the International Headache Society. The International Classification of Headache Disorders: 2nd ed. *Cephalalgia.* 2004;24(suppl 1):9–160
6. Goadsby PJ, Cittadini E, Burns B, Cohen AS. Trigeminal autonomic cephalalgias: diagnostic and therapeutic developments. *Curr Opin Neurol.* 2008;21(3):323–330.
7. Goadsby PJ, Lipton RB. A review of paroxysmal hemicranias, SUNCT syndrome and other short-lasting headaches with autonomic feature, including new cases. *Brain.* 1997;120(1 Pt 1):193–209.
8. Purdy RA, Kirby S. Headache and brain tumors. *Neurol Clin North Am.* 2004;22:39–43.
9. Matharu MS, et al. SUNCT syndrome secondary to prolactinoma. *J Neurol Neurosurg Psychiatry.* 2003;74:1590–1592.
10. Massiou H, et al. SUNCT syndrome in two patients with prolactinomas and bromocriptine-induced attacks. *Neurology.* 2002;58:1698–1699.
11. Silberstein SD, Peres MF. Hemicrania continua. *Arch Neurol.* 2002;59(6):1029–1030.

12. Marmura MJ, Silberstein SD, Gupta M. Hemicrania continua: who responds to indomethacin? *Cephalalgia.* 2009;29(3):300–307.
13. Bahra A, May A, Goadsby PJ. Cluster headache: a prospective clinical study with diagnostic implications. *Neurology.* 2002;58(3):354–361.
14. Goadsby PJ, Boes C. New daily persistent headache. *J Neurol Neurosurg Psychiatry.* 2002;72(suppl 2):ii6–ii9.
15. Pascual J, Iglesias, F., Oterino, A., et al. Cough, exertional, and sexual headaches: an analysis of 72 benign and symptomatic cases. *Neurology.* 1996;46:1520–1524.
16. Evans, RW. The post concussion Syndrome and sequelae of mild head injury. In: Evans RW, ed. *Neurology and Trauma*, 2nd ed, New York: Oxford University Press; 2006:95–128.
17. Silbertstein, SD, Olesen, J, Bousser, M-G, et al. *The International Classification of Headache Disorders*, 2nd ed. (ICHD-II)—revision of criteria for 8.2 Medication-Overuse Headache. *Cephalalgia*, 2005;25:460–465.
18. Saper JR, Silberstein SD, Lipton RB. Turning treatment failure into treatment success. In: Silberstein SD, Lipton RB, Dodick DW, eds. *Wolff's Headache*, 8th ed. New York: Raven Press; 2008.
19. Mokri B. Low cerebrospinal fluid pressure syndromes. *Neurol Clin.* 2004;22(1):55–74, vi.
20. Mokri B, Atkinson, DW, Dodick, GM, Miller, DG. Absent pachymeningeal gadolinium enhancement on cranial MRI despite symptomatic CSF leak. *Neurology.* 1999;53:402–404.
21. Friedman DI. Pseudotumor cerebri presenting as headache. *Expert Rev Neurother.* 2008;8(3):397–407.
22. Quattrone A, Bono, F, Oliveri, RL, Gambardella, D. Cerebral venous thrombosis and isolated intracranial hypertension without papilledema in CDH. *Neurology.* 2001;57:31–36.
23. Purdy RA, Diagnostic Evaluation of Chronic Daily Headache. In: Goadsby PJ, Silbestein SD, Dodick D, eds. *Chronic Daily Headache for Clinicians.* PMPH-USA, 2005.
24. Evans RW. Diagnostic testing for migraine and other primary headaches. *Neurol Clin.* 2009;27(2):393–415.
25. Frishberg BM. The utility of neuroimaging in the evaluation of headache in patients with normal neurologic examinations. *Neurology.* 1994;44:1191–1197.
26. Kruit MC, van Buchem MA, Hofman PA, et al. Migraine as a risk factor for subclinical brain lesions. *JAMA.* 2004;291(4):427–434.
27. Krumholz, A, Wiebe, G, Gronseth, G. Practice parameter: Evaluating an apparent unprovoked first seizure in adults (an evidence-based review). Report of the Quality Standards Subcommittee of the American Academy of Neurology and the American Epilepsy Society. The electroencephalogram in the evaluation of headache. American Academy of Neurology. *Neurology.* 2007;69:1996–2007.
28. Bigal ME, Sheftell, F. D., Rapoport, A. M., et al. MMPI personality profiles in patients with primary chronic daily headache: a case-control study. *Neurol Sci.*2003;24:103–110.

7

Identifying Psychiatric Comorbidity in Refractory Migraine Patients

Donald B. Penzien, PhD, Todd A. Smitherman, PhD, and Jeanetta C. Rains, PhD

Introduction

Psychiatric comorbidity often complicates head pain management and portends a poorer prognosis for headache treatment. The concept of comorbidity indicates that two disease states co-occur to a greater extent than would be expected on a random basis with the implication that there is potential for the diseases to influence one another.[1] Such is the case for migraine and a variety of psychiatric disorders. As described later, epidemiological research confirms increased prevalence of psychiatric disorders among headache patients. The comorbidity of migraine with mood and anxiety disorders is believed to be based in shared pathophysiology. The presence of psychiatric symptoms has been associated with a poorer response to behavioral and pharmacological headache treatments, with implications for the understanding and management of refractory migraine (RM). This chapter describes the association of headache with psychiatric disorders, reviews theories suggesting a physiological basis for their co-occurrence and interdependence, and offers suggestions for initial screening. Effective management of comorbid psychiatric disorders can improve the quality of life for the RM patient, even when the headache itself remains intractable.

Although psychiatric disorders are disproportionately observed among headache patients compared to the general population, the presence of headache should not lead one to assume psychopathology in the average headache sufferer.

An extensive systematic review of the empirical literature examining more than 300 studies of psychological factors and headache found little empirical support for personality stereotypes (i.e., the "migraine personality") in migraine, helping to lay to rest outdated conceptualizations of migraine as a psychosomatic illness.[2] That same systematic review also revealed little evidence of "clinically significant psychopathology" among typical headache sufferers. Although a substantial proportion of the empirical studies ($n = 190$) reported statistically significant differences in the psychological scores of headache sufferers relative to normative controls, the great majority of these studies found headache patients and controls differed only in "less pathological" terms (e.g., the amount of daily stress experienced, the predominant stress coping strategies employed). "Clinically significant psychopathology" is observed among only a minority of *all* headache sufferers including those in the community at large and those who volunteer for research studies.[2,3]

Nevertheless, numerous clinical and community studies have revealed that psychiatric disorders (e.g., depression and anxiety) occur with greater frequency among recurrent headache patients than among the general population and that the prevalence of psychopathology is over-represented among clinical samples of migraineurs.[4–6] Available evidence indicates that patients with elevated psychological symptoms are more likely to seek medical assistance[7]—especially those with chronic daily or refractory headache[8,9] and those with medication-overuse headache.[10] Psychiatric comorbidity is, in fact, relatively commonplace among headache patients who *present for treatment* (especially those presenting to headache specialists) and is an important consideration in headache treatment planning for RM.

Recent epidemiological studies similarly have identified a significant association between migraine and psychiatric disorders.[11] Table 7.1 lists lifetime prevalence rates for selected Axis I psychiatric disorders among migraineurs and clearly shows they are elevated relative to nonheadache controls. The strongest associations are reported for depression and anxiety disorders with at least a threefold increase among migraineurs relative to controls.[3,12] Note, however, that the research studies summarized in the table do not distinguish the presence of migraine among its episodic, chronic daily headache, or treatment-refractory presentations.

Migraineurs are 2.2 to 4.0 times more likely to have depression than individuals in the general population.[11] Migraine also is comorbid with generalized anxiety disorder (odds ratio [OR] 3.5–5.3), panic disorder (OR 3.7), and bipolar disorder (OR 2.9–7.3). Notably, the co-prevalence of major depression is higher in cases of chronic or "transformed" migraine than in episodic migraine (ORs 6.4 vs. 2.7 for all migraineurs),[9] even after controlling for age and gender,[13] with reported comorbidity prevalence rates among chronic migraine samples as high as 57%.[8] Similarly, anxiety disorders are most prevalent among patients with chronic or transformed migraine (ORs 6.9 vs. 3.2 for all migraineurs).[9,13] Panic disorder in particular has been observed in 25% to 30% of patients with chronic migraine versus only 5% to 17% of those with episodic migraine.[8,14]

Table 7-1 Lifetime Prevalence of Migraine and Selected Psychiatric Disorders

Diagnosis	Migraine Group (%)	Control Group (%)	Odds Ratio[b]
Major Depression	34	10	4.5
Dysthymia	9	2	4.4
Bipolar II[a]	4	1	5.1
Manic Episode	5	1	5.4
Panic Disorder	11	2	6.6
Generalized Anxiety Disorder (GAD)	10	2	5.7
Obsessive–Compulsive Disorder (OCD)	9	2	5.1
Phobia	40	21	2.6
Illicit Drug Use	20	10	2.2
Nicotine Dependence	33	18	2.2

Sources: Breslau N, Merikangas K, Bowden CL. Comorbidity of migraine and major affective disorders. *Neurology*. 1994;44(10 suppl 7):S17–22; Merikangas KR, Stevens DE. Comorbidity of migraine and psychiatric disorders. *Neurol Clin*. 1997;15(1):115–123.

[a]The hypomanic episode does not result in marked impairment.

[b]Odds ratios adjusted for sex

A recently published French epidemiological study further confirmed the increased prevalence of psychiatric comorbidity in chronic versus episodic migraine.[15] Among their sample of more than 10,000 participants, 1127 were diagnosed with episodic and 407 with chronic migraine. When compared on various psychological variables (e.g., perceived headache impact, symptoms of depression and anxiety, and use of coping strategies), chronic migraineurs were more likely to experience significant levels of anxiety (66% vs. 48%) and depression (28% vs. 14%).

Epidemiological studies also reveal a gender discrepancy between rates of migraine as well as comorbid psychiatric disorders. For instance, relative to men, women are more likely to receive lifetime diagnoses of both migraine (24% vs. 9%) and major depressive disorder (24% vs. 13%) by age 30, with relative risk increasing among females for migraine in late adolescence for migraine and about age 20 for depression.[3,16] Longitudinal data indicate women are four times more likely to develop migraine and twice as likely as men to develop depression.[3,16] Likewise, women experience considerably higher rates of anxiety disorders than do men.[17]

In a French study of more than 1500 migraineurs (FRAMIG 3), significantly increased migraine-related disability was observed among those with comorbid anxiety as well as those with both depression plus anxiety (but not for those with depression alone).[18] Moreover, the presence of depression or anxiety was associated with significantly compromised health-related quality of life compared to those without either comorbidity, and those with comorbid depression plus anxiety had lower quality-of-life scores compared to those with either condition alone. Several smaller scale studies also have reported that comorbid psychiatric disorders are associated with increased disability and reduced quality of life among migraineurs. In a sample of 144 chronic daily headache (CDH) patients from the United Kingdom, higher levels of depression or anxiety were associated with higher levels of functional impairment, more pessimistic illness beliefs, and more severe headaches.[19] Greater disability and activity restriction and poorer quality-of-life scores likewise were observed among Canadian migraineurs with comorbid depression, bipolar disorder, or anxiety.[20] Finally, Taiwanese outpatients with major depressive disorder scored lower on quality-of-life measures when they also suffered from migraine.[21]

Psychiatric Comorbidity and Migraine Treatment Prognosis

Whereas an astute clinician might expect psychiatric comorbidity to contribute to migraine intractability, this notion has been investigated only rarely. Table 7.2 summarizes current research on psychiatric comorbidity, migraine chronicity, and response to treatment.

One longitudinal study revealed the presence of psychiatric illness (particularly multiple psychiatric diagnoses) was associated with a poor long-term headache prognosis.[22] For patients with two or more psychiatric diagnoses at

Table 7-2 Psychiatric Comorbidity, Response to Treatment, and Migraine Chronification

1. Chronic migraine is more often associated with significant levels of depression and anxiety than episodic migraine.
2. Comorbid psychiatric disorders are associated with increased disability and reduced quality of life.
3. Higher levels of depression and anxiety are associated with more severe headaches.
4. The presence of multiple comorbid psychiatric disorders is associated with poor long-term prognosis.
5. Migraineurs with depression and anxiety report lower satisfaction with acute drug treatment, poorer drug tolerability, long delays before resuming usual activities, and less migraine relief at 2 hours post-medication.
6. Patients with elevated levels of depression and anxiety are less likely to respond to behavioral treatments focused on headache.
7. The presence of a comorbid psychiatric disorder at initial treatment may be associated with long-term relapse, even in patients who initially respond to pharmacotherapy.
8. Behavioral and psychological risk factors predict the transformation of episodic migraine to chronic and daily headaches (chronification of migraine).
9. Psychiatric comorbidity is a risk factor for nonadherence with medical treatment.
10. Migraine and psychiatric disorders share underlying pathophysiological mechanisms, with bidirectional, interdependent effects.

initial evaluation, 57% exhibited no improvement or deterioration in headache at an 8-year follow-up, 29% were improved, and only 14% were headache free. In contrast, patients with no psychiatric disorder exhibited substantially greater headache improvement 8 years after the initial evaluation: Of patients without a psychiatric comorbidity, 7% showed no improvement or deterioration, 53% were improved, and 40% were headache free. The pattern of headache improvement rates among patients with a single psychiatric diagnosis was intermediate but more closely resembled patients without a psychiatric diagnosis: 15% showed no improvement/deterioration, 46% were improved, and 38% were headache free.

The authors of the FRAMIG 3 study[18] similarly reported that psychiatric comorbidities are associated with poorer outcomes after acute migraine treatment. Relative to those without psychopathology, migraineurs with depression and anxiety reported lower satisfaction with acute drug treatment, poorer drug tolerability, longer delays before resuming usual activities, and less migraine relief two hours post-medication. Although not yet empirically established, an obvious potential implication of this work is that identification and treatment of psychiatric disorders among RM sufferers may prove of substantial value with respect to establishing and enhancing their treatment prognoses.

Additional evidence suggests the presence of even moderate levels of psychological symptoms can portend a poorer treatment response for some headache patients,[23–28] and it is likely that more severe psychopathology will further inhibit treatment responsiveness. To date, depression has been the psychological symptom investigators most often have focused upon when attempting to predict outcome with behavioral headache treatments; the evidence indicates patients with elevated levels of depression are less likely to respond to behavioral treatments than are their less symptomatic counterparts.[24,25]

Although evidence is more sparse, patients with high levels of psychological symptoms similarly may fail to respond to at least some abortive and prophylactic migraine medications. For example, Micieli and colleagues[27] found only a greater occurrence of "clinically marked depressive episodes" to distinguish nonresponders from responders to flunarizine. Holroyd and colleagues[26] found that nonresponders to abortive medication obtained higher scores on the Beck Depression Inventory and the Spielberger Trait Anger Scale than patients who responded to abortive pharmacotherapy. In Holroyd's study, no patient with a trait anger score of 25 or higher on the Trait Anger Scale was a responder to abortive medication, while 85% of the patients with anger scores lower than 25 did respond to abortive medication. More recently, post-hoc analysis of a small open label study of an antidepressant medication (nefazodone) for treatment of chronic daily headache found evidence for differential treatment response in depressed versus nondepressed patients.[28] Although baseline headache severity indices did not differ between the two groups, depressed patients showed a mean 85% headache improvement during the third month of treatment versus only 41% headache improvement for non-depressed patients. Finally, another recent study suggested that the presence of a comorbid psychiatric disorder at initial treatment may be associated with long-term (6–7 years) relapse even when is not associated with a poor initial response to drug therapy.[29]

Beyond the evidence that migraineurs with psychopathology may prove more treatment refractory, there is emerging evidence that a number of behavioral/psychological risk factors are associated with transformation or progression of headache from episodic to chronic and daily—in effect, the *chronification* of migraine.[30–33] Available empirical evidence implicates psychological distress as potentially playing an even greater role in migraine chronification than does analgesic overuse/abuse.[34] Clearly, large-scale and long-term longitudinal studies are called for so that we might better understand not only the natural history of migraine over time but also the influence of comorbid psychopathology upon the prognosis and progression of migrainous headache.[35,36]

Although there has been some evidence to the contrary,[37,38] considered as a whole, the extant literature strongly suggests psychiatric disorders not only are more prevalent among patients with chronic and refractory forms of migraine, but that their presence portends a poorer migraine treatment prognosis and may be associated with migraine chronification.

Nature of the Migraine/Psychopathology Relationship

The precise nature of the relationship between migraine and psychiatric disorders remains unclear. Whereas chronic migraine can present as a severely painful and disabling condition, research has not borne out the notion that affective disorders emerge merely as a consequence of the burden of living with this condition. Alternatively, psychiatric comorbidity clearly is a risk factor for nonadherence with medical treatment,[39,40] and the reported high levels of treatment nonadherence among headache patients could play a significant role in the poorer outcomes observed among migraineurs with psychiatric comorbidity. Nevertheless, it seems unlikely that this explanation accounts for a substantial portion of the relationship between psychopathology and RM.

Several longitudinal studies support a bidirectional relationship between migraine and depression, with each disorder increasing the risk of the other.[11,22] It generally is believed that the occurrence of comorbidity most likely arises from shared pathophysiology of migraine and mood disorders, perhaps through serotonergic dysfunction, The temporal relationship between anxiety disorders and migraine has been less well examined,[22] but one investigation of panic disorder and migraine found that the influence appears to occur principally in the headache to panic disorder direction, rather than the reverse,[41] though there is still also evidence of a bidirectional relationship[22] as in seen in depression. Not surprisingly, having both migraine and an anxiety disorder increases one's odds of also having major depression.[42]

Aberrant serotonergic (5-hydroxytryptamine, 5-HT) functioning has been hypothesized as shared a neurochemical mechanism underlying the comorbidity between migraine and affective disorders. Decreased plasma 5-HT between migraine attacks and increased concentrations of 5-HT during attacks consistently have been observed among migraineurs[43–45] leading many to conclude that migraine emerges at least partially as a consequence of reduced serotonergic transmission originating from the brainstem raphe nucleus.[44] Moreover, selective serotonin agonists (triptans) can be highly efficacious for treatment of migraine. Depression and anxiety likewise have been linked to serotonergic dysfunction, and selective serotonin reuptake inhibitors (SSRIs) are treatments-of-choice for most mood and anxiety disorders. Although reduced serotonergic transmission underlies affective disorders as well as migraine, clinical findings suggest that any shared serotonergic functions underlying the pathophysiologies of migraine and psychopathology are complex. Research is needed to clarify the boundary conditions of serotonergic dysfunction in the shared pathogenesis of migraine and affective disorders.

Recent reports also have implicated shared neuropathic mechanisms underlying the comorbidity of migraine and affective disorders.[46,47] The concept of a "limbically augmented pain syndrome" (LAPS) was brought forward by Rome and Rome[48] in a seminal article articulating the extent to which limbic activation could lead to a complicated intertwining and progression of chronic pain (regardless of location) and affective distress over time. According to Maizels,[1] the LAPS can readily be applied to head pain, yielding a conceptualization of migraine as a "neurolimbic disorder." In Maizels' conceptualization, rather than focusing principally on the brain stem sensitization (as widely endorsed in current conceptualizations of migraine pathophysiology), migraine also may involve cortical sensitization. Cady and colleagues[49] similarly have applied the LAPS conceptualization to headache, suggesting cosensitization of sensory and affective components of pain may underlie comorbid migraine/psychopathology relationships, and making reference to neuroplastic processes in corticolimbic structures where an expanding corticolimbic field becomes activated by both nociceptors and psychological stimuli over time. Accordingly, depression and anxiety may contribute to progression of migraine and emotional distress through shared limbic activation and corticolimbic sensitization in susceptible individuals.

Effect on Migraine of Treating Comorbid Psychopathology

The poor headache treatment prognosis associated with psychiatric comorbidity in tandem with their high prevalence among patients with chronic migraine and RM emphasizes the merits of identifying psychopathology and suggests that treatment of psychiatric comorbidity may prove of value toward enhancing outcomes in head pain management. Unfortunately, there is no cogent evidence to date establishing that simply treating psychopathology (i.e., depression or anxiety) necessarily improves migraine outcomes. The lack of findings to indicate treating psychiatric comorbidity improves headache outcomes is not a function of repeated null findings; instead, there simply is a paucity of research addressing this issue. Nevertheless, clinical experience and indirect empirical findings converge to suggest that identification and treatment of comorbid psychiatric conditions is warranted, as psychiatric disorders add impairment and have negative consequences in their own right.[50]

Recognizing Comorbid Psychiatric Disorders

In the following sections, we present the characteristics of selected psychiatric disorders that are prevalent among head pain patients or can prove especially challenging for clinicians. These disorders include depression, panic disorder, somatoform disorders, and selected personality disorders. For information pertaining to management of these and other comorbid psychiatric disorders in headache patients, we recommend works by Griffith and Razavi.[3,16,51] Lipchik, Smitherman, Penzien, and Holroyd;[50] Saper and Lake;[52] and Saper and Sheftell,[53] as well as chapters by Drs. Lake, Saper, and Rosen in this volume.

Depression

Major depressive illness is commonplace, with a lifetime prevalence of more than 20% in women and 10% in men.[54] It has been referred to as "the neglected major illness" because of its consistent under-recognition and the tremendous costs it engenders (more than $44 billion annually in the United States),[55] making it one of the most costly (and deadly) diseases in industrialized countries. The lion's share of the cost of depression is a consequence of inadequate recognition and care of the illness leading to lowered employment productivity. Although it can be a lifelong disorder, the majority of patients with depression can be successfully treated.

The hallmark symptoms of major depressive illness are sad/depressed mood and a loss of interest or pleasure in previously-enjoyed activities (anhedonia). Additional symptoms include feelings of worthlessness or guilt, psychomotor symptoms (e.g., changes in energy, sleep, appetite, and/or weight), difficulty concentrating, and thoughts of death or suicide. The symptoms must interfere with the individual's normal level of functioning to merit a diagnosis; however, not all depressed individuals experience every symptom, and the presence and severity of symptoms varies considerably both between and within patients over time. Depressive illness has a high rate of comorbidity with anxiety disorders and substance abuse. While full-blown depression is not challenging to diagnose, depression may not always be self evident. Systematic inquiry addressing all of the criteria for major depression is the key to accurate diagnosis of depression.

Panic Disorder

Panic disorder is an anxiety disorder characterized by discrete panic attacks, characterized as sudden, intense rushes of fear that include both physiological (e.g., rapid heart rate, trouble breathing, sweating, chest pain, tingling) and cognitive (e.g., feelings of impending doom, fear of death or going crazy) symptoms, as well as and persistent anxiety about having future attacks or about the consequences of the attacks. Panic disorder with or without agoraphobia (technically, "fear of open spaces"; intense fear of leaving home or familiar settings) has a lifetime prevalence of 1.5% to 3.0%, and like major depression, panic disorder has a two to three times greater prevalence in women than in men.[56] Although total prevalence rates for panic disorder are relatively low, associated morbidity is high, with most panic disorder patients experiencing significant social impairment and more than half experiencing comorbid major depression. Panic disorder also commonly co-occurs with other anxiety disorders (e.g., generalized anxiety disorder, phobias, obsessive–compulsive disorder), and frequently is associated with poor health perception, financial dependence, alcohol abuse, and suicide attempts. Patients with panic disorder often present to medical settings seeking diagnosis of their symptoms and amelioration of their distress; unfortunately, this disorder may elude detection or be misdiagnosed because its clinical presentation commonly is mistaken for other more sinister medical conditions, (e.g., cardiac events, respiratory conditions, gastrointestinal disorders).

Somatoform Disorders

Headache sufferers present on occasion with comparatively less prevalent psychiatric disorders such as one of the somatoform disorders (e.g., somatization disorder, conversion disorder, hypochondriasis). The hallmark of somatoform disorders is patient reports of physical symptoms (e.g., pain, gastrointestinal symptoms, urinary or sexual complaints, fatigue, loss of appetite, dizziness) that mimic a medical disease but cannot be traced to a specific physical cause. The comorbidity of migraine and somatoform disorders is not well documented, as these disorders seldom have been addressed in epidemiological or clinical studies of headache patients. However, patients with somatization disorder and undifferentiated somatoform disorder routinely include headaches on their lengthy list of presenting physical complaints. Further, recurrent headache undoubtedly is among the most common physical symptoms among patients diagnosed with somatoform pain disorder (characterized by pain as the predominant focus of clinical attention and wherein psychological factors are judged to play an important role in its onset, severity, exacerbation, or maintenance). When a somatoform disorder is suspected, psychiatric disorders commonly associated with somatic complaints (e.g., depression, anxiety, substance abuse/dependence, personality disorders) should be carefully ruled out. Even when a full-blown somatoform disorder is not present, somatic complaints such as nausea, sleeping trouble, and fatigue are most prevalent among chronic headache types and among individuals with comorbid depression and anxiety,[57] and often must be attended to in clinical practice for optimal treatment results.

Personality Disorders

Personality disorders are characterized by inflexible and pervasive behavioral patterns that often result in significant personal and social difficulties and functional impairment. In general, the maladaptive behavior patterns are enduring and stable, but they can intensify during times of acute distress. No epidemiological studies have addressed the comorbidity of migraine and personality disorders.[52,58] However, since personality disorders can be diagnosed in 10% to 13% of the general population,[59] it is not uncommon for headache treatment providers to encounter patients with these disorders, as they appear particularly common among headache patients who are refractory to usual care. As but one example, headaches were a significant complaint in 60% of the borderline personality disorder patients who presented to a hospital emergency department for acute treatment.[60]

Although seldom examined in the empirical headache literature, there is little question that personality disorders can markedly complicate head pain management simply because of the patient's difficult interpersonal style (e.g., histrionic patients may greatly exaggerate physical complaints, passive/dependent patients may rely excessively on healthcare providers, narcissistic patients may be demanding, borderline patients may be manipulative). From a patient management perspective, the borderline personality disorder is probably the most difficult of the personality disorders. Its essential characteristic is a pervasive pattern of unstable swings in interpersonal relationships, mood, and self-image, and it often is complicated by impulsivity; chronic emptiness or boredom; self-destructive behaviors; inappropriate, intense anger; and frantic efforts to avoid abandonment. Borderline personality disorder is found in approximately 2% of the general population, about 10% of psychiatric outpatients, and close to 20% of psychiatric inpatients, with approximately 75% of patients being female.[56]

Screening for Comorbid Psychiatric Disorders

Because of the high rates of psychiatric comorbidity in headache patients, it is highly recommended that all primary headache patients be screened, at a

Table 7-3 Rationale for Psychiatric Screening in Headache Patients

1. Psychiatric comorbidity can impact headache prognosis and satisfaction with headache treatment and is associated with increased headache-related disability. Anxiety and depression can produce differential response to headache prophylaxis and may indicate use of psychotropic medications to treat the comorbid disorder(s).
2. Psychiatric comorbidity can influence adherence with headache treatment and increase patients' tendencies to experience and report side effects.
3. Psychiatric comorbidity can degrade quality of life and increase health care utilization.
4. The use of antidepressants can trigger mania in patients with unrecognized bipolar disorder.
5. Patients with bipolar disorder and/or history of chemical dependency may have a tendency toward medication overuse or drug-seeking behavior.
6. Recognition of psychiatric comorbidity can be a key component in developing therapeutic doctor–patient relationship.
7. Use of screening tools can improve the patients' recognition of and attention to relevant behavioral/psychiatric factors.
8. Screening tools can be useful in ruling out suspected psychiatric basis for somatic complaints.

Adapted from Maizels M, Smitherman TA, Penzien DB. A review of screening tools for psychiatric comorbidity in headache patients. *Headache.* 2006;46(suppl 3):S98–109.

minimum, for anxiety and depression. Additional imperatives for the psychological screening of migraineurs are listed in Table 7.3. Psychopathology screening is particularly pertinent for headache patients presenting to specialty centers, the population of which often includes large proportions of patients with refractory headache types. Such screening can take several different forms including verbal questioning, administration of disorder-specific or multidimensional screening measures, and utilization of a structured diagnostic interview. In most instances, verbal or brief questionnaire screening is most practical and time-efficient, particularly when such screening assesses the hallmark features of the relevant disorders. Structured diagnostic interviews generally are reserved for confirming a suspected diagnosis or when the clinical presentation is particularly complex. However, more detailed psychiatric assessment often is warranted among patients who are refractory to usual care and who present to headache specialty clinics.

In screening for psychiatric disorders, clinicians must be aware of the overlap of somatic symptoms associated with headache, depression, and anxiety disorders in order to avoid inappropriate or incorrect psychiatric diagnoses.[35,61] Using somatic symptoms such as insomnia, fatigue, or difficulty concentrating as indicators of depression in headache patients may confound the assessment of depression with headache symptoms and severity.[62] Similarly, muscle tension, irritability, and sleep disturbance are commonly reported symptoms in both headache and anxiety disorders. Thus, it is recommended that an initial screen that is positive for psychopathology be followed by a diagnostic workup with an emphasis upon the alternate core symptoms of the potentially identified psychiatric disorder (i.e., for depression: feeling down and loss of pleasure in previously enjoyed activities most days during the past 2 weeks; for anxiety: feeling anxious, panic attacks, excessive rumination/worry during the past 6 months).

Psychopathology Screening Instruments

There is a broad array of well-validated and efficient screening tools designed to facilitate psychological symptom assessment in a variety of contexts, and they are described in detail by Maizels, Smitherman, and Penzien.[61] One of the most useful and well-validated multidimensional screening instruments for the major psychiatric disorders is the PRIME-MD (*Primary Care Evaluation of Mental Disorders*).[63] This 26-item self-administered symptom checklist was developed specifically for use in medical settings to assess for a variety of common psychiatric disorders based upon diagnostic criteria from the American Psychiatric Association's *Diagnostic and Statistical Manual of Mental Disorders* (DSM-IV-TR). The disorders identified by the PRIME-MD include mood disorders (depression, bipolar), anxiety disorders (panic disorder, generalized anxiety disorder), eating disorders, alcohol abuse or dependence, and somatization disorders. The PRIME-MD has been well utilized in many studies including an increasing number addressing primary headache. For example, Schriger and colleagues[64] administered the PRIME-MD to 218 patients presenting to an emergency department with long-standing headache or abdominal or back pain (patients with known psychiatric illness were excluded from the study). Most patients willingly completed the PRIME-MD in a short period of time (median time of 7 minutes), which in turn yielded psychiatric diagnoses among 42% of these patients with primary complaints of pain.

Screening for Depression

Verbal screening for depression is most effective when it focuses on the two hallmark symptoms of depression as they have occurred over the previous 2 weeks: (1) depressed mood and (2) anhedonia or loss of usual interest in activities. Endorsement of either symptom merits further assessment and should be followed by more in-depth questions (including inquiries about suicidal ideation) and/or administration of a depression-specific screening measure.

Four commonly used self-report screening measures for depression are the *Beck Depression Inventory-II* (BDI-II),[65] the *BDI-Primary Care* (BDI-PC),[66] the *Patient Health Questionnaire depression module* (PHQ-9),[67] and the *Quick Inventory of Depressive Symptomatology (16-Item) Self-Report* (QIDS-SR16).[68] These measures have strong psychometric properties, include questions about cognitive (nonsomatic) symptoms of depression, and can each be completed by most patients in 5 minutes or less. Because of its brevity, high predictive value, correspondence with diagnostic criteria of depression, and availability at no cost, the PHQ-9 is perhaps the preferred depression screening tool for primary care and headache clinic settings. The QIDS-SR16 is a relatively new instrument based on the current American Psychiatric Association (DSM-IV-TR) criteria for major depressive disorder; this measure is freely available in the public domain and can also be used to detect changes in symptoms following treatment.[69]

Screening for Anxiety

Screening for anxiety disorders often is more complex than screening for depression owing to the numerous manifestations and disorders of anxiety. The symptom profiles of the various anxiety disorders (panic disorder, generalized anxiety disorder, obsessive–compulsive disorder, phobias, etc.) are somewhat distinct from one another, and anxious patients often do not outwardly appear anxious. In clinical settings, verbal screening for anxiety can nevertheless be informative as long as it is targeted to specific anxiety phenomena. Although symptom constellations and presentations differ across patients, the hallmark symptoms of anxiety generally include chronic, uncontrollable worry or fear; unpleasant sensations of physiological arousal; and/or avoidance behavior. Thus, questioning a patient about difficulty controlling chronic worry, fear of having panic attacks, obsessions/compulsions, or frequent avoidance behaviors is likely to be considerably more informative than asking only about "anxiety" more generally.[70]

Unfortunately, most of the anxiety screening measures designed for use in primary care settings inquire about "global" anxiety symptoms rather than specific anxiety disorders. Two such measures that are psychometric validated and commonly used are the *Beck Anxiety Inventory* (BAI),[71] and the *State-Trait Anxiety Inventory* (STAI).[72] A recently developed instrument that assesses the cardinal features of generalized anxiety disorder and that likewise has been validated for use in primary care settings is the *Generalized Anxiety Disorder 7-item scale* (GAD-7).[73] Beyond generalized anxiety disorder, the GAD-7 also is sensitive to panic disorder, social phobia, and post-traumatic stress disorder.[74]

Readers interested in a more thorough discussion of additional instruments for assessing psychiatric comorbidity, particularly for disorders not reviewed above, should consult Maizels, Smitherman, and Penzien.[61]

Conclusion

Although the study of psychiatric comorbidities and headache disorders is still a relatively young scientific endeavor, existing literature is consistent in finding that depression, anxiety, and some other psychiatric disorders are more prevalent among treatment-seeking headache patients than among those without headache. Elevated rates of psychiatric comorbidity are most strongly associated with chronic forms of headache and those who present to headache specialty clinics, making them of particular interest to individuals who work with patients suffering from RM. Such comorbidities are generally associated with a poorer prognosis and may interfere with headache-specific treatments, although further research is needed to explore the relationship between psychiatric comorbidities and headache treatment outcomes.[75]

In addition to the complexities of RM itself, the clinician who treats RM patients should be attentive to issues of psychiatric comorbidity among these patients. Most notably, symptoms of depression and anxiety, at a minimum, should be assessed through verbal screening, and more formal quantitative assessment using self-report measures and/or diagnostic interviews is certainly merited in those who endorse screening items positively, who have a particularly complex presentation, or who have failed to respond to conventional headache treatment regimens. Because the RM patient is the *sine qua non* patient for fulfilling these characteristics, suspicion of psychiatric comorbidity among these patients should be the rule rather than the exception. Measures have been described that afford accurate identification of psychiatric comorbidities in an expedient fashion. Through recognition of the role of psychiatric comorbidities and concerted efforts to assess them, improved management of RM patients may be achieved.

References

1. Maizels M. Understanding the headache patient with complex comorbidities: a primary care physician's perspective. *Headache.* 2006;46(suppl 3):S160–162.
2. Penzien DB, Rains J, Holroyd KA. Psychological assessment of the recurrent headache sufferer. In: Tollison C, Kunkel R, eds. *Headache: Diagnosis and Treatment.* Baltimore: Williams & Wilkins; 1993:39–49.
3. Breslau N, Merikangas K, Bowden CL. Comorbidity of migraine and major affective disorders. *Neurology.* 1994;44(10 suppl 7):S17–22.
4. Holroyd KA, Stensland M, Lipchik GL, Hill KR, O'Donnell FS, Cordingley G. Psychosocial correlates and impact of chronic tension-type headaches. *Headache.* 2000;40:3–16.
5. Italian Collaborative Group for the Study of Psychopathological Factors in Primary Headaches. Psychiatric comorbidity and psychosocial stress in patients with tension-type headache from headache centers in Italy. *Cephalalgia.* 1999;19:159–164.
6. Puca F, Genco S, Prudenzano MP, et al. Psychiatric comorbidity and psychosocial stress in patients with tension-type headache from headache centers in Italy. The Italian Collaborative Group for the Study of Psychopathological Factors in Primary Headaches. *Cephalalgia.* 1999;19:159–164.
7. Ziegler DK, Paolo AM. Headache symptoms and psychological profile of headache-prone individuals. A comparison of clinic patients and controls. *Arch Neurol.* 1995;52:602–606.

8. Juang KD, Wang SJ, Fuh JL, et al. Comorbidity of depressive and anxiety disorders in chronic daily headache and its subtypes. *Headache.* 2000;40:818–823.
9. Radat F, Swendsen J. Psychiatric comorbidity in migraine: a review. *Cephalalgia.* 2005;25:165–78.
10. Mitsikostas DD, Thomas AM: Comorbidity of headache and depressive disorders. *Cephalalgia.* 1999;19:211–217.
11. Hamelsky SW, Lipton RB. Psychiatric comorbidity of migraine. *Headache.* 2006;46:1327–1333.
12. Breslau N, Davis GC. Migraine, physical health and psychiatric disorder: a prospective epidemiologic study in young adults. *J Psychiatr Res.*1993;27:211–221.
13. Zwart JA, Dyb G, Hagen K, et al. Depression and anxiety disorders associated with headache frequency. The Nord-Trondelag Health Study. *Eur J Neurol.* 2003,10:147–152.
14. Wang SJ, Juang KD, Fuh JL, et al. Psychiatric comorbidity and suicide risk in adolescents with chronic daily headache. *Neurology* 2007,68:1468–1473.
15. Radat F, Lantéri-Minet M, Nachit-Ouinekh F, et al. The GRIM2005 study of migraine consultation in France. III: Psychological features of subjects with migraine. *Cephalalgia.* 2009;29:338–350.
16. Breslau N, Davis GC, Schultz LR, Peterson EL. Joint 1994 Wolff Award Presentation. Migraine and major depression: a longitudinal study. *Headache.* 1994;34:387–393.
17. Craske MG, ed. *Origins of Phobias and Anxiety Disorders: Why More Women than Men?* Boston: Elsevier Science; 2003.
18. Lantéri-Minet M, Radat F, Chautart MH, Lucas C. Anxiety and depression associated with migraine: influence on migraine subjects' disability and quality of life, and acute migraine management. *Pain.* 2005;118:319–326.
19. Page LA, Howard LM, Husain K, et al. Psychiatric morbidity and cognitive representations of illness in chronic daily headache. *J Psychosom Res.* 2004;57:549–555.
20. Jette N, Patten S, Williams J, et al. Comorbidity of migraine and psychiatric disorders—a national population-based study. *Headache.* 2008;48:501–516.
21. Hung CI, Liu CY, Fuh JL, et al. Comorbid migraine is associated with a negative impact on quality of life in patients with major depression. *Cephalalgia.* 2006;26:36–32.
22. Guidetti V, Galli F, Fabrizi P, et al. Headache and psychiatric comorbidity: clinical aspects and outcome in an 8–year follow-up study. *Cephalalgia.* 1998;18:455–462.
23. Blanchard EB, Andrasik F. *Management of Chronic Headaches: A Psychological Approach.* New York: Pergamon Press; 1985.
24. Blanchard EB, Andrasik F, Evans DD, Neff DF, Appelbaum KA, Rodichok LD. Behavioral treatment of 250 chronic headache patients: a clinical replication series. *Behav Ther.* 1985;16:308–327.
25. Jacob RG, Turner SN, Szekely BC, Edelman BH. Predicting outcome of relaxation therapy in headaches: the role of "depression." *Behav Ther.* 1983;14:457–465.
26. Holroyd KA, Holm JE, Hursey KG, et al. Recurrent vascular headache: home-based behavioral treatment vs. abortive pharmacological treatment. *J Cons Clin Psychol.* 1988;56:218–223.

27. Micieli G, Piazza D, Sinforiani E, et al. Antimigraine drugs in the management of chronic daily headaches: clinical profiles of responsive patients. *Cephalalgia.* 1985;5(suppl. 2):221–224.
28. Saper JR, Lake AE 3rd, Tepper SJ. Nefazodone for chronic daily headache prophylaxis: an open-label study. *Headache.* 2001;41:465–474.
29. Mongini F, Keller R, Deregibus A, Raviola F, Mongini T, Sancarlo M. Personality traits, depression and migraine in women: a longitudinal study. *Cephalalgia.* 2003;23:186–192.
30. Bigal ME, Lipton RB. Concepts and mechanisms of migraine chronification. *Headache.* 2008;48:6–15.
31. Lipton RB, Pan J. Is migraine a progressive disease? *JAMA.* 2004;291:493–494.
32. Penzien DB, Rains JC, Lipton RB. Introduction to the Special Series on the Chronification of headache: mechanisms, risk factors, and behavioral strategies aimed at primary and secondary prevention of chronic headache. *Headache.* 2008;48:5–6.
33. Scher AI, Midgette L, Lipton RB. Risk factors for headache chronification. *Headache.* 2008;48:16–25.
34. Siniatchkin M, Riabus M, Hasenbring M. Coping styles of headache sufferers. *Cephalalgia.* 1999;19:165–173.
35. Smitherman TA, Maizels M, Penzien DB. Headache chronification: screening and behavioral management of comorbid depressive and anxiety disorders. *Headache* 2008;48:45–50.
36. Smitherman TA, Rains JC, Penzien DB. Psychiatric comorbidities and migraine chronification. *Curr Pain Headache Rep.* 2009;13:326–331.
37. Heckman BD, Holroyd KA, Himawan L, et al. Do psychiatric comorbidities influence headache treatment outcomes? Results of a naturalistic longitudinal treatment study. *Pain.* 2009.146:56–64.
38. Smitherman TA, Penzien DB. Were we wrong about the role of psychiatric comorbidities in primary headache? *Pain.* 2009;146:11–12
39. Rains JC, Lipchik GL, Penzien DB. Behavioral facilitation of medical treatment for headache--part I: Review of headache treatment compliance. *Headache.* 2006;46:1387–1394.
40. Rains JC, Penzien DB, Lipchik GL. Behavioral facilitation of medical treatment for headache--part II: Theoretical models and behavioral strategies for improving adherence. *Headache.* 2006;46:1395–403.
41. Breslau N, Schultz LR, Stewart WF, Lipton RB, Welch KMA. Headache types and panic disorder. *Neurology.* 2001;56:350–354.
42. Breslau N, Davis GC, Andreski P. Migraine, psychiatric disorders and suicide attempts: an epidemiologic study of young adults. *Psychiatry Res.* 1991;37:11–23.
43. Ferrari MD, Saxena PR. On serotonin and migraine: a clinical and pharmacological review. *Cephalalgia.* 1993;13:151–165.
44. Hamel E. Serotonin and migraine: biology and clinical implications. *Cephalagia.* 2007;27:1295–3000.
45. Schwedt TJ. Serotonin and migraine: the latest developments. *Cephalalgia.* 2007;27:1301–1307.
46. Silberstein SD. Shared mechanisms and comorbidities in neurologic and psychiatric disorders. *Headache.* 2001;41(suppl 1):S11–17.

47. Guidetti V, Galli F. Psychiatric comorbidity in chronic daily headache: pathophysiology, etiology, and diagnosis. *Curr Pain Headache Rep.* 2002;6:492–497.
48. Rome HP, Jr, Rome JD. Limbically augmented pain syndrome (LAPS): kindling, corticolimbic sensitization, and the convergence of affective and sensory symptoms in chronic pain disorders. *Pain Med.* 2000;1(1):7–23.
49. Cady R, Farmer K, Dexter J, Schreiber C. Cosensitization of pain and psychiatric comorbidity in chronic daily headache. *Curr Pain Headache Rep.* 2005;9:47–52.
50. Lipchik GL, Smitherman TA, Penzien DB, Holroyd KA. Basic principles and techniques of cognitive-behavioral therapies for comorbid psychiatric symptoms among headache patients. *Headache.* 2006;46(suppl 3):S119–132.
51. Griffith JL, Razavi M. Pharmacological management of mood and anxiety disorders in headache patients. *Headache.* 2006;46(suppl 3):S133–141.
52. Saper JR, Lake AE 3rd. Borderline personality disorder and the chronic headache patient: review and management recommendations. *Headache.* 2002;42:663–674.
53. Saper JR, Sheftell F. Headache in the abuse-prone individual. In: Olesen J, Tfelt-Hansen P, Welch KMA, eds. *The Headaches* (2nd ed). Philadelphia: Lippincott, Williams & Wilkins; 2000:953–958.
54. Kessler RC, McGonagle KA, Zhao S, et al. Lifetime and 12–month prevalence of DSM-III-R disorders in the United States: results from the National Comorbidity Survey. *Arch Gen Psychiatry.* 1994;51:8–19.
55. Greenberg PE, Stiglin LE, Finkelstein SN, Berndt ER. The economic burden of depression in 1990. *J Clin Psychiatry.* 1993;4:405–418.
56. American Psychiatric Association. *Diagnostic and Statistical Manual of Mental Disorders*, 4th ed., text revision. Washington, DC: American Psychiatric Association; 2000.
57. Maizels M, Burchette R. Somatic symptoms in headache patients: the influence of headache diagnosis, frequency, and comorbidity. *Headache.* 2004;44:983–993.
58. Saper JR. "Are you talking to me?" Confronting behavioral disturbances in patients with headache. *Headache.* 2006;46(suppl 3):S151–156.
59. Weissman MM. The epidemiology of personality disorders: a 1990 update. *J Pers Disord.* 1993;7:44–62.
60. Hegarty AM. The prevalence of migraine in borderline personality disorder. *Headache.* 1993;33:271.
61. Maizels M, Smitherman TA, Penzien DB. A review of screening tools for psychiatric comorbidity in headache patients. *Headache.* 2006;46(suppl 3):S98–109.
62. Holm JE, Penzien DB, Holroyd KA, Brown TA. Headache and depression: confounding effects of transdiagnostic symptoms. *Headache.* 1994;34:418–423.
63. Spitzer RL, Williams JB, Kroenke K, et al. Utility of a new procedure for diagnosing mental disorders in primary care: The PRIME MD 1000 study. *JAMA.* 1994;272:1749–1756.
64. Schriger DL, Gibbons PS, Langone CA, et al. Enabling the diagnosis of occult psychiatric illness in the emergency department: a randomized controlled trial

of the computerized self-administered PRIME-MD diagnostic system. *Ann Emerg Med.* 2001;37:132–140.
65. Beck AT, Steer RA, Brown GK. *Beck Depression Inventory Manual*, 2nd ed. San Antonio, TX: Psychological Corporation; 1996.
66. Beck AT, Guth D, Steer RA, Ball R. Screening for major depression disorders in medical inpatients with the Beck Depression Inventory for Primary Care. *Behav Res Ther.* 1997;35:785–791.
67. Kroenke K, Spitzer RL, Williams JB. The PHQ-9: validity of a brief depression screening measure. *J Gen Intern Med.* 2001;16:606–613.
68. Trivedi MH, Rush AJ, Ibrihim HM, et al. The Inventory of Depressive Symptomatology, Clinician Rating (IDS-C) and Self-Report (IDS-SR), and the Quick Inventory of Depressive Symptomatology, Clinician Rating (QIDS-C) and Self-Report (QIDS-SR) in public sector patients with mood disorders: a psychometric evaluation. *Psychol Med.* 2004;34:73–82.
69. Rush AJ, Trivedi MH, Carmody TJ, et al. Self-reported depressive symptom measures: sensitivity to detecting change in a randomized, controlled trial of chronically depressed, nonpsychotic outpatients. *Neuropsychopharmacology.* 2005;30:405–416.
70. Smitherman TA, Penzien DB, Maizels M. Anxiety disorders and migraine intractability and progression. *Curr Pain Headache Rep.* 2008;12:224–229.
71. Beck AT, Epstein N, Brown G, Steer RA. An inventory for measuring clinical anxiety: psychometric properties. *J Consult Clin Psychol.* 1988;56:893–897.
72. Spielberger CD, Gorsuch RL, Lushene R, Vagg PR, Jacobs GA. *Manual for the State-Trait Anxiety Inventory (Form Y).* Palo Alto, CA: Mind Garden; 1983.
73. Spitzer RL, Kroenke K, Williams JBW, Löwe B. A brief measure for assessing generalized anxiety disorder. *Arch Intern Med.* 2006;166:1092–1097.
74. Kroenke K, Spitzer RL, Williams JBW, Monahan PO, Löwe B. Anxiety disorders in primary care: prevalence, impairment, comorbidity, and detection. *Ann Intern Med.* 2007;146:317–325.
75. Lake AE 3rd, Rains JC, Penzien DB. Headache and psychiatric comorbidity: historical context, clinical implications, and research relevance. *Headache.* 2005:45:493–506.

Section II

Treatment of Refractory Migraine

8

Prophylactic Treatment of Refractory Migraine

Ninan T. Mathew, MD, FRCP(C)

Migraine progresses from the episodic to chronic (Chronic Migraine [CM]) in some patients.[1–3] Migraine patients with an intermediate headache frequency of 6 to 9 days per month are at greater risk for headache chronicity, and this risk is even higher for patients with critical frequency of 10 to 14 headaches days per month.[4] A significant percentage of CM becomes refractory. Two major factors contributing to refractory migraine (RM) are acute medication overuse and psychiatric comorbidities such as depression and anxiety.

General Preventive Strategies

Modifiable and nonmodifiable risk factors have been identified for progression of migraine into chronic refractory stage. Headache frequency, obesity, acute medication overuse, depression, stressful life events, excessive caffeine consumption, snoring, and allodynia are modifiable risk factors.[2] Headache frequency and obesity are among the most important risk factors for migraine progression. In those with high-frequency migraine, medication overuse accelerates the process of chronification, even though some patients can experience refractory CM without medication overuse.[2,4] So, one of the most important strategies in the preventive approach to refractory headache is to address these modifiable risk factors in all patients with migraine particularly, in those who have frequency of six or more per month. Decreasing headache frequency with behavioral and pharmacological interventions, weight loss and maintenance of ideal body weight, and avoiding medications that increase weight, are important strategies. Regular aerobic physical exercise such as walking, jogging, and running as well as relaxation techniques such as biofeedback therapy and yoga should be encouraged. Avoiding medication and caffeine overuse and treating sleep disorders such as snoring, sleep apnea, and insomnia appropriately are essential steps.[5]

Routine screening for depression, anxiety, and bipolar illness is accomplished by utilizing detailed history taking, depression scales, anxiety scales, and mood disorder questionnaires. Once a comorbid psychiatric condition is identified, it is extremely important to treat that condition appropriately along with migraine preventive agents. This leads us to consider rationale combination therapy in RM.

Prevalence and severity of somatic symptoms are greater in patients with chronic headaches, which in turn contribute to disability.[6] Major depressive disorders also coexist in these patients. Non-headache pain conditions such as fibromyalgia or arthritis are more likely to occur in patients with chronic RM.[7,8] Concomitant management of these pain conditions is a must when dealing with RM.

Prophylactic Pharmacotherapy of RM

Rationale Co-Pharmacy or Combination Therapy

RM patients usually come to the physician specialist after having failed three or more individual agents approved for prophylactic therapy such as adrenergic blocking agents, valproate, and topiramate. They might have also tried tricyclic antidepressants such as amitriptyline. At this stage, there is no purpose in going back on those monotherapy approaches unless the physician is convinced that the patient failed the drugs because of inadequate dosage or too short periods of trial. If the patient had failed to respond to monotherapy after an adequate trial (dosage and duration), then there are strong reasons to implement combination therapy. There are a few convincing reasons for combination therapy:

1. Present standard of therapy for many of the chronic medical conditions, such as diabetes, hypertension, and HIV is combination therapy,
2. Combination therapy targets multiple pathophysiological mechanisms, and this approach is very relevant to migraine.
3. Combination therapy can address comorbidities such as depression, anxiety, bipolar illness, fibromyalgia, and insomnia.

Combining drugs can increase the risk of adverse events; however, they can be minimized by careful monitoring of the adverse events and titration of doses or modification of combinations. One of the drawbacks of combination therapy is that until now there were no well-controlled randomized clinical trails to provide evidence-based recommendations. Clinical experience of many expert physicians and a few open level published trials, reviewed in the text that follows, strengthen the argument for combination therapy.

An open-label study that combined a beta-blocker (nadolol or propranolol) and valproate was performed.[9] Patients who had episodic migraine with or without aura and who were previously unresponsive to beta-blockers and valproate in monotherapy were included in the study. Combination therapy with a beta-blocker and valproate was effective in preventing migraines in more than 50% of previously resistant migraine cases. However, combining drugs can increase risk of adverse events, and in this study, almost 20% of the participating patients were unable to tolerate even typically low doses of these medications.

Another open-label study tested the combination of a beta-blocker (nadolol or propranolol) and topiramate in migraine patients, who previously did not respond to either treatment as monotherapy.[10] Approximately 60% of these patients with RM observed at least a 50% reduction in the number of headache days in the third month of treatment as a result of combining therapy. However, 17% of the patients who had previously tolerated each medication as monotherapy discontinued the study early because of adverse events, which included cognitive impairment, paresthesia, depression, and gastrointestinal symptoms.

In another trial of propranolol alone, amitriptyline alone, biofeedback alone, a combination of amitriptyline and propranolol, or the combination of amitriptyline, propranolol, and biofeedback therapy, it was shown that the best results were obtained in chronic migraine by using combination of amitriptyline, propranolol, and biofeedback therapy compared to individual therapies.[11]

The use of tricyclic antidepressant medication, stress management therapy, and combination of these two therapeutic approaches were evaluated for their ability to treat chronic tension type headache in a placebo-controlled study.[12] Although, CTTH is treated primarily with tricyclic antidepressants, some trials have reported a little or no improvement in CTTH with the tricyclic antidepressant amitriptyline. Amitriptyline up to 100 mg per day or nortriptyline up to 75 mg per day was administered either as a monotherapy or in combination with stress management therapy.[12] Stress management therapy utilized both relaxation and cognitive skills for preventing and managing stress and headache. Tricyclic antidepressant medication and stress management therapy each produced larger reductions in headache activity, analgesic medication use, and headache-related disability than placebo with more rapid improvement observed with antidepressant medication. Combining therapies increased the likelihood of producing significant reduction (at least 50%) in headache index.

The National Institute of Neurological Disorder and Stroke (NINDS) is presently conducting a randomized placebo controlled comparative trial of topiramate and propranolol to asses the merits of combination therapy. Until such study results are available, we have to choose the individual medication combinations based on the experience. The purpose of the combination therapy is to improve the efficacy by combining drugs, which have different mechanisms of action.

It is desirable:

1. To choose medications from different therapeutic categories.
2. To treat comorbidities concurrently.

The suggested combinations are:

1. Beta-blockers plus tricyclic antidepressants. This combination is particularly helpful in RM with depression or insomnia.
2. Beta-blockers plus selective serotonin–norepinephrine inhibitors (SNRIs) are useful in patients with RM, depression and fibromyalgia (SNRI—duloxetine or milnacipran are approved for fibromyalgia).
3. Beta-blockers plus topiramate may be useful for increased efficacy and for RM patients, who are obese.
4. Beta-blockers plus valproate in RM patients with cyclothymia and bipolar disorder.
5. Topiramate plus antidepressants. Selection of antidepressants will depend on the type of depression and other comorbidities like insomnia. Tricyclics are preferable if there is insomnia. SNRIs are preferable to selective serotonin reuptake inhibitors (SSRIs) and agents like quetiapine are very useful for patients with cyclothymia, bipolar depression, and insomnia.
6. Topiramate plus pregabalin. When there is migraine and fibromyalgia, this combination may be useful.
7. Topiramate plus SNRIs plus pregabalin in RM with depression and fibromyalgia.
8. Valproate, lithium, or lamotrigine in RM with bipolar illness.
9. Physicians can use their own logical combination provided there are no known drug–drug interactions.

Individual Drugs with Some Evidence of Efficacy

Classes of agents used to treat RM prophylactically include β-adrenergic antagonists, calcium-channel blockers, α_2-adrenergic agonists, serotonin antagonists such as methysergide, antidepressants, nonsteroidal anti-inflammatory drugs, and antiepileptic drugs.[13,14] Unfortunately, the usefulness of these agents is limited because of poor compliance resulting from intolerable side effects, daily dosage administration requirements, and inadequate efficacy.[13] Other than propranolol, valproate, and topiramate, no drug to date has received regulatory approval for patients with migraine.[13,15] Few of the preventive agents typically used to prevent migraine have been evaluated for their effectiveness in treating CM.(16) The efficacy of these agents for the prevention of CM has not been evaluated in large, multicenter, controlled clinical trials.[16] None of the individual medications have been studied in RM. Consequently, there is a great need for further research to develop effective treatments.[13]

Gabapentin

Gabapentin is an antiepileptic medication used for a variety of painful disorders.[13] It is an analog of γ-aminobutyric acid (GABA) and may stimulate the release of GABA, which blocks pain signaling. Gabapentin also binds to voltage-gated calcium channels.[13] Gabapentin has been demonstrated to increase the percentage of headache-free days over placebo by 9.1% ($p = 0.0005$).[17] Headache severity, disability, and quality of life also showed some improvement, as did headache duration when compared with prerandomization.[17] The amount of analgesic use was reduced as a consequence of treatment with gabapentin.[17]

Tizanidine

Tizanidine is an α_2-adrenergic agonist that inhibits the release of norepinephrine in both the brainstem and the spinal cord. It acts as a central muscle relaxant and also has antinociceptive effects.[14] The effectiveness of tizanidine over placebo in a study on patients with chronic daily headache (CDH) was assessed using the headache index (calculated as the sum of the products of the number of headache days, average intensity, and duration of each headache during each 4-week interval, divided by 28 days), as the primary end point.[14] Tizanidine was shown to reduce the overall headache index compared with placebo and to reduce the average number of headache days per week, severe headache days per week, average headache intensity, peak headache intensity, and mean headache duration.

Fluoxetine

Fluoxetine is an SSRI that downregulates serotonin receptors, thereby increasing synaptic serotonin.[13] Fluoxetine has been demonstrated to be moderately effective in treating CDH, such that it caused a significant improvement in overall mood and a modest decrease in headache frequency.[18]

Amitriptyline

Amitriptyline downregulates serotonin receptors, increases the levels of synaptic norepinephrine, and enhances endogenous opioid receptor actions.[13] Although amitriptyline is used to treat CDH, adverse effects may limit its use or prevent increasing the dose to a therapeutic level.[19] The efficacy of combining amitriptyline and fluoxetine compared with amitriptyline alone was assessed in patients with CDH.[19] Although amitriptyline alone, as well as in combination with fluoxetine, caused an overall decrease in the reported headache indexes at the end of the study, no significant improvement over the effect of amitriptyline was observed by combining it with fluoxetine.[19] This lack of difference may be due to the small number of study participants and the relatively short duration of the study.[19]

Valproate

Although the mechanism by which valproate improves migraine symptoms is unclear, previous studies have demonstrated its effectiveness in migraine prophylaxis.[20] The efficacy and tolerability of valproate on CDH was assessed in a prospective, double-blind, randomized, placebo-controlled study.[21] Valproate reduced the level and frequency of pain in patients with CDH compared with placebo. In addition, when comparing two of the subgroups of CDH, 500 mg twice daily of valproate was more effective in treating CM than chronic tension-type headache (CTTH). The incidence of adverse effects in this study was lower than previously reported for valproate.

Topiramate

Topiramate blocks voltage-sensitive sodium channels and voltage-activated calcium channels, inhibits glutamate release, and increases GABA levels.[13] Extensive studies have demonstrated that topiramate is a safe, effective, and well-tolerated drug for migraine prophylaxis.[20,21] Topiramate is associated with a wide range of side effects, including paresthesia, fatigue, anorexia, nausea, diarrhea, weight loss, dizziness, taste perversion, and difficulty with memory and concentration.[22] In another study, topiramate treatment resulted in a significant reduction in the number of monthly migraine days in the medication overuse subpopulation, although analgesic use did not decrease in the topiramate group compared with the placebo group.[23] This study suggests that it may not be necessary to withdraw patients with CM from medication overuse before initiating preventive treatment.[23] However many experts feel that the above claim is not fully substantiated because the majority of those patients overused triptans rather than opioids or butalbital compounds. A different study demonstrated that topiramate had a very good tolerance profile when doses lower than those typically used in epilepsy management were given to patients with CM.[24] A dose of daily topiramate 50 mg significantly reduced the 28-day headache frequency compared with placebo. This demonstrated that low doses of topiramate can be effective at reducing headache frequency in patients with CM with medication overuse.[24] Higher doses of topiramate (approximately 100 mg per day) have also been shown to be effective at reducing the average monthly migraine headache days in patients with CM.[16]

Botulinum Toxin Type A

Botulinum toxin type A (BoNT-A) is a focally acting protein that inhibits the release of acetylcholine from presynaptic nerve endings and blocks the release of nociceptive mediators, such as substance P, glutamate, and calcitonin gene-related peptide.[13] Reduction of peripheral nociceptive mediators may cause a reduction in central sensitization by reducing inflammatory signals to sensitized regions of the brain. The biologic effects of BoNT-A are reversible and last for approximately 3 months.

The ability of BoNT-A to treat migraine effectively has been evaluated in many studies with different subsets of migraine patients. The effectiveness of BoNT-A in the treatment of CM without medication overuse has been evaluated.[25] Patients were excluded from the study if they were taking triptans more than 3 days per week, ergotamine more than 2 days per week, dihydroergotamine more than 2 days per week, or any combination of these medications for more than 3 days per week. Analgesic use was restricted to 2 opioids and 10 simple analgesic tablets per week or 9 combination analgesics per week. Caffeine consumption in excess of 500 mg per day was another criterion for exclusion from the study. The injection of 100 units of BoNT-A into five sites (glabella, temporal, frontal, suboccipital, and trapezius) using a fixed dose resulted in significant reductions in migraine episodes in the patients with CM receiving BoNT-A, without the complication of medication overuse. The high level of safety and tolerability of BoNT-A as a preventive CM therapy was demonstrated by the low number of adverse events in this study.

The effectiveness of BoNT-A injection for patients with refractory CM was assessed in a different study. The patient-selection criteria required the participants to have tried tree classes of prophylactic medications for at least 1 year with no improvement.[26] Doses of 250 units of BoNT-A were injected into 15 sites, and patients were followed for 4 months. Pain intensity and frequency of headaches decreased during the study, demonstrating the effectiveness of BoNT-A to treat RM.

A 2005 study to assess BoNT-A in patients with CDH did not discriminate as to specific CDH subtype but included any combination of migraines, with or without aura, migrainous/probably migraine, and frequent episodic migraine.[27] In addition, many patients in the study were overusing acute medications and/or taking concurrent prophylactic headache treatments. BoNT-A use in this study did not statistically meet the predetermined primary efficacy measure of the number of headache-free days per month. However, a statistically significant higher percentage of BoNT-A patients, compared with placebo patients, had at least a 50% decrease in frequency of headache days by day 180. This exploratory study suggested that the number of headache-free days per 30-day period may not be the optimal end point for detecting a treatment response for patients in this headache population.

When the effectiveness of BoNT-A in CM was assessed without concomitant prophylaxis, BoNT-A decreased by at least half, compared with baseline, the frequency of headaches in more than 50% of the patients after three injection sessions.[28] Statistically significant decreases in headache frequency and headache severity were observed between BoNT-A and placebo for most time points from day 180 through day 270. Consequently, this subgroup analysis demonstrated that BoNT-A is an effective treatment for patients with CDH who are not taking other preventive headache medications.

Two phase 3, double-blind, placebo-controlled studies, (PREEMPT 1 and PREEMPT 2) evaluated efficacy and safety of botulinum toxin type A (BoNT-A) in CM sufferers with or without medication overuse.[29] One thousand three hundred and eighty-four adults were randomized to injections. The primary endpoint for PREEMPT 1 was change from 28-day baseline to the 28-days ending with week 24 for headache days. The primary endpoint for PREEMPT 2 was change in headache episodes from baseline 28-days to the 28-days ending with week 24.

A large decrease for the frequency of headache days from baseline, with statistically significant between group difference favoring BoNT-A over placebo, was observed in both PREEMPT 1 ($p = 0.006$) and PREEMPT 2, $p < 0.001$. For the frequency of headache episodes, a significant difference favoring BoNT-A was observed in PREEMPT 2 ($p = 003$), whereas no between group significant difference was observed in PREEMPT 1.

Pooled analyses significantly favored BoNT-A at all timepoints for key endpoints, headache days ($p < 0.001$) and headache episodes ($p = 0.009$), and 5/6 secondary endpoints in one or both trials. BoNT-A was safe and well tolerated with few treatment related AEs and discontinuations.[29]

These phase 3 trial results establish BoNT-A as an effective and safe prophylactic treatment for patients with CM, including those who overuse acute headache medications.[29]

Predictors of response to BoNT-A were evaluated in a recent study of patients with CDH, specifically with CM and CTTH.[30] It has been reported previously that patients with imploding (pain is felt from the outside to the inside of the head) or ocular (pain is localized around or behind the eye) headaches responded to BoNT-A, whereas patients with exploding (painful buildup inside the head) headaches did not.[31] The terms "imploding" and "exploding" are rather confusing and inconsistent when described by the patients and therefore are not reliable as predictors of response. To isolate factors that might predict response to BoNT-A in CDH, patients with CM or CTTH, which form the majority of CDH disorders, received at least two injections of BoNT-A 100 units at 12- to 15-week intervals, using fixed-sites, fixed-dose, and "follow-the-pain" approaches.[30] Patients were divided into responders (≥50% reduction in both headache frequency and migraine disability assessment scale scores compared with baseline) and non-responders (<50% reduction.[30] A larger proportion of patients with CM (76.1%) responded to BoNT-A than did patients with CTTH (36.4%).[30] In CM, treatment response was associated with a high incidence of unilateral headache and allodynia, such that scalp and muscle allodynia were seen in 82% and 61% of treatment responders, respectively. Non-responders had 12% and 18% scalp and muscle allodynia, respectively.[30] Specifically, the presence of scalp allodynia, muscle allodynia, and unilateral headache appeared to be predictors for response to BoNT-A in patients with CM, whereas muscle allodynia in patients with CTTH may be a predictor of responsiveness to BoNT-A.[30]

BoNT-A versus. Topiramate in 2008 CM Study

In a study to assess the effectiveness of BoNT-A versus topiramate to treat CM, patient selection included those individuals with CM, no medication overuse, and age between 18 and 65 years.[32] After randomization, one group received either a BoNT-A injection (maximum 200-unit dose at baseline visit and at month 3 only) or an oral placebo, and the other group received topiramate (100 mg/day, with an optional 4-week titration to 200 mg/day) or a placebo injection. Both groups were assessed at intervals of 1, 3, 6, and 9 months. The percentage improvement was reported as marked, moderate, or mild, and all treatments had a similar effect. At month 6, both groups had significantly fewer headaches compared with baseline, with BoNT-A showing a larger decrease than topiramate. By month 9, however, both treatment groups demonstrated an equivalent reduction in headache days per month. A higher number of patients in the topiramate group opted out due to adverse events (53% vs. 25%).

BoNT-A versus Divalproex in 2005 Headache Study

Inclusion criteria for this study involved men and women ages 18 to 65 years with EM (between 3 and 15 migraine days/month) or CM (>15 migraine days/month), with stable headache severity and pattern.[33] The overall duration of the study was 10.5 months, including 1 month of baseline screening, one 3-month treatment cycle, one 6-month treatment cycle, and a final safety visit. After the baseline period, eligible patients were randomized (1:1) to receive either BoNT-A or divalproex. The BoNT-A group received a total of 100 units of BoNT-A injections and placebo-divalproex tablets orally. Eleven muscle areas were injected by the "follow-the-pain" approach: the procerus, corrugators, frontalis, temporalis, splenius capitis, sternocleidomastoid, trapezius, occipitalis, and masseter. Injection sites and dosages were determined on an individual basis, depending on each patient's symptom profile. Patients in the divalproex group received 250 mg twice a day orally and a series of saline injections (placebo-BoNT-A). After the first week, the divalproex dose was increased up to 500 mg twice a day if deemed necessary and tolerable.

This study demonstrated that prophylactic treatment with either BoNT-A or divalproex in patients with EM or CM significantly reduced disability associated with these types of headaches.[33] Both treatments showed significant improvements in migraine disability scores and reductions in headache days and headache index. A possible trend in decreased headache severity was also observed with BoNT-A. Compared with divalproex, BoNT-A had a more favorable tolerability profile, with fewer reported adverse events and a lower percentage of patients discontinuing treatment.

In this study comparing BoNT-A and divalproex for prophylactic treatment of EM or CM, significantly fewer adverse events possibly related to treatment were reported for the patients receiving BoNT-A injections compared with the divalproex group.[33] The most frequently reported adverse events for the BoNT-A group were eyelid (26.7%) and/or eyebrow (16.7%) drooping (blepharoptosis), and the divalproex group reported nausea/gastrointestinal discomfort (41.2%), hair loss (17.2%), and fatigue/sleepiness (31.0%). A significantly greater proportion of the divalproex group (27.6%) discontinued the study because of adverse events compared with the BoNT-A group (3.3%). Although the majority of adverse events were transient and no more than moderate in severity for both treatment groups, the adverse events leading to leaving the study in the BoNT-A group were nausea and irregular breathing, whereas hair loss, fatigue, tiredness, tinnitus, disorientation, nausea, weight gain, edema, numbness, tremors, decreased appetite, and elevated liver enzymes were the adverse events leading to discontinuation in the divalproex group.

Thus, evidence is rapidly accumulating to recommend botulinum toxin type A as an effective treatment with less adverse events than topiramate and valproate for RM. Treatments have to be repeated every 3 to 4 months. Apart from the proven efficacy, the most important aspect of the treatment is the lack of any serious side effects. Further studies as to the reason why some patients do not respond and more research of predictors to response are important.

Device-Based Treatments

Because of unsatisfactory control of headache with pharmacotherapy in RM, some investigators have turned their attention to device-based treatments.

Patent Foramen Ovale Closure in Migraine

Clinical series have reported that up to 48% of patients with migraine with aura may have patent foramen ovale (PFO) with right-to-left shunt (RLS). In an uncontrolled series, closure of PFO resulted in prevention of migraine in 29% of patients, as well as substantial improvement in all features of migraine in 59% of patients.[34] However, to date there has been no randomized prospective controlled positive data published to substantiate the claim that closure of PFO is an effective preventive measure for migraine. Moreover, three such trials were terminated in 2008 by their sponsors.[35] At present, PFO closure as a measure of migraine prevention cannot be recommended.

Occipital Nerve Stimulation

A review of uncontrolled case series showed successful use of occipital nerve stimulation (ONS) in the management of intractable headache, including CDH and may affect the trigeminocervical complex neurons.[36]

Current status of ONS was reviewed by Peroutka.[35] Over the past few years, ONS has been suggested to be a potential treatment option for a variety of intractable primary headache disorders. Preliminary results from the occipital nerve stimulation for the treatment of chronic migraine headache were reported to be possibly effective against refractory chronic migraine in February 2009. An investigational device was tested in 68 patients suffering severe headaches at least 15 days each month despite conventional treatments. The device was implanted surgically in the abdomen, with electrical leads threaded up the patient's back and terminating adjacent to the occipital nerve at the base of the skull. This study represents the first double-blind controlled trial of ONS for intractable headache.

Responses were defined as either a decline in headache days per month of at least 50% or a drop in overall pain intensity of at least 3 points. After 3 months of treatment in a randomized trial, 39% of patients with adjustable stimulation achieved clinically significant responses compared with zero patients assigned to conventional medical management, according to the Principal Investigator of the study. However, the adjustable stimulation failed to show significant advantages in some efficacy outcomes, such as number of headache days per month ($p = 0.06$) and overall pain intensity ($p = 0.09$). Adverse effects in the study included electrode lead migration in 12 patients and worsened headaches in 9% of the adjustable-stimulation group and 41% of those assigned to preset stimulation. In summary, this study shows relatively modest reductions in headache frequency and severity in a very difficult to treat patient group. Future studies appear warranted.

Indeed, at least two additional ONS studies are ongoing. One of these is a Phase 3 study that is planned to enroll 179 subjects. Data from these studies, however, are unlikely to be available within the next 2 years.

More encouraging results with ONS were reported in 6 patients with hemicrania continua, using a second generation ONS device known as Bion.[37] While the role of ONS in RM is not yet clear, it appears that it is more useful in strictly unilateral headache conditions like hemicrania continua. Further study results are awaited. Refining implantation techniques and improving the equipment technology are required to improve the utility of this approach.

Essential Steps of Prophylactic Therapy of RM

- Correction of modifiable risk factors of migraine progression
- Stop medication overuse
- Detoxify
- Treat acute attacks adequately early
- Rationale combination therapy (co-pharmacy) taking into account comorbidities
- Continuing behavioral and life style adjustments—biofeedback, exercise, diet
- Botulinum toxin type A—repeated
- Continuing care

Vagal Nerve Stimulation

Vagal nerve stimulation (VNS) is another technique being explored for its possible use to alleviate headache pain. VNS, which is approved to treat seizures, may provide an activating or inhibiting effect downstream of the nucleus tractus solitarius, which projects to the trigeminal nucleus caudalis.[38] The results of a small study suggested that VNS may have a prophylactic effect on migraine, with 8 out of 10 patients showing at least a 50% reduction of monthly headache frequency.[38] Larger and more accurate studies are needed to assess further the usefulness of this technique as a preventive migraine treatment.

Transcranial Magnetic Stimulation

Transcranial direct current stimulation has demonstrated that short-term homeostatic plasticity is altered in patients with visual aura between attacks.[38]

A randomized, double-blind, parallel group, sham-controlled study evaluating the efficacy and safety of noninvasive nonrepetitive TMS for acute preemptive treatment during the aura phase of migraine was completed in 2008.[35] The device, about the size of a hair dryer, was positioned against the back of the head, and subjects pushed a button to administer the magnetic pulse. Of the 201 subjects enrolled, 102 received a genuine TMS device, and 99 were given an identical-appearing sham device that vibrated and made a clicking noise when activated but did not deliver a magnetic pulse. In the results analyzed for 164 patients, 39% using TMS were pain-free at 2 hours after treatment, as compared with 22% of those using the sham device. No treatment-related serious adverse events were reported.

Prophylactic benefits of repeated TMS or its long-term sequela have not been studied in RM patients and warrant investigation.

References

1. Mathew NT, Reuveni U, Perez F. Transformed or evolutive migraine. *Headache.* 1987;27:102–106.

2. Bigal ME, Rapoport AM, Sheftell FD, Tepper SJ, Lipton RB. International classification of headache disorders revised criteria for chronic migraine; field testing in a headache specialty clinic. *Cephalalgia.* 2007;27:230–234.
3. Lipton RB, Bigal ME. Looking to the future; research designs for study of headache research progression. *Headache.* 2008;48:58–66.
4. Katsarava Z, Schneeweiss S, Kurth T, et al. Incidence and predictors for chronicity of headache in patients with episodic migraine. *Neurology.* 2004;62:788–790.
5. Scher AI, Lipton RB, Stewart WF. Habitual snoring as a risk factor for chronic daily headache. *Neurology.* 2003;60:1366–1368.
6. Tietjen GE, Brandes JL, Digre KB, et al. High prevalence of somatic symptoms and depression in women with disabling chronic headache. *Neurology.* 2007;68:134–140.
7. Scher AI, Stewart WF, Lipton RB. Comorbidity of headache with other pain syndromes. *Headache.* 2006;46:1416–1423.
8. De Tommaso M, Sardaro M, Serpino C, et al. Fibromyalgia comorbidity in primary headaches. *Cephalalgia.* 2009;29:453–464.
9. Pascual J, Leira R, Lainez JM. Combined therapy for migraine prevention? Clinical experience with a beta-blocker plus sodium valproate in 52 resistant migraine patients. *Cephalalgia.* 2003;23:961–962.
10. Pascual J, Rivas MT, Leira R. Testing the combination beta-blocker plus topiramate in refractory migraine. *Acta Neurol Scand.* 2007;115:81–83.
11. Mathew NT. Prophylaxis of migraine and mixed headache. *Headache.* 1981;20:105–109.
12. Holroyd KA, O'Donnell FJ, Stensland M, et al. Management of chronic tension-type headache with tricyclic antidepressant medication, stress management therapy and their combination; a randomized controlled trial. *JAMA.* 2001;285:2208–2215.
13. Mathew NT. The prophylactic treatment of chronic daily headache. *Headache.* 2006;46:1552–1564.
14. Saper JR, Lake AE III, Cantrell DT, Winner PK, White JR. Chronic daily headache prophylaxis with tizanidine: a double-blind, placebo-controlled, multicenter outcome study. *Headache.* 2002;42:470–482.
15. Bigal ME, Krymchantowski AV. Emerging drugs for migraine prophylaxis and treatment. *Med Gen Med.* 2006;8:1–16.
16. Silberstein SD, Lipton RB, Dodick DW, et al. The Topiramate Chronic Migraine Study Group. Efficacy and safety of topiramate for the treatment of chronic migraine: a randomized, double-blind, placebo-controlled trial. *Headache.* 2007;47:170–180.
17. Spira PJ, Beran RG. Australian Gabapentin Chronic Daily Headache Group Gabapentin in the prophylaxis of chronic daily headache: a randomized, placebo- controlled study. *Neurology.* 2003;61:1753–1759.
18. Saper JR, Silberstein SD, Lake AE III, Winters ME. Double-blind trial of fluoxetine: chronic daily headache and migraine. *Headache.* 1994;34: 497–502.
19. Krymchantowski AV, Silva MT, Barbosa JS, Alves LA. Amitriptyline versus amitriptyline combined with fluoxetine in the preventative treatment of transformed migraine: a double-blind study. *Headache.* 2002;42:510–514.
20. Mathew NT, Saper JR, Silberstein SD, et al. Migraine prophylaxis with divalproex. *Neurology.* 1995;52:281–286.

21. Yurekli VA, Akhan G, Kutluhan S, Uzar E, Koyuncuoglu HR, Gultekin F. The effect of sodium valproate on chronic daily headache and its subgroups. *J Headache Pain.* 2008;9:37–41.
22. Fontebasso M. Topiramate for migraine prophylaxis. *Expert Opin Pharmacother.* 2007;8:2811–2823.
23. Diener HC, Bussone G, Van Oene JC, Lahaye M, Schwalen S, Goadsby PJ: TOPMAT-MIG-201(TOP-CHROME) Study Group. Topiramate reduces headache days in chronic migraine: a randomized, double-blind, placebo-controlled study. *Cephalagia.* 2007;27:814–823.
24. Silvestrini M, Bartolini M, Coccia M, Baruffaldi R, Taffi R, Provinciali L. Topiramate in the treatment of chronic migraine. *Cephalalgia.* 2003;23:820–824.
25. Freitag FG, Diamond S, Diamond M, Urban G. Botulinum toxin type A in the treatment of chronic migraine without medication overuse. *Headache.* 2008;48:201–209.
26. Menezes C, Rodrigues B, Magalhä E, Melo A. Botulinum toxin type A in refractory chronic migraine: an open-label trial. *Arq Neuropsiguiatr.* 2007;65:596–598.
27. Mathew NT, Frishberg BM, Gawel M, Dimitrova R, Gibson J, Turkel C: BOTOX CDH Study Group. Botulinum toxin type A (BOTOX) for the prophylactic treatment of chronic daily headache: a randomized, double-blind, placebo-controlled trial. *Headache.* 2005;45:293–307.
28. Dodick DW, Mauskop A, Elkind AH, DeGryse R, Brin MF, Silberstein SD: BOTOX CDH Study Group, Botulinum toxin type A for the prophylaxis of chronic daily headache: subgroup analysis of patients not receiving other prophylactic medications: a randomized double-blind, placebo-controlled study. *Headache.* 2005;45:315–324.
29. Dodick DW, et al. OnabotulinumtoxinA for Treatment of Chronic Migraine: PREEMP 2 Trial Double-Blind Phase. (2009). Poster presented at: 14th International Headache Congress, September 10–13, 2009, Philadelphia, PA.
30. Mathew NT, Kailasam J, Meadors L. Predictors of response to botulinum toxin type A (BoNTA) in chronic daily headache. *Headache.* 2008;48:194–200.
31. Jakubowski M, McAllister PJ, Bajwa ZH, Ward TN, Smith P, Burstein R. Exploding vs. imploding headache in migraine prophylaxis with botulinum toxin A. *Pain.* 2006;125:286–295.
32. Mathew NT. A double-blind comparison of botulinum toxin type A (BoNTA) and topiramate for the prophylactic treatment of transformed migraine headaches: a pilot study. Presented at the 12th Congress of the European Federation of Neurological Societies: August 23–26, 2008;Madrid, Spain.
33. Blumenfeld AM, Schim JD, Chippendale TJ. Botulinum toxin type A and divalproex sodium for prophylactic treatment of episodic or chronic migraine. *Headache.* 2008;48:210–220.
34. Morandi E, Anzola GP, Angeli S, Melzi G, Onorato E. Transcatheter closure of patent foramen ovale: a new migraine treatment? *J Interv Cardiol.* 2003;16:39–42.
35. Peroutka SJ. Clinical trials update 2008: The year in review. *Headache.* 2009;49:796–802.
36. Jasper J, Hayek S. Implanted occipital nerve stimulators. *Pain Physician.* 2008;11:187–200. Review.

37. Burns B, Watkins L, Goadsby PJ. Treatment of hemicrania continua by occipital nerve stimulation with a bion device. Long-term follow up of a crossover study. *Lancet Neurol.* 2008;7:1001–1012.
38. Lenaerts ME, Oommen KJ, Couch JR, Skaggs V. Can vagus nerve stimulation help migraine? *Cephalalgia.* 2008;28:392–395.
39. Antal A, Lang N, Boros K, Nitsche M, Siebner HR, Paulus W. Homeostatic metaplasticity of the motor cortex is altered during headache-free intervals in migraine with aura. *Cereb Cortex.* 2008;18:2701–2705.

9

Acute and Urgent Treatment of Refractory Migraine

Brian E. McGeeney, MD, MPH

Evaluating Acute and Urgent Treatment Needs in Patients with Refractory Migraine

The patient with (RM) typically is more knowledgeable and experienced with acute and abortive therapies than the average migraineur. In most cases, however, their experience has been disappointing and frustrating. Such patients often have tried numerous types of medication for the treatment of individual headache attacks, only to find them ineffective, incompletely effective, or unreliable.

For these reasons, it is especially important to review the prior medication history of a patient with apparently RM in detail, with particular attention to previously tried doses and treatment timing. It is especially useful to

> Evaluating the Adequacy of Previous *Acute Treatment in Patients with Apparently Refractory Migraine*
>
> - Were highly effective medications used first, or reserved for use if less potent treatment failed?
> - Was combination therapy attempted?
> - Were nonoral formulations tried?
> - Was the patient instructed to treat the headache early, while pain was still mild?

elicit the patient's perceptions of previous treatment trials, and to understand the treatment strategies that have been tried. In some cases, it will be apparent that appropriate classes of medication have not been tried, that doses have been suboptimal, or that high-yield treatment formulations have not been used. Armed with this information, more aggressive and targeted therapy can be attempted, with a gratifying amount of success in many instances.

In other cases a careful history makes clear that all appropriate methods and types of treatment have been tried, but with disappointing or inconsistent results. In this situation, patients benefit from expert guidance in making the necessary difficult choices about treatment tradeoffs and limits. For most migraine patients, the choice of acute therapy is made by deciding on an appropriate balance among outcomes, side effects, tolerability, overuse concerns, patient preference, comorbidities, concurrent medication use, and availability. This is true for the patient with RM as well, but a larger emphasis has to be placed on avoidance of long-term side effects or complications. In particular, even though patients with RM often have severe and disabling headaches, limits on safe medication use may mean that not all attacks can be aggressively treated. It may also mean that therapies with side effects ordinarily deemed unacceptable in the average migraineur (such as sedation) have a primary place in the treatment plan.

This is the main point of difference between acute therapy in patients with RM and acute therapy in patients with ordinary episodic migraine that is treatment-responsive. In treatment-responsive patients with episodic attacks, aggressive therapy of headaches early in their course is encouraged. For them, the benefits of definitive, timely treatment outweigh the potential drawbacks of early treatment. In patients who have RM, however, advice about how to manage acute attacks of headache must be carefully tailored to the individual patient's circumstances.

Patients with relatively infrequent attacks of treatment-refractory headache may well benefit from earlier, more aggressive treatment of individual attacks. They may need encouragement to use the highest possible dose of a drug or a combination of drugs, sometimes in parenteral formulations. In the case of patients whose treatment-refractory headaches are very frequent, however, this advice can make things worse. It is very likely to lead to medication overuse and consequent worsening of headache. These patients are in the unenviable position of having to pick and choose which headaches they will treat, and sometimes must settle for treating bad headaches with less effective or less well tolerated medications that at least are not likely to provoke medication overuse headache or other complications.

Treatment Principles, Challenges, and Goals

An acute treatment plan is a joint agreement between provider and patient. In addition to the need to limit the types and frequency of treatments, there are a number of additional challenges in deciding on an appropriate treatment strategy in patients with RM. Patients with comorbid depression, anxiety, or strong memories of catastrophic treatment failures may find it difficult to delay or limit treatment. Patients who do not understand or accept limits on medication use or expect immediate relief from any level of pain are likewise prone to overuse medications. Patient education and management of patient expectations thus are critical elements in determining treatment outcomes; patients (and providers) with unrealistic expectations of treatment benefit are likely to be dissatisfied.

The goals of acute and urgent treatment of migraine are a return to baseline function and elimination of pain. However, complete pain relief and complete restoration of function may not be achievable in the RM patient. More modest treatment goals are appropriate in these circumstances. An acceptable acute care plan in these cases might be one that does not render the patient pain-free but nonetheless reduces the use of urgent or emergency department (ED) care and reliance on telephone calls or clinic visits. An acceptable plan would also minimize patient disability and avoid drug use patterns that increase the risk of medication overuse headache.

Acute Treatment Goals in Refractory Migraine

- Must be realistic.
  - Complete pain relief may not be possible.
  - Return to baseline function may not be achievable in all attacks.
- Must balance short-term pain relief with longer term goals of disease management.
  - Patients with frequent attacks may have to pick and choose which attacks they treat aggressively.
  - Less convenient but more effective nonoral medications may be necessary; the side effect burden of treatment may be relatively high.

Acute treatment plans are generally not static. They must be reviewed often, and altered depending on changes in patient circumstances and drug response. Regular follow-up visits to review management are thus advisable, even if a plan seems to be working well. Stratified care is recommended in deciding on treatment for individual headache attacks. This means assignment of treatment based on disability; in other words, migraine-specific and stronger medications will be used in patients whose attacks are associated with moderate to severe disability (often the case in patients with RM), whereas patients with mild attacks causing minimal disability might be treated with nonspecific medications and treatment escalated as needed.

A number of factors must be borne in mind when making plans for acute treatment of migraine. The choice of medication is influenced by comorbidities such as vascular disease, hypertension, Raynaud's phenomenon, and peptic ulcer disease. Most acute treatment plans should include second-line agents, sometimes called "rescue" therapy, to be used if initial attempts at treatment are unsuccessful. Here the goal is to minimize the need for ED or urgent care. Choosing an appropriate route of administration is also important, because formulation has a large impact on the effectiveness, convenience, and acceptability of treatment. In general, reliance on oral formulations risks a reduced drug effect from reduced stomach emptying and slowed absorption that have been demonstrated to occur during acute migraine.

As noted in the preceding text, careful, tailored counseling about frequency of medication use is required. Overuse of analgesics or other acute headache drugs can increase the risk of headache worsening over time, or even cause a series of headaches in quick succession. This type of withdrawal or "rebound" headache must be distinguished from headache recurrence, which is the same headache coming back as medication wears off. A good rule of thumb is that use of acute medications for migraine should be limited to no more than 2, or at the very most 3, days a week, ideally leaving 5 days during which no acute medications are used. This is thought to minimize the risk of developing medication overuse headache, which is strongly related to frequency of use. Even if patients fail to meet this goal of 2 to 3 days a week, it is important that they are reminded of it and continue efforts to limit drug intake. Patients who do not accept the concept of medication overuse are more difficult to manage.

Monitoring Acute Treatment in Patients with Refractory Migraine

- Review the treatment plan at regular follow-up visits.
- Encourage patients to keep a diary of treatment frequency and types.
- Monitor emergency department visits and other health care use as a rough guide to success.
- Reinforce educational messages about appropriate medication use.
    - Drugs associated with medication overuse headache should be limited to 2 to 3 days of use/week.

The Limits of Currently Available Therapy

Here it must be acknowledged that many RM patients perceive a short-term benefit from medication "overuse," if it allows them to escape severe pain or maintain their level of function at work or home. This tension between the short-term goal of pain relief and the long-term goal of avoiding complications of medication use is almost always present in RM. Often the short-term goals are more compelling for the patient, while the longer term goal of disease management is uppermost in the caregiver's mind. Not infrequently, these different points of view can lead to substantial disagreement between patient and doctor, usually centering on disagreements about how much and what kind of medication can or should be used.

> The Limits of Current Therapy
>
> - Recommended limits on use of acute medications are based on imperfect evidence.
> - They may not be realistic or appropriate in every case.
> - Deviation from recommended amounts and types of medication may sometimes be the best that can be accomplished in a particular patient.
>   - This is best determined in consultation with other headache experts and after aggressive conventional therapy has been exhausted.

It is helpful to remember that any recommended limit on medication use is, in the end, arbitrary and based on theoretical and research evidence about the "average" patient with migraine. An individual patient's susceptibility to medication overuse headache may be higher or lower than that of the average patient, and the threshold of medication use required to cause medication overuse headache must vary considerably from patient to patient or even within a single patient over a lifetime of headaches. There remain many patients, then, with RM for whom alternative goals and deviation from usual limits of treatment may be defensible or represent the best that can be accomplished for a particular patient at a particular time. Such determinations, however, are best made after conventional attempts at treatment have been exhausted and efforts have been made to adhere to such limits.

For practical purposes, it is helpful to divide acute medications into two broad categories: those that are associated with (and likely cause) medication overuse headache and those that are not known to cause rebound headache. The former category includes combination analgesics, triptans, ergots and opioids, while the latter category includes medications such as the dopamine antagonists or lidocaine nasal drops. Therapeutic options devoid of the potential to cause medication overuse headache are used more frequently in the RM population. Many headache experts allow patients with RM to use these drugs on a relatively liberal "as needed" basis, with the goal of minimizing the need for more specific medications that can cause medication overuse headache.

Patients with RM often respond poorly to acute treatment, so that combination treatment using drugs with different mechanisms of action are also an important part of acute therapy. Acute therapy in the patient with RM also may emphasize the use of injectable or other nonoral formulations of drugs to a greater extent than is the case in patients with easy-to-treat headaches. This is because when acute treatment is failing or has failed, promoting sleep may be the best option. Although this is not always practical, in many cases it is a better option than continued pain. When asleep one is not in pain. Upon awakening the headache may well have run its course.

Acute treatment options are commonly considered to be either nonspecific agents, which do not have a mechanism of action specific to migraine, or

Acute Treatment Options Unlikely to Cause Medication Overuse Headache

- Diphenhydramine
- Dopamine antagonists
- Intranasal lidocaine
- Intravenous magnesium sulfate
- Occipital nerve blocks

specific medications that work on underlying disease mechanisms unique to migraine. Nonspecific choices for treatment include NSAIDs or opioids; specific medication choices include the triptans, ergots, or the soon-to-be approved calcitonin gene–related peptide antagonists. It must be stressed that specific migraine abortive agents have been reported to relieve non-migraine headaches in some circumstances, so that response to treatment should not be considered diagnostic of migraine.

With few exceptions, patients with RM should be encouraged to keep a headache diary or calendar to monitor headache frequency and use of medication. Sample calendars and instructions for use are available at the website of the American Headache Society at www.americanheadachesociety.org. A calendar provides a useful record of consumption and if kept carefully can allow the provider to account for every pill prescribed.

The Major Categories of Acute Treatment for Migraine

This section reviews each of the major categories of acute treatment, with an emphasis on special considerations when using them to treat RM.

Nonsteroidal Anti-inflammatory Drugs

Nonsteroidal anti-inflammatory drugs (NSAIDs) are the most commonly used medications for acute headache treatment, and remain useful in the RM population, often given with other medications (Table 9.1).[1] All NSAIDs work at least in part by inhibiting cyclooxygenase, reducing prostaglandin synthesis both in the central nervous system (CNS) and outside the blood–brain barrier.

Clinical experience suggests that parenteral administration results in particularly good outcomes. Ketorolac, the only NSAID available in the United States for intravenous (IV) or intramuscular (IM) administration, may be beneficial even if the patient has already taken oral NSAIDs. IV aspirin, available in Europe and Japan, also has been shown useful in acute migraine. Parenteral ketorolac is a first line agent in urgent treatment settings, 15 mg to 30 mg may be given IV or 30 to 60 mg IM. Benefit may be due to the relatively high concentration of NSAID that reaches the CNS. Some patients, especially

Table 9-1 Nonsteroidal Anti-inflammatory Drugs

Non-oral Formulations
Ketorolac: 15 mg–30 mg IV/30 mg–60 mg IM
Indomethacin: 50-mg suppository
Oral Formulations
Naproxen: 500–1000 mg
Aspirin: 500–1000 mg
Ibuprofen: 600–800 mg
Flurbiprofen: 100 mg
Mefenamic acid: 500 mg
Piroxicam: 20 mg
Celecoxib: 200–400 mg

IV, intravenous; IM, intramuscular.

those with previous healthcare experience, may be able to use intramuscular ketorolac at home. The drug comes in prefilled syringes, eliminating the need for complex preparations for use.

However, the majority of patients will not be able to self-administer parenteral NSAIDs at home. Rectal administration of NSAIDs in suppository formulation might be considered in these cases. Compounded suppository formulations of indomethacin (50 mg) are a good acute treatment or rescue therapy option, especially when first-line oral administration fails or is inadvisable.

The major side effect of NSAIDs is gastrointestinal intolerance and bleeding. The risk of gastrointestinal bleeding is not eliminated by nonoral therapy, although abdominal pain and nausea might be. When NSAIDs are contraindicated because of the risk of gastrointestinal bleeding, celecoxib, a selective cyclooxygenase-2 (Cox-2) inhibitor can be considered for use, at a dose of 100 to 400 mg orally. Cox-2 inhibitors, however, may carry other risks, notably an increased risk for cardiovascular events.

The NSAIDs with the most consistent clinical trial evidence for the treatment of acute migraine are aspirin, ibuprofen, naproxen sodium, flurbiprofen, diclofenac sodium, and tolfenamic acid.[2–5] A proprietary over-the-counter aspirin/acetaminophen/caffeine combination has received U.S. Food and Drug Administration approval for migraine treatment on the basis of positive placebo-controlled randomized trials.[6] There are no head-to-head comparative trials, however, so the choice of individual NSAID is based on clinical considerations such as prior patient experience with the drug, desired onset of action, cost, and the availability of nonoral formulations.

Acetaminophen is generally included in the NSAID family, despite a relative lack of anti-inflammatory effect. Experience and some head-to-head trials against aspirin suggest that acetaminophen is not as effective for acute migraine treatment as other NSAIDs, although it is superior to placebo.

Ergotamine and Its Derivatives

Ergotamine has been used to treat migraine for over 85 years, and is available in tablet, suppository, nasal, and parenteral forms, sometimes combined with caffeine.[7] Because of concerns about potentially additive side effects, current drug labeling recommends against taking ergots within 24 hours of triptan use. Ergotamine and its derivatives did not undergo the same level of clinical trial evaluation as did the triptans, so the evidence base supporting their use in migraine is less extensive.[8] Ergotamine and its derivatives are not as widely used as they were just a few decades ago, but some members of this family can be especially useful in patients with RM.

This is particularly true of the ergot derivative dihydroergotamine (DHE). Its long half-life makes it very useful for patients who experience headache recurrence. It is administered nasally or parenterally, and produces less nausea and peripheral constriction than ergotamine. It also is a weaker arterial vasoconstrictor, although venous constriction is similar. Nasal DHE is commonly used in outpatient management when triptans or other primary treatments fail to produce benefit.

The ergots work well in combination with NSAIDs. Ergotamine has a somewhat selective vasoconstrictive effect on cranial vasculature but still affects extracerebral arteries, the vasoconstriction being serotonin receptor mediated. Ergotamines are also agonists at α-adrenergic and dopaminergic receptors, and it is this activity that is responsible for undesirable effects such as nausea. The duration of action of ergots is longer than that of the triptans but their oral bioavailability is low, around 1% of an administered dose, compared with the 2% to 3% bioavailability of suppository forms, and 40% bioavailability of nasal DHE. Of particular importance to patients with RM, ergotamine and caffeine suppositories are useful rescue treatments. Patients may even be trained to self-administer subcutaneous (SC) or IM DHE as an acute treatment. DHE is not, however, available in prefilled syringes or as an autoinjector, making it less convenient to use.

Repetitive, scheduled administration of IV DHE 0.5 mg to 1 mg every 8 hours (for up to 72 hours), along with an antiemetic such as metoclopramide, is extremely useful for prolonged migraine attacks. This strategy is often used in conjunction with other therapies in patients who are being withdrawn from overused medications. This method of treatment is sometimes called the "DHE protocol" or "Raskin protocol," in honor of its originator Dr. Neil Raskin. Its use is practical only in patients who are hospitalized or who can be treated in an outpatient infusion center.[9] Some headache experts try to replicate the use of scheduled parenteral DHE on an outpatient basis. In this strategy, patients use the nasal spray formulation of 1 mg DHE every 8 hours for up to 3 days. There is no formal evidence to support or refute this practice, but it is likely to be at least as safe as use of the parenteral formulation.

The DHE protocol often provides relief even for refractory patients, provided that the side effects of DHE can be tolerated. In urgent care, a single dose of 0.5 mg of IV DHE can be very effective, but must be preceded by administration of an antiemetic to counteract its tendency to produce nausea or vomiting. The IV DHE is administered by slow IV push or can be infused over half an hour in 50 mL to 100 mL of 5% dextrose solution. After administration of IV DHE, some patients may gain sufficient control of their headache to be discharged home to continue with the use of nasal DHE twice daily for a short time, at the discretion of the treating provider.

Ergotamine levels may be significantly increased when the drug is used with potent cytochrome P450 (CYP) 3A4 inhibitors such as ketoconazole, protease inhibitors, and macrolide antibiotics (e.g., clarithromycin). It is best to avoid this medication combination.

Isometheptene Combinations

The combination of isometheptene, dichloralphenazone, and acetaminophen in capsules (Duradrin/Epidrin) has been used for decades to treat migraine and tension-type headache. This combination was statistically significantly but modestly effective against placebo in two out of three clinical trials. In clinical practice, it is not thought to be as helpful as triptans or ergotamine. Therefore, it plays a limited role in the treatment of patients with RM.[10–12]

Butalbital Combination Products

Butalbital is available compounded with acetaminophen or aspirin with or without caffeine and with or without codeine. It has not been well studied in migraine but paradoxically is one of the most commonly used prescription drugs for headaches of all kinds. There are no randomized, placebo-controlled studies demonstrating the effectiveness of butalbital-containing agents for the acute treatment of migraine.

U.S. Headache Consortium treatment guidelines recommend that the use of butalbital containing analgesics should be limited and carefully monitored in all patients with migraine. This is because of concerns about dependence syndromes, medication overuse headache, and the possibility of a withdrawal syndrome that can include seizures. Butalbital is particularly likely to be overused, despite the fact that most clinicians believe it is less helpful for headache than specific drugs such as the triptans. One reason for this may be the sedative and antianxiety properties of the drug. This makes it attractive to headache patients who have concomitant anxiety disorders or sleeping problems. Overuse may be especially likely in migraine patients, because affective disorders and migraine share genetic predispositions.

Triptans

The triptans are all selective 5-hydroxytryptamine $(5\text{-HT})_{1B/1D}$ agonists and produce headache relief without producing significant sedation.[1] Even with parenteral administration of an adequate dose, however, not all migraineurs are triptan-responsive. Triptans are thought to work by inhibition of dural plasma protein extravasation and central transmission of trigeminal impulses. However, the main mechanism responsible for its clinical effect is probably constriction of dilated extracerebral cranial blood vessels.

Seven triptans are available in the United States. All have the same mechanism of action but differ in oral bioavailability and other pharmacokinetic parameters. If one triptan is not effective after two attempts, it is worth trying another one. See Table 9.2 for recommendations regarding administration and dosing. Some triptans are marketed in several different strengths; as a general rule, the maximum recommended dose should be tried in a patient with RM before concluding that the drug is ineffective. As mentioned previously, triptans should not be administered within 24 hours of ergotamine use to avoid precipitating synergistic side effects.

The RM patient typically has tried triptans, unless they are contraindicated. Most clinical trials of triptans were conducted in patients with episodic migraine whose response to medication is better than that of patients with more frequent or complex headache problems. As with most drugs, nonoral formulations of triptans are generally more effective than comparable oral doses of the drug. Sumatriptan is the only triptan available for parenteral administration, in a 6- or 4-mg dose. Rectal formulations of triptans are not available in the United States, but rectal sumatriptan is popular in Europe. Two triptans, zolmitriptan and sumatriptan, are available in nasal spray formulations. Triptans are generally well tolerated. Adverse events of triptans include chest discomfort and dizziness. Triptans are contraindicated in patients with known coronary artery disease or those who are at high risk for occult cardiac disease on the basis of risk factors.

Other contraindications to triptans include uncontrolled hypertension and pregnancy. Triptans minimally increase blood pressure, thought to be related to peripheral vasoconstriction. Drug interactions are a topic of particular importance in treating patients with RM, who may be taking many medications. Those of particular relevance in the case of triptans include interactions with beta-blockers and some psychiatric medications. The use of

Table 9-2 Triptans

Sumatriptan[a]: 50-mg/100-mg tablet, 5-mg/20-mg nasal spray, 4-mg/6-mg subcutaneous injection
Zolmitriptan: 2.5-mg/5-mg tablet/orally disintegrating tablet, 5-mg nasal spray
Eletriptan: 20-mg/40-mg tablet
Almotriptan: 6.25-mg/12.5-mg tablet
Frovatriptan: 2.5-mg tablet
Naraptriptan: 1.25-mg/2.5-mg tablet
Rizatriptan: 5-mg/10-mg tablet/oral disintegrating tablet

[a]Sumatriptan is also available in a fixed combination tablet with naproxen sodium of 85 mg sumatriptan/500 mg naproxen sodium.

propranolol, for example, increases the level of rizatriptan; it is suggested that in patients using propranolol the dose of rizatriptan should be reduced by half. Eletriptan should not be used with potent CYP 3A4 inhibitors such ketoconazole and clarithromycin. Zolmitriptan levels are increased when used with cimetidine or quinolone antibiotics (which inhibit CYP1A2) and it is suggested to limit zolmitriptan to 5 mg in a day in this circumstance. Sumatriptan, zolmitriptan, and rizatriptan should not be used with monoamine oxidase-A inhibitors.

The U.S. Food and Drug Administration has issued a public health advisory about the risk of serotonin syndrome when triptans are used with selective serotonin reuptake inhibitors (SSRIs) and selective serotonin-norepinephrine reuptake inhibitors (SSNRIs). Although serotonin syndrome can occur with use of only one of these medications, it is probably more common when combinations are used. The symptoms of serotonin syndrome vary in type and severity and can include confusion, sweating, hypertension, altered mental status, hyperreflexia, muscle jerks or stiffness, and seizures.

Patients with RM are probably more likely than other headache patients to be using combinations of serotonergic drugs. The drugs might be needed for prophylaxis of migraine, or may be used to treat affective disorders such as depression that are commonly comorbid with migraine.

Patients with RM may need help from their caregivers to weigh the potential harms and benefits of these drug combinations. It is important to view the risks in the perspective of the patient's individual situation. One estimate of the risk is that the annual onset of new cases of serotonin syndrome in patients taking both SSRIs and triptans is less than 3 in 10,000. Although the relative risk of serotonin syndrome in patients using combinations of serotonergic drugs is elevated, the absolute risk remains low. Thus, for many patients the benefits of continued use of some of these combinations may be judged worth the benefit. It is prudent, though, to make sure these patients are aware of the potential risk and informed of the symptoms of serotonin syndrome. Triptans with a longer duration of action might be more likely to induce serotonin syndrome. For patients who need to use more than one serotonergic drug, then, it may be wise to avoid using the two triptans with the longest half-lives, which are frovatriptan and naratriptan.

In clinical practice, it is not uncommon to encounter patients who report that they are "allergic" to triptans. True life-threatening anaphylactic reactions to triptans are exceedingly rare. In most cases, careful questioning will reveal that the patient experienced an adverse reaction but not an allergic reaction to the drug. Some patients, for example, will have flushing, chest pressure, or chest pain with parenteral administration of sumatriptan. Although extensive experience shows that these "triptan sensations" are usually transient and not serious, this event may be frightening for the patient or caregivers. Some such patients are told they should not use this class of medications again, which in turn may translate in their mind to the idea that they have a drug allergy.

Table 9-3 Triptans: Drug Interactions and Adverse Events

- True allergic reactions to triptans are rare; most reported "allergies" turn out to be tolerability problems. Patients may benefit from a retrial of a different dose, formulation or another triptan.
- Do not use eletriptan in patients on CYP 3A4 inhibitors such as clarithromycin or ketoconazole.
- Sumatriptan, rizatriptan, and zolmitriptan should not be used with monoamine oxidase A inhibitors.
- Reduce the dose of zolmitriptan in patients on cimetidine or quinolones.
- Reduce the dose of rizatriptan in patients on propranolol.
- Serotonin syndrome is a rare but serious potential problem when triptans are used in combination with other drugs that raise serotonin levels.
  - Since the problem is rare, the benefits of combination treatment may outweigh risks; these patients should be closely monitored.
  - Combinations of more than two serotonergic drugs should be avoided if possible; triptans with longer half-lives (naratriptan and frovatriptan) may increase risk.

Patients who have had such reactions to a triptan often do not experience them again on rechallenge with the drug. Because triptans can be such an important part of a treatment regimen for migraine, it is often worth trying a different triptan, perhaps in an oral rather than parenteral formulation, or at a lower dose. This might not be worthwhile in patients who have many treatment choices, but it can be very important in patients with apparently RM who have limited treatment options. Finally, many patients who understand that the triptan sensations are not dangerous may learn to tolerate or even welcome them as a sign that the drug is beginning to work. Table 9.3 summarizes drug interactions and adverse events associated with triptans.

Dopamine Antagonists

Dopamine antagonists (Table 9.4) are an especially useful class of drugs in the care of patients with RM. They have long been used for headache treatment because they treat nausea and may provide some analgesia for headache beyond their antiemetic action.[13] Dopamine antagonists are used frequently as first-line agents in urgent care or the ED with considerable success. They are also useful accessory treatments in outpatient settings.

Nonoral routes of administration are generally preferred for these drugs, in part because nausea makes oral absorption uncertain. In urgent or ED settings, intravenous administration of drugs is ideal. IM administration is also an option. On an outpatient basis where this is not practical, rectal suppositories may prove useful. It is important to remember that patients who report failure with an oral form of a medication might still respond to nonoral preparations.

Most of the dopamine antagonists are available in nonoral formulations. Intravenous administration provides the fastest and most reliable onset of

Table 9-4 Dopamine Antagonists

Medication	Dose
Metoclopramide:	5–10 mg IV/IM, 20 mg PR
Prochlorperazine:	5–10 mg IV/IM, 25 mg PR
Promethazine:	10 mg IM, 25 mg PR, 25–50 mg PO
Chlorpromazine:	12.5–37.5 mg IV, 25 mg–75 mg IM
Haloperidol:	4–6 mg IV/IM
Domperidone:	10–40 mg PO, 30–60 mg PR
Droperidol:	2.5 mg IV/PO, 5 mg IM
Olanzapine:	2.5–5 mg PO
Ziprasidone:	40–60 mg PO

IV, intravenous; IM, intramuscular; PR, per rectum; PO, per os (oral).

action, although side effects may also be increased.[14] Side effects vary depending upon which dopamine antagonist is used. They include sedation, akathisia, and hypotension. The different dopamine antagonists have variable activity on the cholinergic, serotonergic, and histamine systems, with large variation in affinity for the dopamine receptor. The mechanism of action for dopamine antagonists in migraine is unknown. Side effects are dependent on the receptor affinities. Older drugs may be particularly likely to cause extrapyramidal symptoms such as dystonia and akathisia. The side effect of akathisia is sometimes missed by providers, so vigilance is important. Tardive dyskinesia has occurred in patients using dopamine antagonists chronically for migraine. The risk with intermittent use is not known, but it is recommended to limit use to no more than 2 days a week. Strong α-adrenergic antagonism from some neuroleptics can result in postural hypotension. Many dopamine antagonists also carry a risk of cardiac QTc interval prolongation and are contraindicated in those with cardiac disease.

Prochlorperazine

A randomized double-blind study of prochlorperazine 10 mg IV compared with placebo showed that 74% of those who received prochlorperazine obtained complete headache relief within 60 minutes and 14% obtained partial relief (88% complete or partial relief).[15] This was in contrast to complete or partial relief in 45% of patients taking placebo. Head-to-head clinical trials of prochlorperazine 10 mg IV have demonstrated superior headache relief to IV magnesium, IV ketorolac, and IV sodium valproate.[16–18] Akathisia is a common side effect, which can be avoided or treated with the coadministration of diphenhydramine.

Parenteral prochlorperazine is a first-line agent in the ED when treating acute migraine. Prochlorperazine is often used on an outpatient basis as a second-line "rescue" agent for patients whose first-line therapy is occasionally unsuccessful. In the RM patient, however, it may be a reasonable first-line therapy, because it is not thought to produce medication overuse headache.

Although the significant sedative side effects of the dopamine antagonists are considered unacceptable on a regular basis in patients with occasional migraine, they may be acceptable in patients who have few other choices for treatment. Twenty-five-milligram rectal prochlorperazine suppositories are especially useful because they can be used at home even when patients are vomiting, sometimes obviating the need for an ED visit.

Metoclopramide

Metoclopramide has been particularly popular in Europe, where it is often combined with a nonsteroidal anti-inflammatory agent. It is valued for its significant prokinetic effects, which are thought to help promote absorption of other oral medications. Gastric emptying and absorption are believed to be impaired during migraine attacks; this belief is based on a study using effervescent aspirin.[19] Between attacks, patients had normal absorption characteristics. In a follow-up study, metoclopramide was shown to help normalize the absorption of effervescent aspirin in the setting of migraine.[20] It is suggested that oral metoclopramide added to a triptan results in an additional benefit.[21] The majority of metoclopramide trials use a 10-mg dose, easily administered parenterally in urgent care. A meta-analysis of parenteral metoclopramide for acute migraine concluded that this is an effective acute migraine treatment.[22]

Unlike other dopamine antagonists, metoclopramide does not usually cause sedation, so it can be used when patients are at work or otherwise must be able to function.

Other Dopamine Antagonists

Promethazine has weak dopamine antagonism, strong anticholinergic and antihistaminic effects, and is a useful first or second-line agent in the refractory migraineur. The main side effect is drowsiness, which can be helpful in inducing sleep during a migraine attack. The weak dopamine antagonism results in a considerably reduced risk of extrapyramidal symptoms, making this a good choice for patients who did not tolerate other similar drugs.

A double-blind placebo controlled trial of chlorpromazine (0.1 mg/kg) for migraine was performed on 128 randomized participants.[23] The chlorpromazine group had a significant improvement in pain compared to placebo beginning as early as 30 minutes. Drowsiness (a common side effect) and postural hypotension (from adrenergic antagonism) were adverse events more commonly experienced in those given chlorpromazine.

Haloperidol has strong dopamine receptor binding and is not particularly sedating owing to its weak anticholinergic and antihistaminic effects. One recent double-blind placebo controlled study of haloperidol showed benefit for a 5-mg infusion of haloperidol in patients with migraine pain.[24] After infusion, the mean visual analog scale score went from 7.7 to 2.2 in the haloperidol group compared with a drop from 7.2 to 6.3 in the placebo group.

Haloperidol appears to be an effective medication for migraine, but it may not be a first choice compared with others in the group because it seems to more commonly cause akathisia.

Domperidone is similar to metoclopramide in antiemetic and prokinetic effects but has reduced extrapyramidal side effects, probably because it does not easily pass the blood–brain barrier. Domperidone has not been studied in a double-blind placebo-controlled fashion for migraine. It is not approved or available in the United States but is sometimes used in other countries; occasionally U.S. patients obtain the drug from outside the country. Contraindications include cardiac disease, as there may be QTc prolongation.

Droperidol is a potent antidopaminergic medication popularly used as an antiemetic. It has mild antagonism against histamine and serotonin receptors. Although never approved by the U.S. FDA for a migraine indication, intravenous droperidol was widely used by headache specialists to treat migraine in the ED. The clinical impression was that is was extraordinarily useful, particularly in patients who did not respond well to other drugs. However, the FDA recently issued a "black box" warning for droperidol because of the risk of QTc prolongation and torsade de pointes. Both side effects are rare, and emerged in post-marketing surveillance. A head to head study of droperidol compared with prochlorperazine was performed in ED patients with headache. Results showed similar efficacy, suggesting that prochlorperazine is a reasonable alternative to droperidol.[25] Droperidol remains an option, however, for migraine patients without cardiac problems and a normal electrocardiogram. A commonly used dose is 2.5 mg PO or IV, which can be repeated.

Benzodiazepines

Benzodiazepines can be effective as acute treatment of headache because they provide sedation, but they do not have any significant analgesic benefits. They are not first-line agents for most migraine patients because of side effects, their danger in overdose or in drug combinations, and their association with dependence and addiction syndromes. In patients with RM, though, some of these drawbacks may be deemed acceptable in certain patients. Benzodiazepines can, for example, help promote much-needed sleep in a patient with a prolonged headache, and reduce the need for other sedative medications that are even less desirable, such as opioids. In an outpatient, diazepam 5-mg tablets or suppositories may be used. In urgent care settings, intravenous options exist and should generally be used with other therapies.

Corticosteroids

Corticosteroids are not first-line agents for outpatient treatment of acute headache, but may be very useful to treat prolonged or particularly severe headaches. Although they do not have immediate benefit, clinical experience suggests they may reduce the risk of headache recurrence or interfere with mechanisms that maintain or prolong headache. Their use must be limited, however, to minimize the risk of steroid side effects such as osteonecrosis. A common practice is to allow patients to use steroid "rescue therapy" only six to eight times a year. There is no evidence to suggest that one steroid is more effective than another, or to suggest what dose is best. In the absence of such evidence, a common practice is to use Decadron 4 mg tid for 2 to 3 days, or to use a prepackaged prednisone taper (e.g., a Medrol dosepack).

There is good quality evidence of benefit from steroid treatment of acute migraine in the ED setting. A meta-analysis showed that single dose parenteral dexamethasone, added to conventional abortive therapy, decreased the risk of headache recurrence by 26%, with a number-needed-to-treat of 9. There were no differences between intravenous or intramuscular administration. The dose of dexamethasone varied from 10 to 25 mg.[26] Because single doses of steroids are well tolerated, this treatment should be strongly considered in patients with RM who present for urgent or emergency care. However, the possibility of cumulative side effects should be considered in patients who have frequent ED visits or who also use steroids at home for abortive therapy of migraine or for other conditions. It would be prudent to limit any use of steroids to no more than six to eight times a year. The mechanism of benefit is presumed to be suppression of inflammatory processes that are involved in migraine and its recurrence.

Opioids

The use of opioids to treat migraine is controversial. A full discussion of this matter is beyond the scope of this chapter. In the case of patients with RM, opioids may sometimes be used (albeit reluctantly, in most cases) when specific medications are contraindicated, not tolerated, or ineffective. Opioid use is associated with the development of medication overuse headache, and at relatively low frequencies of use. Thus, it is desirable to avoid or minimize their use when possible. The use of opioids in headache therapy varies enormously throughout the world. Opioids are perhaps more commonly used in the United States, possibly reflecting greater availability, experience with the use of opioids for other conditions, and high expectations from patients regarding pain relief.

The decision to use opioids is somewhat dependent on whether the healthcare provider views their use as detrimental, beneficial, or neutral in the longer term. Once opioids have been added to the regimen of a patient with RM, it can be difficult to stop or limit use. Newly emerging evidence suggests that opioids may produce hyperalgesia and other permanent neurological changes.[27] Nonetheless, for many patients with RM, and for many reasons, acute treatment of headaches with opioids will be needed. Treatment is more likely to be successful, and overuse avoided, when the caregiver and patient set and adhere to mutually discussed limits on use. In most cases, use should not be entirely contingent on pain; it is probably better to allow use up to an

Table 9-5 Opioids

Morphine: 2 mg IV, 5 mg IM, or instant release 10 mg orally
Hydromorphone: 2-mg/4-mg tablets, 3-mg suppository
Oxycodone: 5-mg tablets
Codeine: 30–60 mg orally, often combined with acetaminophen
Methadone: 5-mg tablets
Fentanyl: 50–100 μg IV

IV, intravenous; IM, intramuscular.

agreed-upon amount and then treat additional headaches with nonspecific or sedative medicines, perhaps anti-dopaminergic agents.[28]

There is a much stronger case to be made for the use of opioids in pregnant patients with RM. Although they have many drawbacks, intermittent use of opioids is not convincingly associated with an increased risk of fetal malformations. The naturally occurring opioids morphine and codeine are commonly used but result in more allergic reactions and side effects than synthetic opioids. Morphine can result in histamine release and can even cause headache. Meperidine intramuscularly is often used in the United States but is particularly noted for overuse potential and with repeated administration can cause seizures.[29] It is best avoided. Options for outpatient treatment include hydromorphone 3-mg suppositories and the oral options listed in Table 9.5. Butorphanol nasal spray is not widely used because it proved to have significant abuse potential and causes dysphoria and other poorly tolerated side effects.

Other Treatments

Valproic acid 500 to 1000 mg IV is sometimes used to treat acute migraine, even though evidence of benefit is mixed. It is not a first-line treatment, however. Propofol IV has been used to treat acute headache in those refractory to other therapies but requires the intensive monitoring used for conscious sedation.[30] Lidocaine infusions have been used for severe migraine, but this needs further study before routine use can be recommended.[31] There is better evidence for the use of 4% lidocaine solutions administered by nasal dropper. This relieved acute migraine in about half of patients who received it.[32] Diphenhydramine 10 to 50 mg IM/IV (also used orally) is used by some headache specialists for acute treatment of headache, but has not been extensively studied. In one comparative trial a combination of diphenhydramine and trimethobenzamide was well tolerated but not more effective than sumatriptan.[33]

Occipital nerve blocks may also be helpful for acute treatment of migraine. Occipital nerve blocks can be easily performed in an outpatient setting. A combination of an anesthetic such as lidocaine, in combination with a steroid, is injected into the area of the greater occipital nerve. The mechanism of action in migraine is not certain. Such blocks are not associated with the development of medication overuse headache. Although their benefit in acute migraine has not been extensively studied, small preliminary case series and open label studies do support their use and they are well tolerated with very few contraindications to use.[34] Intravenous magnesium sulfate has some preliminary evidence of benefit in acute headache. It is well tolerated, with the major contraindication to use being renal insufficiency.[35] Like lidocaine, diphenhydramine, dopamine antagonists, and occipital nerve blocks, it is unlikely to produce medication overuse headache.

Evidence-Based Treatment Guidelines

Evidence-based consensus guidelines regarding acute treatment of migraine have been issued by the U.S. Headache Consortium. Initially published in 2000, at time of this writing they are due to be updated and revised.[36] The majority of the evidence on which these guidelines are based was developed in clinical trials that excluded patients with refractory or chronic migraine. For this reason, acute treatment decisions in refractory migraine involve a substantial amount of expert, clinical judgment because the high quality evidence needed to guide therapy does not yet exist.

References

1. Silberstein SD, Freitag FG, Bigal ME. Migraine treatment. In: Silberstein S, Lipton RB, Dodick DW, eds. *Wolff's Headache and Other Head Pain*, 8th ed. New York. Oxford University Press; 2008:177–292.
2. Boureau F, Joubert JM, Lasserre V, et al. Double-blind comparison of an acetaminophen 400 mg-codeine 25 mg combination versus aspirin 1000 mg and placebo in acute migraine attack. *Cephalalgia*. 1994;14:156–161.
3. Kloster R, Nestvold K, Vilming ST. A double-blind study of ibuprofen versus placebo in the treatment of acute migraine attacks. *Cephalalgia*. 1992;12:169–171.
4. Hakkarainen H, Vapaatalo H, Gothoni G, et al. Tolfenamic acid is as effective as ergotamine during migraine attacks. *Lancet*. 1979;2:326–328.
5. Sargent JD, Baumel B, Peters K, et al. Aborting a migraine attack: naproxen sodium versus ergotamine plus caffeine. *Headache*. 1988;28:263–266.
6. Lipton RB, Stewart WF, Ryan RE Jr, et al. Efficacy and safety of acetaminophen, aspirin, and caffeine in alleviating migraine headache pain: three double-blind, randomized, placebo-controlled trials. *Arch Neurol*. 1998;55: 210–217.
7. Mair HW. L'ergotamine inhibitteur du sympathique etudie en Clinique, comme moyen d'exploration et comme agent therapeutique. *Rev Neurol*. 1926;33:1104–1108.
8. Scott AK. Dihydroergotamine: a review of its use in the treatment of migraine and other headaches. *Clin Neuropharmacol*. 1992;15:289–296.
9. Raskin NH. Repetitive intravenous dihydroergotamine as therapy for intractable migraine. *Neurology*. 1986;36:95–997.

10. Ryan RE. A study of Midrin in the symptomatic relief of migraine headache. *Headache.* 1974;14:33–42.
11. Diamond S, Medina JL. Isometheptene—a nonergot drug in the treatment of migraine. *Headache.* 1975;15:211–213.
12. Diamond S. Treatment of migraine with isometheptene, acetaminophen, and dichloralphenazone combination: a double-blind, crossover trial. *Headache.* 1976;15:282–287.
13. Tfelt-Hansen P, Young WB, Silberstein SD. Antiemetic, prokinetic, neuroleptic, and miscellaneous drugs in the acute treatment of migraines. In: Olesen J, Goadsby PJ, Ramadan NM, Tfelt-Hansen P, Welch KMA, eds. *The Headaches*, 3rd ed. (Philadelphia: Lippincott Williams & Wilkins; 2006:505–514.
14. Siow HC, Young WB, Silberstein SD. Neuroleptics in Headache. *Headache.* 2005;45:358–371.
15. Jones J, Sklar D, Dougherty J, White W. Randomized double-blind trial of intravenous prochlorperazine for the treatment of acute headache. *JAMA.* 1989;261:1174–1176.
16. Ginder S, Oatman B, Pollack M. A prospective study of i.v. magnesium and i.v. prochlorperazine in the treatment of headaches. *J Emerg Med.* 2000;18:311–315.
17. Seim MB, March JA, Dunn KA. Intravenous ketorolac vs intravenous prochlorperazine for the treatment of migraine headaches. *Acad Emergency Med.* 1998;5:573–576.
18. Tanen DA, Miller S, French T, Riffenburgh RH. Intravenous sodium valproate versus prochlorperazine for the emergency department treatment of acute migraine headaches: a prospective, randomized, double-blind trial. *Ann Emerg Med.* 2003;41:847–853.
19. Volans GN. Absorption of effervescent aspirin during migraine. *BMJ.* 1974;4:265–269.
20. Volans GN. The effect of metoclopramide on the absorption of effervescent aspirin in migraine. *Br J Clin Pharmacol.* 1975;2:57–63.
21. Schulman EA, Dermott KF. Sumatriptan plus metoclopramide in triptan-nonresponsive migraineurs. *Headache.* 2004;44:446–447.
22. Colman I, Brown MD, Innes GD, et al. Parenteral metoclopramide for acute migraine: meta-analysis of randomised controlled trials. *BMJ.* 2004;329:1369–1373.
23. Bigal ME, Bordini CA, Speciali JG. Intravenous chlorpromazine in the emergency department treatment of migraines. A randomized controlled trial. *J Emerg Med.* 2002;23:141–148.
24. Honkaniemi J, Liimatainen S, Rainesalo S, Sulavuori S. Haloperidol in the Acute Treatment of Migraine: A Randomized, Double-Blind, Placebo-Controlled Study. *Headache.* 2006;46:781–787.
25. Miner JR, Fish SJ, Smith SW, Biros MH. Droperidol vs. prochlorperazine for benign headaches in the emergency department. *Acad Emerg Med.* 2002;8:873–879.
26. Colman I, Friedman BJ, Brown MD, et al. Parenteral dexamethasone for acute severe migraine headache: meta-analysis of randomized controlled trials for preventing recurrence. *BMJ.* 2008;336(7657):1359, doi:10.1136/bmj.39566.806725.BE

27. Ballantyne JC, Mao J. Opioid therapy for chronic pain. *N Engl J Med.* 2003;349:1943–1953.
28. Chou R, Fanciullo GJ, Fine PG, et al. Clinical guidelines for the use of chronic opioid therapy in chronic noncancer pain. *J Pain.* 2009;10:113–130.
29. Ziegler DK. Opioids in headache treatment. Is there a role? In: Mathew NT, ed. *Neurologic Clinics of North America*, Vol. 15. Philadelphia: Saunders;1997:199–207.
30. Krusz JC, Belanger J. Propofol—a highly effective treatment for acute headaches. *Cephalalgia.* 1999;19:358 (Abstr).
31. Hand PJ, Stark RJ. Intravenous lignocaine infusions for severe chronic daily headache. *Med J Aust.* 2000;172:157–159.
32. Maizels M, Scott B, Cohen W, Chen W. Intranasal lidocaine for the acute treatment of migraine. *JAMA.* 1996;276: 319–321.
33. Friedman BW, Hochberg M, Esses D, et al. A clinical trial of trimethobenzamide/diphenhydramine versus sumatriptan for acute migraines. *Headache.* 2006;46(6):934–941.
34. Ashkenazi A, Young WB. The effects of greater occipital nerve block and trigger point injection on brush allodynia and pain in migraine. *Headache.* 2005;45(4):350–354.
35. Cete Y, Dora B, Ertan C, Ozdemir C, Oktay C. A randomized prospective placebo-controlled study of intravenous magnesium sulphate vs. metoclopramide in the management of acute migraine attacks in the Emergency Department. *Cephalalgia.* 2005;25(3):199–204.
36. U.S. Headache Consortium Guidelines available at www.americanheadachesociety.com/professionalresources accessed 6/14/2009

10

Medication Overuse Headache in Refractory Migraine and Its Treatment

Stewart J. Tepper, MD, and Deborah E. Tepper, MD

Introduction

Medication overuse headache is the most common secondary cause of the daily or near-daily headaches that affect up to 70% of patients seeking care in specialty headache practice.[1–3] In the case of medication overuse headache, the headache is secondary to the frequent use of immediate-relief headache or pain medications. In everyday clinical practice, clinicians and patients alike often use the term "rebound" headache to describe headache that results from medication overuse, and we use that term in this chapter as well. It is not, however, an officially recognized term, but because it is descriptive and efficient it remains in common use.

Many patients with medication overuse headache have profound disability and poor quality of life. They are also at risk for the non-headache complications of frequent use of acute medications. These include gastrointestinal bleeding or renal impairment from nonsteroidal anti-inflammatory drugs, or dependence and addiction syndromes that may develop with opioids or barbiturates. If the diagnosis of medication overuse headache is missed, an important chance for improvement is lost, and patients may incorrectly be labeled refractory to treatment. Thus, the possibility of medication overuse headache should be carefully considered in any patient who appears to have refractory migraine (RM).

Recognizing Medication Overuse Headache in Patients with RM

Many patients with RM use large amounts of acute medication, but it can be difficult to determine whether medication overuse plays a role in their headache problem. The current *International Classification of Headache Disorders-II* (ICHD-II) diagnostic criteria for medication overuse headache (Table 10.1) require both that the headaches develop or worsen in the context of medication overuse, and that the headaches improve upon withdrawal of the overused medication.[4]

In many cases, however, it is not possible to reconstruct the amount and type of acute medication that was being used at the time headaches worsened. Some patients do not improve after medication withdrawal. Others are unwilling to attempt it or are unsuccessful in their attempts. This is not surprising, since medication withdrawal can require a significant investment of time and effort and temporarily results in absence from or reduced effectiveness at work or domestic responsibilities. Still other patients do not have access to a physician with the expertise or time required to supervise successfully what can be a lengthy, complex withdrawal process.

Many patients with apparently treatment-refractory headaches who are using large amounts of acute medication report that they have attempted medication withdrawal, but that their headaches did not improve. It is often difficult to be certain that they were withdrawn from all potentially offending medications or that the duration of withdrawal was adequate. Even when medication withdrawal is done correctly and maintained for long periods of time, improvement in headaches may occur slowly or not at all. Patients and their physicians are often reluctant to commit to the substantial effort necessary for medication withdrawal when there is no certainty of success, or when they perceive that it has already been unsuccessfully attempted.

The classification committee of the International Headache Society recognized these problems, particularly the difficulty caused by the requirement that medication overuse headache can be diagnosed only in retrospect, after withdrawal produces improvement in headaches. "This means that when patients have it, it cannot be diagnosed."[5] The committee also recognized that medication withdrawal may not always produce improvement in headaches, even when it may have been the initial cause of headache worsening. This, they suggested, might be due to permanent changes that are caused by medication overuse.

Table 10-1 ICHD-II Diagnostic Criteria for Medication Overuse Headache

A. Headache present on ≥15 days/month fulfilling criteria C and D
B. Regular overuse for >3 months of one or more drugs that can be taken for acute and/or symptomatic treatment of headache
C. Headache has developed or markedly worsened during medication overuse.
D. Headache resolves or reverts to its previous pattern within 2 months after discontinuation of overused medication.

Table 10-2 Proposed Revised ICHD-2 Criteria for the Diagnosis of Medication Overuse Headache (currently contained in the Appendix)

A. Headache on ≥15 days/month
B. Regular overuse for >3 months of ≥1 acute/symptomatic treatment drugs:
   1. Ergotamine, triptans, opioids, or combination analgesic medications ≥ on 10 days/month on a regular basis for >3 months
   2. Simple analgesics or any combination of ergotamine, triptans, analgesics, or opioids on ≥ 15 days/month on a regular basis for >3 months without overuse of any single class alone
C. Headache has developed or markedly worsened during medication overuse.[5]

As a means of dealing with the problem of a diagnosis that can be made only in retrospect, alternate criteria for the diagnosis of medication overuse headache have been proposed and are likely to be adopted in the next revision of the ICHD; Table 10.2). At present, they are in the Appendix of that document, and it is hoped that researchers will field-test them and report back to the committee. The proposed criteria for medication overuse headache would not require improvement in headache as a condition of diagnosis, but rather would assume a default diagnosis of medication overuse headache in any headache patient whose acute medication use exceeds a certain threshold. This default diagnosis, the classification committee suggests, will encourage doctors to "do the right thing"—namely, withdraw their patients from medication: "Further, not all patients improve after discontinuation of rebound medications. That is, patients who become chronic due to medication overuse may become intractably chronic. However, even those who don't improve after withdrawal may become responsive to previously ineffective prophylaxis. A default diagnosis of medication overuse headache in all patients with medication overuse would encourage doctors globally to take the most important clinical step in caring for these patients, namely to detoxify patients as the first step in treatment.[5]

At a population level, the economic, medical, and social consequences of frequent headaches are enormous. Compared to patients with an episodic pattern, those whose headaches evolve and transform over time to chronic headaches miss more work or school and are less productive. They also require more primary care visits, neurologist or headache specialist visits, pain clinic visits, and emergency room visits. Direct and indirect per-year per-patient costs were 4.4-fold greater for patients with frequent migraine ($7750) compared with episodic migraine ($1757).[6–8] Thus, appropriate treatment of patients whose migraine frequency has increased as a result of medication overuse can be highly cost effective from the perspective of society and payers as well as from the perspective of the patient.

The Historical Context of Medication Overuse Headache

Dreisbach was the first to label headaches resulting from an abrupt decrease in caffeine intake "withdrawal headaches."[9] Ergotamine overuse headache

Table 10-3 Mathew's Diagnostic Criteria for Transformed Migraine[21]

- The headache is not a chronic daily headache that develops de novo in a previously headache-free subject.
- One of the following must exist:
  - A prior history of migraine by International Classification of Headache Disorders II criteria[28]
  - A period of escalating headache frequency
  - Concurrent superimposed attacks of episodic migraine that fulfill the International Classification of Headache Disorders criteria

was first described by Wolfson, Graham, Moister, and colleagues in 1949.[10,11] Peters and Horton also noted that ergotamine tartrate seemed to cause dependence and withdrawal headaches, for which they coined the term "rebound headaches."[12]

In 1982, Kudrow[13] and Isler[14] reported that rebound headache could be caused by overuse of simple analgesics, and that withdrawal of the analgesics led to reversion of frequent or daily headaches to episodic migraine, an observation confirmed by Rapoport and colleagues.[15–17] Dichgans et al referred to the rebound headache as "chronic analgesic-induced headache,"[18] and Mathew and colleagues in one study referred to it as "drug-induced refractory headache."[19]

Another term used to describe rebound headache was "transformed migraine," also coined by Mathew et al. (Table 10.3), describing the condition in which episodic migraine turned into chronic daily headache (CDH)[20,21] They did not distinguish, however, between secondary transformation due to overuse of medications (referred to in the ICHD-II as Medication Overuse Headache), and transformation for no apparent reason (termed chronic migraine in the Classification).

At present, the second edition of the ICHD-II) recognizes two major forms of CDH:

1. Chronic Migraine (CM), a complication of migraine, and a primary headache disorder, and
2. Medication Overuse Headache, a secondary headache disorder.

Chronic migraine, the primary headache disorder, was initially defined as migraine headache occurring on 15 days or more per month for longer than 3 months, that is, CDH reaching migraine level in the absence of medication overuse. The revised criteria for chronic migraine require (1) previous history of episodic migraine, (2) CDH, (3) reaching migraine levels on 8 days or more per month or responding to migraine-specific medications such as triptans on those days, and (4) no medication overuse.[5] Note that chronic migraine is neither the same as transformed migraine, which included both primary and secondary chronic headaches, nor the same as medication overuse headache, as chronic migraine is exclusively a primary headache disorder.[22]

The Clinical Presentation of Medication Overuse Headache

The severity, location, quality, and associated symptoms of head pain in medication overuse headache vary considerably within and between patients. Thus, it is the quantity, more than the quality, of the headaches that suggests the diagnosis. Medication overuse headaches often demonstrate a predictable, drug-dependent rhythmicity. Headaches improve after medication intake but return, often worse, when medication wears off—the feature that gives rise to the popular and descriptive term of "rebound" headaches. They are often worst in the morning; they may even awaken the patient prematurely from sleep, perhaps because patients go for longer periods without medication during sleep than they do during their waking hours, and thus are more prone to experience the falling drug levels that provoke headache.

There is a clinical impression that patients with medication overuse headache often have neck pain. Some may seek help specifically for neck pain and receive muscle relaxants. When these patients are withdrawn from the overused acute headache medications, however, the neck pain usually remits over a period of months but can still recur with episodic headaches. This neck pain is generally not a symptom of a primary neck disorder; rather, it is a part of the headache problem and as with the headaches is exacerbated by medication overuse.

Patients with medication overuse headache also commonly have concomitant depression or anxiety disorders. These disorders are known to be comorbid with migraine of any kind, but are particularly common in those with chronic forms of the disorder. Effective treatment of coexistent depression or anxiety does not usually have an impact on headaches, although it can improve a patient's ability to cope with headaches or improve their adherence to treatment. There are antidepressants (tricyclics [TCAs] and monoamine oxidase inhibitors [MAOIs]) which cross over and treat both migraine and depression, and there are psychotropic classes (serotonin norepinephrine reuptake inhibitors [SNRIs]) which can treat depression, anxiety, and migraine. However, targeting just the psychiatric comorbidity is often not effective in treating the headaches.

In the authors' experience, most patients with medication overuse headache report nonrestorative sleep. Poor sleep may be due to the caffeine component of combination analgesics that are being overused, but may also reflect a daily acute drug withdrawal syndrome. The sleep problems may also be part of a depressive disorder. Whatever the cause, sleep often improves after patients have successfully discontinued overused medications. When it does not, a primary sleep disorder should be considered, but the default assumption should be that, as with neck pain, sleep disturbance is a part of the syndrome of medication overuse headache.

Patients with medication overuse headache may report autonomic signs or symptoms such as rhinorrhea, nasal stuffiness, or lacrimation. These may result

Box 10-1 The Clinical Presentation of Medication Overuse Headache

- Headache symptoms are highly variable.
- Quantity more than quality of headaches should suggest the diagnosis.
- The headache pattern may show drug-dependent rhythmicity of attacks.
  - These may awaken patients from sleep or be worst on awakening.
  - Often associated with neck pain, autonomic signs and symptoms mistaken for sinus problems, depression/anxiety, or nonrestorative sleep

from medication withdrawal, especially opioids. They are often attributed to sinus disease, however, and patients with medication overuse headache are at risk of undergoing unnecessary sinus procedures or being prescribed antibiotics, decongestants, and other inappropriate medications. Decongestants, in particular, are vasoconstrictors and thus can actually produce and prolong medication overuse headache. They should be withdrawn if used regularly. Once again, it is best to assume that the autonomic signs and symptoms are features of medication overuse that may remit with detoxification and appropriate treatment.

The Clinical Impact of Medication Overuse Headache and Withdrawal of Overused Acute Medications (see Box 10.5)

Many headache experts believe that preventive medications for migraine are less effective in patients who are overusing acute headache medications, and that sensitivity to prophylactic treatment is improved after withdrawal of the offending drugs. The same problem of lack of response seems to occur with migraine-specific acute medications. Triptans and ergots fail in patients with rebound, and medication overuse headache may be the most important reason for clinical failure of acute migraine-specific drugs. On the other hand, detoxification frequently results in a restoration of the episodic headache pattern, restoration of the effectiveness of preventive medications, and restoration of clinical response to migraine-specific medications such as triptans. Thus, withdrawal from overused acute care drugs is often considered a crucial step in treatment, and one that is expected to alter clinical outcome. Spontaneous remission of medication overuse headache is not thought to occur in the absence of removal of overused medications continued for several months.[2,23–28]

Finally, a clinical observation may be useful. Because medication overuse headache is common, it is the most likely diagnosis when a patient complaining of CDH seeks medical care. The more diagnoses previously suggested, the more medications tried, the more procedures a patient with CDH has incurred, the more likely the diagnosis is medication overuse. Assuming that medication overuse headache is the default diagnosis in CDH is a high-yield clinical strategy because medication overuse headache is generally treatable.

The evidence that medication withdrawal by itself improves treatment response comes largely from observational studies in which patients with frequent headaches and frequent medication use who undergo medication withdrawal have improvements in headache compared with their own baseline. Very few of these studies include a control group of patients who do not undergo medication withdrawal and who are comparable in other ways to patients who do undergo withdrawal. In addition, in most cases medication withdrawal regimens are accompanied by alterations in prophylactic regimens, institution of alternative methods of headache control, or even hospitalization, making it difficult to isolate the specific effects of medication withdrawal. Because it would be difficult to do a randomized, blinded trial, we are left with the circumstantial evidence from observational studies and case reports. Not all patients who develop frequent headaches do so because of medication overuse, and not all patients with daily headaches will improve after medication withdrawal. There are, though, many other reasons to discontinue or minimize acute medication use, as most of the drugs involved have other undesirable side effects such as sedation, gastric irritation, or dependence and addiction syndromes.

One especially compelling reason deserves particular comment: long-term use of large amounts of acute medications in the absence of apparent headache benefit can make it difficult for patients and doctors to establish a harmonious working relationship. Clinicians almost invariably feel uncomfortable prescribing large amounts of potentially habit-forming or other acute care medications to patients who are not clearly deriving benefit, as is the case in RM, which by definition is poorly responsive to treatment.

If the drugs used include barbiturates or opioids, doctors worry that they are contributing to the development of dependence and addiction syndromes, without substantial improvements in pain or function to compensate for this risk. They may delay or resist refilling prescriptions, with the result that the patient may become anxious and demanding, and display behaviors interpreted as drug-seeking. These might include obtaining prescriptions from multiple sources, or hoarding and stockpiling drugs. Over time, as tolerance to the drugs develops or headaches worsen, dose escalation and deteriorating patient function may further compound caregiver anxiety. Constant tussles and disagreements about the appropriate level of medication use ensue, and interfere with attention to other aspects of the headache problem.

Many patients with apparent RM report difficulty establishing a long-term, satisfactory working relationship with a caregiver. Some have been repeatedly discharged from care. Almost always a careful inquiry will show that the root cause of these failed relationships is disagreement about the amount and type of medication needed to treat the patient's headaches. Repeated unsatisfactory interactions with caregivers are a serious barrier to headache improvement. For this and other reasons, it is usually worthwhile to attempt medication withdrawal in patients who appear to have RM and who are using large amounts

Box 10-2 Reasons to Attempt Medication Withdrawal in Patients with Apparent Refractory Migraine

- Medication withdrawal may restore response to previously ineffective acute and preventive medication.
- Previous attempts at withdrawal may have been inadequate in scope or duration.
- Medication withdrawal has other beneficial effects even if headaches do not improve:
  - It reduces the risk of medical complications of frequent acute medication use, such as gastrointestinal bleeding, renal insufficiency, or addiction or dependence syndromes.
  - It reduces the likelihood of unproductive clinician–patient disagreements about medication and allows a focus on treatment of the underlying headache problem.

of acute medication. Gaining control over the type and amount of acute medication use in patients with apparent RM almost always pays other dividends even if the hoped-for headache improvements do not occur.

What Causes Medication Overuse Headache?

It is not clear how medication overuse causes headache escalation over time. Theories include central sensitization, kindling, basement membrane leakage, and habituation and dependence.

Central Sensitization

One theory proposes that medication overuse produces structural and functional changes in the trigeminal nucleus caudalis, resulting in a decrease in the pain threshold and an increase in receptive fields. These changes bring about a decrease in platelet serotonin (5-hydroxytryptamine, 5-HT) and upregulation of 5-HT_{2A} excitatory receptors[29], probably from increased neuronal firing. Increased platelet production of nitric oxide leads to more vasodilation. Levels of neuroinflammatory peptides such as substance P and nerve growth factor in the cerebrospinal fluid (CSF) and nerve growth factor also increase.

In this theory, repeated episodes of peripheral vasodilation and neurogenic inflammation during migraine attacks sensitize nociceptors and reduce threshold for future headaches. Repetitive and inadequate treatment of pain with analgesics can induce central pain activation, slowly change pain processing, and result in CDH. Central activation may affect the pain pathways or the cell bodies in or around the periaqueductal gray.[30–36]

How does repetitive under-treatment begin? Patients who self-medicate using over-the-counter or non-specific medications to treat severe migraine obtain partial relief followed by recurrence of the same attack, so they are likely to repeat treatment over the duration of the migraine, which can be days long. When the patient gets another migraine several days later, the overuse of the analgesics begins again. If frequency of analgesics climbs to 10 or more days a month (or even to less than that in the case of butalbital or opioids), medication overuse headache may result.

Kindling

This theory suggests that a process similar to kindling in epilepsy could generate medication overuse headache. Repeated intermittent neuronal activity would lead to a "neuronal memory" and a change in the 5-HT system associated with a lowered threshold for headaches.

Basement Membrane Leakage

Recurrent episodes of migraine may lead to progressive damage to the integrity of the basement membrane, allowing leakage of inflammatory substances. Cumulative damage could result in chronic firing of neurons, loss of the blood–brain barrier, and chronic headache.[37]

Withdrawal, Habituation, and Dependence

In this theory, the daily headaches are merely a complex withdrawal phenomenon, with the headache on a given day resulting from withdrawal from the medications taken over the previous several days. The circadian rhythmicity of medication overuse headache, and its tendency to awaken patients from sleep or be present in the morning, would be explained by withdrawal during the night. Autonomic features would also be explained by withdrawal.

How Much Acute Medication Does It Take to Generate Medication Overuse Headache?

The production of medication overuse headache appears to require an interaction of three factors: (1) a genetic predisposition to migraine, (2) a high baseline frequency of headache, and (3) use of acute medication that exceeds a particular threshold of frequency. The idea that medication overuse headache only develops in those with a genetic predisposition to migraine is supported by studies showing that if non-migraineurs take daily opioids or analgesics or anti-inflammatories, they never develop daily headache. In contrast, if migraineurs take acute medicine daily, even for reasons other than headaches (such as for ulcerative colitis or arthritis) they can develop daily headache.[38,39]

Two studies, one population-based, and one clinic-based, demonstrate that a high baseline frequency of headache increases the risk that headaches will become even more frequent over time. Scher and colleagues followed patients with 180+ headaches per year, n = 1,134, and controls (two to 104 headaches per year, $n = 798$) and interviewed them two times over an average 11 months of

Box 10-3 Possible Causes of Medication Overuse Headache

- Central Sensitization
- Kindling
- Basement Membrane Leakage
- Withdrawal, habituation and dependence

follow-up. The more headaches that the episodic subjects had at baseline, the greater was their risk of developing CDH.[40]

Researchers in a German headache clinic likewise found that the number of headache days per month at the beginning of a year indeed predicted the likelihood of developing CDH by the end of the year. Patients with 6 to 9 headache days per month had an odds ratio (OR) of 6.2 for developing CDH over a year compared to patients starting off the year with 0 to 4 headache days per month. Patients starting off the year with 10 to 14 headache days per month had an OR of 20 for developing CDH over the year compared to those starting the year with 0 to 4 headache days per month.[41]

Not all medications are equally likely to cause medication overuse headache, and patients probably have a range of susceptibility to developing it. Opinions vary about which drugs and what doses can produce medication overuse headache. Some information on these matters, however, can be gleaned from the few studies that have been done. Limmroth and colleagues interviewed 96 patients with at least 10 days of headache per month to gain information about diagnosis, drugs, doses, and frequency of use. Patients were categorized by whether they overused ergots, triptans, or analgesics and the "mean critical duration of medication overuse until onset of medication overuse headache" was reported. The duration of use prior to the development of medication overuse headache was shortest in patients overusing triptans (1.7 years), followed by those patients overusing ergots (2.7 years), and longest of all in patients who had overused analgesics (4.8 years).[42]

The researchers also calculated the mean "critical monthly intake frequency" in cases that had developed medication overuse headache from particular drugs. This turned out to be 18 single dosages per month for triptans, 37 single dosages per month for ergots, and 114 single dosages per month for analgesics. Their recommendation was to restrict triptan use to a maximum of 10 single dosages per month (see Table 10-4).

The issue raised by Limmroth and colleagues as to whether different medications cause different phenotypes of daily headache is unresolved. For example, they reported that in triptan overuse headache, 39.5% developed an increase in the frequency of their migraine attacks, 26.3% developed a migraine-like daily headache, and 34.2% developed a tension-type daily headache. Créac'h and colleagues described pure triptan intake medication overuse headache as less severe and more intermittent. Because most patients with medication overuse headache consume combinations of medications

Table 10-4 Commonly Used Acute Headache Medications: Dose and Duration of Use Before Medication Overuse Headache (MOH)

Drug	Average Duration of Use Before Development of MOH (years)	Mean Critical Monthly Intake Frequency
Analgesics	4.8	114 doses
Ergots	2.7	37 doses
Triptans	1.7	18 doses

Data adapted from ref. 42.

and caffeine, it may be difficult to ever resolve the question of what quantity of medication use is necessary to produce medication overuse headache for every possible medication or combination of medications.[43]

In the largest study of its kind, Bigal and colleagues surveyed 24,000 subjects in a population-based study. From this group, they identified 8219 who had migraine and who returned a follow-up survey. This survey revealed 6805 with episodic migraine, and 209 with transformed migraine. The study confirmed that medication class, frequency of use, and headache frequency modified the likelihood for transformation.[44]

Use of opioids and barbiturates is associated with an overall increased risk of transformed migraine even when frequency of use is relatively low. For barbiturates, which are primarily consumed in the United States in the form of butalbital-containing combination medications, frequency of intake as low as 5 days per month was associated with increased risk of headache transformation; for opioids the frequency of use at 8 to 10 days per month was associated with increased risk for medication overuse headache. The very low frequency of use of barbiturate necessary to trigger medication overuse headache is a particular concern given that butalbital-containing combination medications were the most frequently used drugs associated with medication overuse headache in a survey of rebound patients in a tertiary headache center.[44] (See Table 10-5.)

Somewhat surprisingly, infrequent use of nonsteroidal anti-inflammatory drugs appeared to be protective against the development of more frequent headache. However, once frequency of use climbed above 10 days per month, nonsteroidal anti-inflammatory medications did seem to induce medication overuse headache.

The evidence is mixed regarding the effects of frequent use of aspirin as well. Post hoc analyses of data from two randomized trials of older men, done to evaluate the use of daily low-dose aspirin for cardioprotection, suggested a beneficial effect on migraine.[45,46] Post hoc analyses from the Nurses' Health Study, however, did not support a similar effect in women.[47] These data are consistent with observational studies and other small randomized trials of aspirin for prophylaxis of migraine. From a clinical perspective, these data suggest that low-dose use of aspirin, if necessary for cardiovascular or cerebrovascular

Table 10-5 The Association of Selected Drugs and Substances with Medication Overuse Headache

Drug	Associated with MOH?	Comments	Recommendations
Combination analgesics	Yes	For barbiturate-containing drugs, even low levels of use associated with MOH; other undesirable effects include sedation and risk of addiction/dependence syndromes	Avoid barbiturate-containing combination medications if possible. If used, limit to less than 5 days/month.
Caffeine	Yes	Dietary and medicinal caffeine consumption appears to be a modest risk factor for the development of frequent headache in patients with episodic headache; young women may be at higher risk than others. Patients may not report non-medicinal intake of caffeine unless asked[48]	May work through similar mechanisms as other vasoconstrictors, so by analogy limiting use to less than 10 days/month seems prudent. Abstinence from dietary caffeine may be wise.
Decongestants	Yes	Patients may not report use of over the counter decongestants such as pseudephedrine	Effects probably similar to those of caffeine; consider limiting use to less than 10 days/month.
Ergots	Yes	Dihydroergotamine is thought less likely to induce MOH	Effects probably similar to those of triptans; consider limiting use to less than 10 days/month.
NSAIDs	Risk is dependent upon frequency of use; evidence is conflicting for different types of NSAIDs	Use less than 10 days/month may be protective; use above 10 days/month is associated with MOH. In 2 randomized trials, low dose aspirin in cardioprotective doses was associated with migraine improvement in men; in 1 study in women it was not.	Limit use of most NSAIDs to less than 10 days/month; low daily doses of aspirin may improve migraine in men. Use of low-dose daily aspirin in women should not be discouraged if needed for reasons other than migraine.
Opioids	Yes	Even low levels of use associated with MOH; other undesirable effects include sedation and risk of addiction/dependence syndromes	Avoid if possible. If used, consider limiting to 8–10 days of use per month.
Triptans	Yes	Shorter duration to MOH onset than other drugs but with pure triptan overuse, headaches may be less severe and more intermittent than with other drugs or combinations of drugs	Limit use to 10 doses per month in most circumstances.

Note: Most patients use more than one type of medication for acute treatment of headaches. In addition to the above limits, the total number of acute treatment days/month should be limited to less than 15.

prevention, is probably unlikely to provoke or aggravate migraine, and may even have a beneficial effect.

Below 10 days of use per month, triptans were neither protective against medication overuse headache nor associated with headache transformation. However, as with nonsteroidal anti-inflammatory medications, triptan use above 10 days of use per month seemed to induce medication overuse headache.

Thus, barbiturates and opioids are best avoided in acute migraine, and use of nonsteroidal anti-inflammatory drugs and triptans should be kept below 10 days per month. This same admonition seems prudent for combined analgesics.

The revised IHS consensus on diagnostic criteria for medication overuse headache (at present contained in the Appendix and not yet officially adopted) suggests that combined use of any of these symptomatic medications can produce medication overuse headache. Therefore, in calculating intake for a particular patient, days of combined analgesic use should be added to days of triptan, barbiturate, and opioid use, and if the total exceeds 10 days per month, considerable risk for transformation to medication overuse headache can be assumed.[5]

Treatment of Medication Overuse Headache

An Ounce of Prevention

The best approach to medication overuse headache is to prevent it from happening, that is, to carefully limit medication use while patients still have episodic migraine. Inadequate treatment of episodic migraine may lead patients to overuse medication, and increase the risk of medication overuse headache. In migraine patients whose attacks are apparently refractory to acute treatment, it is worth examining whether treatment attempts have been adequate.

Outcomes for episodic migraine are better when highly effective migraine-specific medications are used first-line in patients with significantly disabling migraine, rather than forcing them to first try simple over the counter medications or non-specific prescriptions. In one study, patients who were started on these low-end therapies and then stepped up to more specific treatment if needed had less favorable outcomes in terms of migraine relief and disability than those who were prescribed triptans first-line if manifesting significant migraine disability.[49]

One clinical goal of treatment that might reduce the risk of medication overuse headache or the development of chronic migraine is to aim for a sustained pain-free response when treating acute migraine; in other words, a "one-and-done" treatment. For example, a patient who has one migraine a week lasting up to 72 hours and who uses a triptan or ergot at headache onset might be pain free two hours later with no recurrence of headache. This adds up to 4 days of treatment per month. The same patient, however, using nonspecific or over the counter analgesics for a headache, might experience only partial relief of the headache along with several recurrences over 3 days, and would end up using acute medication 12 days a month. That level of use elevates the risk of developing medication overuse headache and may cause the patient and clinician to inaccurately assume that the patient is refractory to treatment. Clinical tricks to maximize the likelihood of a sustained pain-free response in a patient with episodic migraine include (1) using the optimal dose of triptan or dihydroergotamine (DHE) in optimal formulation, (2) administering the triptan or DHE early in an attack when pain is still mild (<30 minutes into the attack), and (3) adding a nonsteroidal anti-inflammatory drug to the triptan.

The second important step to prevent medication overuse is to know when to intervene with daily preventive medications to keep the number of headache days per month below 10 days per month. Ideally, daily prophylaxis should reduce migraine frequency and duration by at least 50%. Some patients who were previously refractory to aggressive acute therapy will find that optimal response to acute treatment is restored once they are on appropriate prophylactic treatment.

A headache diary is necessary to provide an accurate record of headache days and the number of days of acute treatment for migraine. If the number of days of headache or acute medication use is 10 per month or above, preventive treatment should probably be recommended. Even when patients have 6 to 10 headache days per month, especially if significant disability is associated with the migraines, prophylaxis should be considered.

Therefore, the two principal strategies for preventing rebound are to limit the use of triptans to fewer than 10 days per month for patients with disabling migraine, and consider the use of prophylactic treatment when headache frequency and frequency of acute medications use climb to or approach 10 days per month.

Outpatient Treatment of Medication Overuse Headache

The treatment of medication overuse headache is based on three principles: (1) absolute detoxification from the overused medications without substitute of yet another rebound drug, (2) establishment of daily preventive medication, and (3) establishment of as-needed treatment for the severe episodic migraines with strict limits on frequency of use.

This regimen can be accomplished in many cases on an outpatient basis, even in many patients whose headaches have been labeled refractory. Patients who can usually be treated as outpatients include those who have a shorter duration of medication overuse, use only one to two substances at low doses, and who have support of family or friends and/or are highly motivated themselves. Outpatient treatment can take one of two forms: a slow wean or an abrupt discontinuation with some sort of pharmacological bridge therapy.

Box 10-4 Principles of Medication Overuse Headache Treatment

- Discontinuation of the overused medications without substitution of other drugs that cause medication overuse headache
- Institution of prophylactic treatment, even if seemingly ineffective in the past
- Identification of appropriate acute treatment for severe interval attacks of headache with strict limits on frequency of use.

Before initiating any treatment, it is important to educate the patient about the expected course and outcome of medication withdrawal. This necessitates differentiating overuse, abuse, dependence, and addiction. It is important to reassure patients (when appropriate) that the need for medication withdrawal or detoxification does not mean they are drug abusers or addicts. Rather, medication overuse headache should be described as an inadvertent habituation to medication in patients who are desperate for relief from their migraines.

Education includes setting appropriate expectations about treatment benefits. Improvement in headache almost always requires time, and patients should be told that headaches may get worse for several weeks before they get better. Explain the importance of sticking to a program and the need for long-term follow-up. Arrange for frequent visits during the analgesic washout period to provide emotional support and encouragement and monitor medication use and side effects of withdrawal (1–3 months). Finally, educate family and significant others to enhance support.[50,51]

In addition to education, non-pharmacological management is extremely helpful in treating medication overuse headache patients, both as an outpatient and in more intensive settings. Behavioral management techniques have been shown to produce additional benefits beyond pharmacotherapy alone, and a psychologist improves outcomes dramatically when treating medication overuse headache.

Trained psychologists can help with evaluation and treatment of comorbid psychiatric conditions. They also can treat with biofeedback training, stress management techniques, relaxation therapies, and cognitive–behavioral therapies. In general, a shift of locus of control from practitioner to patient is important as the patient takes responsibility for treatment.[51]

There are helpful nondrug interventions not requiring a psychologist. They include counseling on diet, exercise, and sleep hygiene, and time management. Dr. Fred Sheftell suggests such strategies as setting aside "my time," and the use of a headache calendar.[52] Headache calendars or diaries help monitor possible triggers, medication intake and effect, as well as frequency, intensity, and duration of headaches. This nonpharmacological regimen encourages active participation on the part of the patient, instead of the passive role, as when treatments are done to the patient.

Box 10-5 Educating Patients with Medication Overuse Headache About Medication Withdrawal

- The need for withdrawal does not mean they are drug addicts.
- Headaches may worsen in the short-term with gradual improvement thereafter.
- Full benefits may not be noted for several months, during which abstinence from the offending medication(s) remains necessary.
- Complete remission of headache is not expected; rather the goal is a decrease in frequency, severity, and response to treatment.
- Understanding and cooperation from family, friends, and employers increases the chance of long-term success.

Slow Outpatient Treatment of Medication Overuse Headache

With slow outpatient detoxification, prevention is established before or during the acute medication wean. A "quit date" is set for stopping the acute medicines from which time no low level headaches are treated. New acute medicines are added with limits. The wean of acute medicines, including caffeine, should generally take about 4 to 6 weeks. Thus, it is useful to write out an example (Table 10.6). Preventive daily medications are added during the wean, starting at the lowest possible dose to avoid side effects and increasing over the same period. As noted, some care providers establish prophylaxis before the wean.

The migraine-specific acute medication is initiated around week 4, which is usually the quit date for treating low-level headaches, and the new acute medication is limited to 2 days per week. If the patient is refractory, a course of steroids can be helpful, although the literature has been controversial in this regard.[53–55]

Rapid Outpatient Treatment of Medication Overuse Headache

This approach is not an appropriate strategy for patients on high-dose butalbital or opioids (≥ 3 tablets per day). Rebound medications are abruptly discontinued with quick initiation of preventive medication. While this requires an acceptance of a higher rate of side effects, it also results in a more rapid exit from withdrawal headaches and a faster recovery. A bridging medicine, often steroids, is used for 5 to10 days to blunt the withdrawal and treat resulting headaches. By the time the bridging medication is stopped, the patient is on prophylaxis. Acute migraine-specific medication is then provided with strict limits on frequency of use (Table 10.7).

Table 10-6 Slow Outpatient Treatment of Medication Overuse Headache

1. Slowly taper offending medications and caffeine over about 5 weeks.
2. Add preventive medications; start at lowest possible dosage to avoid side effects and increase over 2–4 weeks. Options include:
   - Tricyclic (e.g., nortriptyline): Start at 10 mg PO qhs, with a maximum target of 50–75 mg PO qhs. Add 10–25 mg per week.
   - Beta-blocker (e.g., nadolol): Start at 40 mg and increase weekly to maximum of 80 mg per day.
   - Valproate (not in women of child-bearing age or patients withdrawing from butalbital with liver induction): Start at 250 mg PO b.i.d. Increase slowly, aiming for a dose of 500–1000 mg per day or
   - Topiramate, increase by 25 mg PO qhs weekly to 100 mg PO qhs.
3. Initiate migraine-specific acute treatment for severe headache: For example, triptans for migraines, maximum 2 days per week (unless being withdrawn from triptans) OR dihydroergotamine
4. If the patient is refractory, a course of steroids may be helpful, for example, dexamethasone 4 mg tid for 3–5 days.

Table 10-7 Rapid Outpatient Treatment of Medication Overuse Headache

Not an appropriate strategy for patients on high-dose butalbital or opioids (≥3 tablets per day)

1. Stop offending medications—day 1
2. Initiate a bridge therapy for 6–10 days. Examples include
   - Naproxen: 500 mg b.i.d.; Nabumetone: 750 mg per day
   - Prednisone: 60 mg qd (days 1 and 2), 40 mg qd (days 3 and 4), 20 mg qd (days 5 and 6); 6 days total therapy
   - Triptans: Sumatriptan: 25 mg t.i.d. or Naratriptan 2.5 b.i.d. for 10 days or until the patient is 24 hours headache-free, whichever comes first; (not FDA-approved use of triptans)
   - Ergots: DHE nasal spray b.i.d. or t.i.d. for 5–10 days
3. Initiate preventive medications quickly (2 days). Examples would be:
   - Nortriptyline 25 mg qhs (day 1), 50 mg qhs (day 2)
   - Nadolol 40 mg qd (day 1), 80 mg (day 2)
4. Initiate acute medication for severe headache: Triptan for migraine, maximum 2 days/week
5. If the patient is refractory, a course of steroids may be useful.

Infusion Therapy and Multidisciplinary Intensive Treatment of Medication Overuse Headache (Table 10.8)

Certain centers are now offering intensive, multidisciplinary day-hospital outpatient treatment of medication overuse headache (Instituto Neurologico "C Besta" in Milan and the Cleveland Clinic). As with inpatient treatment

Table 10-8 Day-Hospital or Inpatient Treatment of Medication Overuse Headache

1. Abruptly discontinue rebound medications if possible, or quickly taper if necessary—Caution with discontinuing benzodiazepines or barbiturates
   - For barbiturates: phenobarbital should be used to prevent barbiturate-withdrawal syndrome and risk of seizure
   - 50–100 mg butalbital = 30 mg phenobarbital
2. Initiate parenteral bridge therapy: repetitive intravenous (IV) dihydroergotamine (IV aspirin in Germany) coadministered with neuroleptic +/– IV valproate, ketorolac, steroids, and ondansetron
3. Initiate preventive medications rapidly
4. Provide multidisciplinary education and treatment
5. Discharge on prophylaxis with as-needed acute medication limited to 2 days per week.

(Chapter 18), this approach is reserved for patients who have failed conventional outpatient treatment, have multiple medical and psychiatric comorbidities, and/or are using high doses of medications. Thus, the more refractory the patient, the more likely it is that a multidisciplinary approach with infusion capability may be needed.

This regimen for aggressive treatment includes rapid discontinuation of rebound medications, and, where possible, use of parenteral bridging medications (rather than the oral bridging medications that are appropriate for conventional outpatient treatment). Infusion and medication weaning is combined with intensive, coordinated attention from a variety of practitioners (including the disciplines of Neurology, Internal Medicine, Psychology, Physical and Occupational Therapies, and Skilled Nursing) with appropriate additional referrals. Apart from the day-hospital settings, infusions as a bridge to wean patient in medication overuse headache are generally feasible only in an inpatient unit.

A wide variety of protocols and medications have been suggested to aid in withdrawing patients from overused medications. A full review of these strategies is beyond the scope of this chapter, but interested readers are referred to the original publications.[56–60]

Prognosis of Medication Overuse Headache

Most patients with medication overuse headache who undergo detoxification improve, often remitting to episodic migraine The likelihood of improvement is increased by the simultaneous addition of preventive daily medication with the acute medication wean.[60,61] A meta-analysis of all English language studies on medication overuse headache using drug withdrawal with and without prophylaxis from 1966 to 1998 by Zed and colleagues found that acute drug wean by itself resulted in improvement in 45% to 60% of patients, while, during the first year, drug detoxification plus prophylaxis improved 72% to

85% of patients. Recidivism can occur, but 50% to 66% maintained improvement at 3 to 5 years.[24]

Time to improvement is not clearly established, but detoxification for at least 3 months is probably necessary. Some patients improve in the first one to two months, and one case report exists of a patient requiring 6 months before the daily headache stopped.[62] Careful explanation to patients as to time necessary for improvement is very important. Failure to allow enough time for transformation back to episodic migraine is a common clinical mistake and cause for mislabeling these patients as refractory

The evidence that inpatient multidisciplinary treatment with infusion is effective in a substantial portion of patients with apparently refractory headache is quite clear.[63,64] Up to 78% improved acutely at the Michigan Head-Pain and Neurological Institute inpatient program. The authors of that study noted that maintenance of improvement likely depended on multiple post-discharge factors, including continued and continuous follow-up, patient adherence, and home or work environment. The addition of behavioral treatment in intensive treatment is also extremely helpful.[65,66]

The risk of relapse should be paramount in the care provider's mind when treating medication overuse headache and predicting outcomes. Follow-up cohort studies of outcomes after withdrawal are listed in Table 10.9, and as noted above, recidivism is common. Careful follow-up is therefore crucial for good prognosis.

Not all migraineurs exposed to frequent symptomatic medications develop medication overuse headache. The revised ICHD criteria carry the requirement that the headaches should worsen with the increased use of the acute medication. There are clearly migraine patients taking daily acute medicines who do not develop medication overuse headache, either because the acute medications are given on a scheduled basis[72] or because these patients are not inherently susceptible to medication overuse headache.

Nor do all patients with medication overuse headache improve after appropriate wean and treatment. It is important to make sure that detoxification is absolute and in place long enough (months), but even then, some patients remain truly chronic and refractory. It is likely that either the headaches are not due to medication overuse, or that these patients have suffered permanent damage to their pain modulatory systems. An analogy might be a patient with

Table 10-9 Controlled Prospective Studies of Long-Term Outcome in Medication Overuse Headaches Who Have Undergone Drug Withdrawal

1. $n = 103$ patients, within 4 years, 48.5% of patients had recidivism and medication overuse headache again[68]
2. $n = 102$ patients, 4-year relapse rate of almost 71%[69]
3. $n = 98$ patients, 1-year relapse rate 38%[70]
4. $n = 240$ patients, 1-year relapse 40%. This study found a significant difference in the relapse rate for triptans (19%) versus analgesic overuse (58%); $p \leq .0015$.[71]

long-standing tuberculosis treated for a year with antitubercular medications and "cured" but nonetheless left with permanent residual lung damage and abnormal pulmonary function tests.

The good news is that, as noted in the extensive meta-analysis referred to above by Zed and colleagues, the majority of patients with medication overuse headache improve, even when followed for 3 to 5 years. This is the prognosis for adequately treated medication overuse headache patients, even those initially labeled refractory.

Conclusions

Frequent use of nonspecific medication in the face of disabling migraine often leads to medication overuse headache. The likelihood of developing medication overuse headache is linked to the frequency of headache days per month, the frequency of intake of acute medications, and to the class of acute medications. Barbiturates and opioids are the medications most likely to produce medication overuse headache at relatively low frequencies of use.

Medication overuse headache patients can usually be treated effectively, even if they carry the label of being refractory, with detoxification as the first step in treatment. Detoxification should include *absolute* removal of offending medications for at least 3 months, institution of a tolerable preventive medication regimen, and limited acute use of triptans or DHE for migraines with severe headache pain, not to exceed 10 days per month of as-needed use. Weaning of medication, establishment of prophylaxis, and the establishment of acute medication limits can often be accomplished as an outpatient over 4 to 6 weeks. More severely affected patients, with higher doses of medications for longer periods and multiple comorbid medical and psychiatric comorbidities, may require treatment in multidisciplinary headache programs with inpatient facilities or day hospital programs with parenteral infusion capabilities.

Most patients with medication overuse headache will revert to an episodic migraine pattern after proper treatment. Treatment of allegedly RM patients who have unrecognized or inadequately treated medication overuse headache, and who respond to treatment, is a life-changing event for the patient. For the caregiver, it is one of the most gratifying experiences in headache management.

References

1. Rapoport A, Stang P, Gutterman DL, et al. Analgesic rebound headache in clinical practice: data from a physician survey. *Headache.* 1996;36:14–19.
2. Mathew NT. Transformed migraine, analgesic rebound, and other chronic daily headaches. *Neurol Clin.* 1997;15:167–186.
3. Bigal ME, Sheftell FD, Rapoport AM, Tepper SJ, Lipton RB. Chronic daily headache: Identification of factors associated with induction and transformation. *Headache.* 2002;42:575–581.

4. Silberstein SD, Olesen J, Bousser MG, et al.; International Headache Society. The International Classification of Headache Disorders, 2nd Edition (ICHD-II)--revision of criteria for 8.2 Medication-overuse headache. *Cephalalgia.* 2005;25:460–465.
5 Headache Classification Committee: Olesen J, Bousser M-G, Diener H-C, et al. New Appendix Criteria open for a broader concept of chronic migraine. *Cephalalgia.* 2006; 26:742–746.
6. Schwartz BS, Stewart WF, Lipton RB. Lost workdays and decreased effectiveness associated with headache in the workplace. *J Occup Environ Med.* 1997;39:320–327.
7. Meletiche DM, Lofland JH, Young WB. Quality-of-life differences between patients with episodic and transformed migraine. *Headache.* 2001;41:573–578.
8. Munakata J, Hazard E, Serrano D, et al. Economic burden of transformed migraine: results from the American Migraine Prevalence and Prevention (AMPP) Study. *Headache.* 2009;49:498–508.
9. Dreisbach RH. Experimental caffeine withdrawal headache. *J Pharmacol Exp Ther.* 1940;69:283.
10. Wolfson WQ, Graham JR. Development of tolerance to ergot alkaloids in a patient with unusually severe migraine. *N Engl J Med.* 1949;241:296–298.
11. Moister FC, Stanton JR, Freis ED. Observations on the development of tolerance during prolonged oral administration of dihydroergocornine. *J Pharmacol Exp Ther.* 1949;96:21.
12. Peters GA, Horton BT. Headache: with special reference to the excessive use of ergotamine preparations and withdrawal effects. *Mayo Clin Proc.* 1951;26:153–161.
13. Kudrow L. Paradoxical effects of frequent analgesic use. *Adv Neurol.* 1982;33:335–341.
14. Isler H. Migraine treatment as a cause of chronic migraine. In: Rose FC, ed. *Advances in Migraine Research and Therapy.* New York: Raven Press;1982:159–164.
15. Rapoport AM, Sheftell FD, Weeks RE, Baskin SM. Analgesic rebound headache. In: Proceedings of the 12th Meeting of the Scandinavian Migraine Society 1983:37–38 [Abstr].
16. Rapoport A, Weeks R, Sheftell F, Baskin SM, Verdi J. Analgesic rebound headache: theoretical and practical implications. *Cephalalgia.* 1985;5(Suppl 3): 448–449 [Abstr].
17. Rapoport AM, Weeks RE, Sheftell FD, Baskin SM, Verdi J. The "analgesic washout period": a critical variable in the evaluation of headache treatment efficacy. *Neurology.* 1986;36(Suppl 2):100–101 [Abstr].
18. Dichgans J, Diener HC, Gerber WD, Verspohl EJ, Kukiolka H, Kluck M. Chronic analgesic-induced headache [in German]. *Dtsch Med Wochenschr.* 1984;109:369–373.
19. Mathew NT, Kurman R, Perez F. Drug induced refractory headache—clinical features and management. *Headache.* 1990;30:634–638.
20. Mathew NT, Stubits E, Nigam MR. Transformation of migraine into daily headache: analysis of factors. *Headache.* 1982;22:66–68.
21. Mathew NT, Reuveni U, Perez F. Transformed or evolutive migraine. *Headache.* 1987;27:102–106.

22. *International Classification of Headache Disorders*, 2nd ed. *Cephalalgia.* 2004;24(Suppl 1): 1–160.
23. Mathew NT. Medication misuse headache. *Cephalalgia.* 1998;18 (Suppl 21):34–36.
24. Zed PJ, Loewen PS, Robinson G. Medication-induced headache: overview and systematic review of therapeutic approaches. *Ann Pharmacother.* 1999;33:61–72.
25. Diener HC, Katasarva Z. Analgesic/abortive overuse and misuse in chronic daily headache. *Curr Pain Headache Rep.* 2001;5:545–550.
26. Tepper SJ. Debate: analgesic overuse is a cause, not consequence, of chronic daily headache. Analgesic overuse is a cause of chronic daily headache. *Headache.* 2002;42:543–547.
27. Tepper SJ, Rapoport AM, Sheftell FD, Bigal ME. Chronic daily headache—an update. *Headache Care.* 2004;1:222–245.
28. Dodick DW. Clinical practice. Chronic daily headache. *N Engl J Med.* 2006;354:158–165.
29. Srikiatkhachorn A. Chronic daily headache: a scientist's perspective. *Headache.* 2002;42:532–537.
30. Burstein R, Cutrer MF, Yarnitsky D. The development of cutaneous allodynia during a migraine attack: clinical evidence for the sequential recruitment of spinal and supraspinal nociceptive neurons in migraine. *Brain.* 2000;123 (pt 8):1703–1709.
31. Srikiatkhachorn A, Maneesri S, Govitrapong P, Kasantikul V. Derangement of serotonin system in migrainous patients with analgesic abuse headache: clues from platelets. *Headache.* 1998;38:43–49.
32. Srikiatkhachorn A, Puangniyom S, Govitrapong P. Plasticity of 5-HT_{2A} serotonin receptor in patients with analgesic-induced transformed migraine. *Headache.* 1998;38:534–539.
33. Srikiatkhachorn A, Tarasub N, Govitrapong P. Acetaminophen-induced anti-nociception vis central 5–HT_{2A} receptors. *Neurochem Int.* 1999;34:491–498.
34. Srikiatkhachorn A, Tarasub N, Govitrapong P. effect of chronic analgesic exposure on the central serotonin system: a possible mechanism of analgesic abuse headache. *Headache.* 2000;40:343–350.
35. Bigal ME, Lipton RB. Concepts and mechanisms of migraine chronification. *Headache.* 2008;48:7–15.
36. Scher AI, Lipton RB, Stewart W. Risk factors for chronic daily headache. *Curr Pain Headache Rep.* 2002;6:486–491.
37. Moskowitz MA. Neurogenic versus vascular mechanisms of sumatriptan and ergot alkaloids in migraine. *Trends Pharmacol Sci.* 1992;13:307–311.
38. Wilkinson SM, Becker WJ, Heine JA. Opiate use to control bowel motility may induce chronic daily headache in patients with migraine. *Headache.* 2001;41:303–309.
39. Bahra A, Walsh M, Menon S, Goadsby PJ. Does chronic daily headache arise de novo in association with regular use of analgesics? *Headache.* 2003;43: 179–190.
40. Scher AI, Stewart WF, Ricci JA, Lipton RB. Factors associated with the onset and remission of chronic daily headache in a population-based study. *Pain.* 2003;106:81–89.

41. Katsarava Z, Schneeweiss S, Kurth T, Kroener U, Fritsche G, Eikermann A, Diener HC, Limmroth V. Incidence and predictors for chronicity of headache in patients with episodic migraine. *Neurology.* 2004;62:788–790.
42. Limmroth V, Katsarava Z, Fritsche G, Przywara S, Diener HC. Features of medication overuse headache following overuse of different acute headache drugs. *Neurology.* 2002;59:1011–1014.
43. Créac'h C, Radat F, Mick G, Guegan-Massardier E, Giraud P, Guy N, Fabre N, Nachit-Ouinekh F, Lanteri-Minet M. One or several types of triptan overuse headaches? *Headache.* 2009;49:519–28.
44. Bigal ME, Serrano D, Buse D, Scher A, Stewart WF, Lipton RB. Acute migraine medications and evolution from episodic to chronic migraine: a longitudinal population-based study. *Headache.* 2008;48:1157–1168.
45. Buring JE, Peto R, Hennekens CH. Low-dose aspirin for migraine prophylaxis. *JAMA.* 1990;264:1711–1713.
46. O'Neill BP & Mann JD. Aspirin prophylaxis in migraine. *Lancet.* 1978; 2:1179–1181.
47. Bensenor I, Cook N, Lee I-M, Chown M, Hennekens C, Buring J. Low-dose aspirin for migraine prophylaxis in women. *Cephalalgia.* 2002;21:175–183.
48. Scher A, Stewart WF, Litpon RB. Caffeine as a risk factor for chronic daily headache: a population-based study. *Neurology.* 2004;63(11):2022–2027
49. Lipton RB, Stewart WF, Stone AM, Láinez MJ, Sawyer JP; Disability in Strategies of Care Study group. Stratified care vs step care strategies for migraine: the Disability in Strategies of Care (DISC) Study: A randomized trial. *JAMA.* 2000;284:2599–2605.
50. Frediani F, Cannatà AP, Magnoni A, Peccarisi C, Bussone G. The patient with medication overuse: clinical management problems. *Neurol Sci.* 2003;24(suppl 2):S108–111.
51. Lipchik GL, Nash JM. Cognitive-behavioral issues in the treatment and management of chronic daily headache. *Curr Pain Headache Rep.* 2002;6:473–479.
52. Sheftell FD. Management of Analgesic Overuse Syndromes. *In*: Special Challenges for the Management of Acute Pain. Postgraduate Medicine 1996;100:October (Special Report):40 - 47.
53. Pageler L, Katsarava Z, Diener HC, Limmroth V. Prednisone vs. placebo in withdrawal therapy following medication overuse headache. *Cephalalgia.* 2008;28:152–156.
54. Ribeiro RT, Carriço LA, Bezerra ML, Villa TR, Pereira MM. Prednisone in withdrawal therapy following medication overuse headache. *Cephalalgia.* 2008;28:999–1000.
55. Tepper SJ. A primary care approach to migraine and chronic headache. *Primary Care Rep.* 1996; 2:151–160.
56. Drucker P, Tepper SJ. Daily sumatriptan for detoxification from rebound. *Headache.* 1998;38:687–690.
57. Krymchantowski AV, Moreira PF. Out-patient detoxification in chronic migraine: comparison of strategies. *Cephalalgia.* 2003;23:982–993.
58. Sheftell, FD, Brunton SA, Coon TL, Hutchinson SL, Kaniecki RG. Chronic daily headache: understanding and treating a common malady. *Family Practice Recert.* 2004;6:25–36.

59. Raskin NH. Repetitive intravenous dihydroergotamine as therapy for intractable migraine. *Neurology.* 1986;36:995–997.
60. Loder E, Biondi D. Oral phenobarbital loading: a safe and effective method of withdrawing patients with headache from butalbital compounds. *Headache.* 2003;43:904–909.
61. Linton-Dahlof P, Linde M, Dahlof C. Withdrawal therapy improves chronic daily headache associated with long-term misuse of headache medication: aretrospective study. *Cephalalgia.* 2000;20:658–662.
62. Warner JS. Time required for improvement of an analgesic rebound headache.*Headache.* 1998;38:229–230.
63. Freitag FG, Lake A 3rd, Lipton R, Cady R, Diamond S, Silberstein S; US Headache Guidelines Consortium, Section on Inpatient Treatment Chairpersons. Inpatient treatment of headache: an evidence-based assessment. *Headache.* 2004;44:342–360.
64. Lake AE 3rd, Saper JR, Hamel RL. Comprehensive inpatient treatment of refractory chronic daily headache. *Headache.* 2009;49:555–562.
65. Lake AE 3rd, Saper JR, Madden SF, Kreeger C. Comprehensive inpatient treatment for intractable migraine: a prospective long-term outcome study. *Headache.* 1993;33:55–62.
66. Saper JR. Pearls from an inpatient headache unit. *Headache.* 2008;48:820–827.
67. Hoodin F, Brines BJ, Lake AE 3rd, Wilson J, Saper JR. Behavioral self-management in an inpatient headache treatment unit: increasing adherence and relationship to changes in affective distress. *Headache.* 2000;40:377–383.
68. Fritsche G, Eberl A, Katsarava Z, Limmroth V, Diener HC. Drug-induced headache: long-term follow-up of withdrawal therapy and persistence of drug misuse. *Eur Neurol.* 2001;45:229–235.
69. Pini LA, Cicero AF, Sandrini M. Long-term follow-up of patients treated for chronic headache with analgesic overuse. *Cephalalgia.* 2001;21:878–883.
70. Katsarava Z, Limmroth V, Finke M, Diener HC, Fritsche G. Rates and predictors for relapse in medication overuse headache: a 1-year prospective study. *Neurology.* 2003;60:1682–1683.
71. Zidverc-Trajkovic J, Pekmezovic T, Jovanovic Z, Pavlovic A, Mijajlovic M, Radojicic A, Sternic N. Medication overuse headache: clinical features predicting treatment outcome at 1-year follow-up. *Cephalalgia.* 2007;27:1219–1225.
72. Sheftell FD, Rapoport AM, Tepper SJ, Bigal ME. Naratriptan in the preventive treatment of refractory transformed migraine: a prospective pilot study. *Headache.* 2005;45:1400–1406.

11

Psychopharmacological Treatment of Refractory Headaches

Noah Rosen, MD

Introduction

Among the large percentage of the population who suffer from headaches, there is a subgroup of primary or secondary headaches that are refractory. The majority appear to be comprised of individuals who suffer from refractory migraine (RM). These patients may experience disability and often have prolonged episodes. They may seek care initially in primary care centers but ultimately gravitate toward headache specialty clinics.

In the recent proposed definition for refractory (RM), patients must meet the *International Classification of Headache Disorders* (ICDH) criteria for migraine or chronic migraine. In addition, the headache must have a significant impact on quality of life, despite modification of triggers, lifestyle changes, and trials of appropriate acute abortive and preventive treatments.[1] These individuals may suffer from an increased frequency of headache, disability from pain and other associated headache features, and frustration from their lack of adequate relief. Comorbid illnesses can often impact headache treatment.[2] As discussed in other chapters in this volume, individuals with headache disorders are at a higher risk of other psychiatric comorbid illnesses.

These disorders may influence the headache condition or be influenced by the headache disorder and may complicate care. Increasing headache frequency amplifies both the risk and intensity of depression and anxiety.[3] Chronic daily headache (CDH) more associated comorbid conditions than episodic migraine.[4] At least one study has suggested that the rate of comorbid psychiatric disease in chronic daily headache may be greater than 90%.[5] There is some suggestion that early life anxiety may predict migraine and mood disorders later on in life.[6] The onset of anxiety disorder tends to precede the age at onset of these other conditions and, in fact, may represent a continuum of illness. The mean age of onset for anxiety is 12 years, 15 years for migraine, and 17 years for depression.[7] However, there is no clear relationship between new episodes of anxiety or major depression and migraine attack frequency.

Psychiatric Conditions with an Increased Incidence in Patients with Migraine

- Major depression
- Bipolar I (manic episodes)
- Bipolar II (hypomanic episodes)
- Dysthymia
- Generalized anxiety disorder
- Social phobia
- Panic disorder
- Obsessive–compulsive disorder

The basic neuronal anatomy and neurotransmitters that are most likely involved in migraine are also involved in the pathogenesis of mood and anxiety disorders. The frontal lobe, anterior cingulate gyrus, and deep limbic structures are involved in both headache and mood.[8] Serotonin, dopamine, and norepinephrine play key roles in the development of headache and associated nausea as well as mood and anxiety disorders. Further research is required to elucidate these mechanisms. Although it is common to see adjustment disorder with depressed features in response to stressful life circumstances (such as illness), these often do not meet the criteria for major depressive episodes. The relationship between mood disorders and migraine is bidirectional with either potentially being the initial presentation in the individual being treated. Even if the direction of the relationship is ambiguous, that does not necessarily prevent us from trying to identify and treat these conditions in order to holistically help our patients.[9]

The initial step of treatment is appropriate diagnosis. The psychiatric comorbidities are sometimes missed, not addressed, or are inappropriately treated. The gold standard for diagnosis of a psychiatric disorder is a Structured Clinical Interview with a qualified professional. Other tests such as Mini-International Neuropsychiatric Interview are available, but are time consuming and not appropriate for general screening, particularly in the primary care office. More focused tests, such as the Beck Depression Index or the Hamilton

Anxiety Scale, are available, and can be used as a screening tool for diagnosis and to follow progression. It is not unusual for a practitioner to have "a sense" of the patient's disorder before any specific testing. These tests then may lead to appropriate diagnoses and an increased likelihood that the patient will receive appropriate treatment.

The comfort level in treating psychiatric conditions will vary with the individual professional. Most patients with depression and anxiety are treated by their primary care physician; relatively few see qualified mental health practitioners. However, when Axis I psychiatric conditions are comorbid with refractory headache conditions, appropriate pharmacological care can be particularly complicated. The headache practitioner derives a distinct benefit by working hand in hand with a mental health practitioner,[10] particularly when dealing with psychopharmacological treatments.

The treatments of headache disorders, especially those that are refractory, often involve a host of pharmacological options. In general, these include abortive and preventive treatments, and management of comorbid disorders, which may influence the frequency, severity, or overall disability associated with RM. Patients with refractory headaches and comorbid depression, anxiety, bipolar illness, or other psychiatric conditions often require complicated treatment. A medical regimen should be tailored not only to the condition, but also to the individual. When considering preventive treatments, the physician typically will make a decision based on the headache subtype, relative drug efficacy, adverse event profile, patient preference, and comorbid (or coexistent) condition.[11] In utilizing psychopharmacological agents, the choice may be influenced by relative efficacy in treating the headache condition and the psychiatric condition, as well as taking into account the possible interactions with other medications.

Sometimes a single agent may be utilized for multiple conditions. However, sometimes this requires significant consideration, as it may lead to medication that is not the best choice for either condition. Further, this strategy can sometimes be complicated if multiple practitioners are adjusting the same medication to manage one disease without regard to another comorbid condition. Sometimes two (or more) medications may be a better option, but that then raises potential issues of medication interactions and raising the risks of polypharmacy.

The choice of preventive treatment for RM may also complicate the care of the psychiatric condition. In choosing preventive medications for the refractory patient, the practitioner needs to be concerned not only of the possible benefit of psychiatric medications, but also the potentially significant negative outcomes that our preventive choices may lead. There is some evidence suggesting that beta-blockers may worsen depression (or at least worsen some of the core constituents of depression such as fatigue, hypersomnia and weight gain.)[12] The use of certain antidepressants in a patient with underlying bipolar disorder may spontaneously trigger a manic (or hypomanic) episode even in someone who has not previously displayed those behaviors. This is sometimes referred to as "bipolar III" and is an iatrogenic condition caused by our choice of medications.

Even abortive medications need to be considered in a patient with comorbid psychiatric disorders and headaches. There may be a small risk of serotonin syndrome in patients using either selective serotonin reuptake inhibitors (SSRIs) or serotonin norepinephrine reuptake inhibitors (SNRIs) in conjunction with triptan medications or other abortive medications such as tramadol. Only a small number of cases have been reported, but this may actually represent an underreporting of the true incidence.[13] With all triptan medications now bearing this warning, the question often arises in the clinical setting of patients who require polypharmacy. While the evidence at hand suggests the risk is minimal, it is an important discussion to have with patients and may further determine the psychopharmacological strategies that are utilized for the individual.

Considering the range of medications that fall under the auspices of the term "psychopharmacology," there is a large host of very different drugs. We may simplify this list by categorizing them based on their target illnesses: antidepressants, anxiolytics, antipsychotics, mood stabilizers, and medications used for attentional disorders. Each of these subcategories includes drugs that may be chemically very distinct and affect a range of different neuronal receptors. In this chapter, we review the full range of psychopharmacological agents, addressing their use not only for the treatment of the psychiatric conditions, but also the role they may play in the treatment of the primary headache condition. We review the pharmacology of each class and assess the evidence that supports these medications as treatment for refractory headache disorders. A full review of these medications may not be possible, but we will hit the "high points" with regard to classification, utility, side effects, and dosing regimens.

Basics of Psychopharmacology

1. Be certain of your diagnosis and your target symptoms.
2. Determine the most appropriate and simplest medication regimen.
3. Work collaboratively with the patient.
4. Set reasonable goals for treatment.
5. Start low and increase doses slowly to avoid adverse events.
6. Have a method for measuring treatment outcomes.
7. Foster collaboration with mental health professionals.

Antidepressants

Depression is an extremely common problem, both in the general population and in the select group of individuals with refractory headache. The 1-year prevalence of depression in the general population is approximately

7.3 per 100. Lifetime prevalence is about 10%.[14] Among the migraine population, the 1-year prevalence of depression is approximately 14.7 per 100.[15] In 1992 Breslau et al. demonstrated that the lifetime prevalence of depression in the migraine population approached 35%.[16] Other studies suggest that the odds ratio of migraine and major depression are between 2.2 and 4.0.[17] Further, patients with migraine with or without major depression are at a higher risk of suicide than those without migraine.[18]). The lifetime prevalence of depression in migraine, probable migraine, and control patients was of 28.1%, 19.5%, and 10.3%, respectively.[19] Breslau et al. demonstrated that depression over a 2-year period, raised the incidence of migraine and presence of migraine raised the incidence of depression.[20] A cross-sectional analysis by Zwart et al. of 50,000 people suggested that increased frequency of migraine was predictive of a higher incidence of both depression and anxiety disorders.[21]

Larger epidemiological studies of the RM population have yet to be done. This is in part due to the fact that there is still yet to be a consensual agreement as to the operating term "refractory." Some work has been done looking at patients with chronic daily headache, predominantly chronic migraine, and have suggested that the incidence of depression is greater than that in the population alone. This does not necessarily correlate with the refractory population and more work needs to be done in this area.

Antidepressant medications are some of the most commonly prescribed medications in the United States and in the world. Some of the medications commonly used today have been around for more than 50 years, while many others have been developed over the last 20 years. In general, antidepressant medications fall into select groups: tricyclic antidepressants (Table 11.1), selective serotonin reuptake inhibitors (SSRIs; Table 11.2), serotonin and norepinephrine reuptake inhibitors (SNRIs; Table 11.3), monoamine oxidase inhibitors (MAOIs; Table 11.4), and atypical or other medications such as norepinephrine dopamine reuptake inhibitors (Table 11.5). The relative efficacy of these medications with regard to both their antidepressant effect and antinociceptive effects is much debated. Very few studies have been done comparing classes or individual agents in a head to head fashion. Agents were instead compared using results of placebo-controlled trials. Some experts argue that newer antidepressant agents are not necessarily more effective, but instead have a lower side effect profile leading to improved patient adherence to medication plans and better outcomes.[22]

A number of these medications are used for other purposes beyond major depression. Some have been found useful for anxiety disorders, obsessive–compulsive disorders, and eating disorders such as anorexia. Side effects can be effective for other conditions seen in this group (e.g., the use of tricyclics for enuresis). Many of these agents have demonstrated an effect on headache disorders as well, including tension-type headache and migraine. It is unclear how these medications prevent headache but it does appear to be separate from their effect on depression.

Table 11-1 Tricyclic Antidepressants

Generic Name	Trade Name	Available Dose Size	Reported Doses	Blood Levels Can Be Obtained
Amitriptyline	Elavil	10, 25, 50, 75, 100, 125, 150 mg	10–300 mg	+
Amoxapine		25, 50, 100, 150 mg	50 mg bid to 600 mg/day	–
Clomipramine	Anafranil	25, 50, 75 mg	25–250 mg	–
Desipramine	Norpramin	10, 25, 50, 75, 100, 150 mg	25–300 mg	+
Doxepin		10, 25, 50, 75, 100, 150 mg; 10 mg/mL	25–300 mg	–
Imipramine	Tofranil	10, 25, 50, 75, 100, 125, 150 mg	25–300 mg	+
Nortriptyline	Pamelor	10, 25, 50, 75; 10 mg/5 mL solution	25–150 mg	+
Protriptyline	Vivactil	5, 10 mg	2.5–20 mg tid	–+
Trimipramine	Surmontil	25, 50, 100 mg	25–300 mg	–

Tricyclic antidepressants are among the best researched migraine preventive treatments. However, only a few of them have had large random controlled studies. Several of them have not been studied at all, and it would not be prudent to assume a class effect, particularly given the wide range of neuroreceptor targets that these medications affect.

Among all of these medications, amitriptyline is the best researched with regards to migraine. However, it also has one of the worst side effect profiles. Studies demonstrate that amitriptyline is at least as effective as propranolol in decreasing migraine frequency and separates significantly from placebo with a 60% to 75% response rate (response is defined as a decrease of headache frequency by at least 50%.[23] In one study, the addition of an SSRI did not change the efficacy in headache prophylaxis.[24] The effect of amitriptyline has been replicated and, although it is not approved by the U.S. Food and Drug Administration (FDA) for the prophylaxis of migraine or tension type headache, it is one of the most commonly prescribed preventive treatments. Other, more limited, evidence exists for imipramine, doxepin, nortriptyline, and desipramine.[25] To date, no evidence has been collected for protriptyline, which has a very different side effect profile than other tricyclic medications.

The most likely mechanism of action of tricyclics is reducing serotonin synthesis in the brainstem raphe nuclei. However, other mechanisms including an effect on norepinephrine may also play a role. Tricyclics are sometimes called "dirty" medications owing to the wide range of neurotransmitter receptors affected, including acetylcholine, histamine, serotonin, norepinephrine, and α_1- adrenergic. This wide profile may in part explain their efficacy, but

Table 11-2 Selective Serotonin Reuptake Inhibitors

Generic Name	Trade Name	Available Dose Size	Reported Doses	Notes
Fluoxetine	Prozac, Sarafem	10, 20, 40 mg, 20 mg/5 mL solution	10–80 mg daily	All SSRIs now have a black box warning for possible increase in suicidal behavior in children, adolescents, and young adults.
Sertraline	Zoloft	25, 50, 100 mg, 20 mg/mL solution	25–200 mg daily	
Fluvoxamine	Luvox	25, 50, 100, 150 mg ER	50–150 mg bid	
Paroxetine	Paxil	10, 20, 30, 40; 12.5, 25 ER; 10 mg/5 mL	20–75 mg daily	
Citalopram	Celexa	10, 20, 40 mg; 10 mg/5 mL solution	20–60 mg daily	
Escitalopram	Lexapro	5, 10, 20 mg; 5 mg/5 mL solution	10–20 mg daily	

also explains their significant side effects. Anticholinergic effects include sedation, dry mouth, dry eyes, and urinary retention. Antihistaminergic effects include weight gain and sedation and α_1-adrenergic effects can lead to impotence and orthostatic hypotension. So, while these medications may be potent antidepressants and antinociceptive agents, they also bear a number of limiting side effects.

Currently the most commonly prescribed medications for depression and anxiety disorders are the selective serotonin reuptake inhibitors.[26] Zimelidine (Zelmid, Normud) was the first SSRI, developed in the 1970s and marketed in 1982. However, it was removed from worldwide markets because of the risk of Guillain-Barré syndrome and a particular hypersensitivity reaction. Fluvoxamine (Luvox) was developed later in the 1970s, and released in Switzerland (1984) and in the United States (1994). Fluoxetine (Prozac) was developed later, released in Belgium (1986) and in the United States (1987), making it the first available SSRI in the United States. The other SSRIs came out over the next decade and rapidly became blockbuster medications.[27]

Because of the response of migraines to earlier antidepressants and the speculated serotonergic underpinnings, these new medications were also studied as to their effect on migraine prophylaxis. Unfortunately, the results were not as brisk as with the tricyclic medications already available. Fluvoxamine, fluoxetine, and citalopram have the most data available but have demonstrated relatively low efficacy.[28] This may be different when looking at a more chronic or refractory population, but those larger studies have

Table 11-3 Serotonin Norepinephrine Reuptake Inhibitors

Generic Name	Trade Name	Available Dose Size	Reported Doses	Notes
Desvenlafaxine	Pristiq	50, 100 mg ER	50–100 mg	
Duloxetine	Cymbalta	30, 60 mg	30–60 mg	
Venlafaxine	Effexor	25, 37.5, 37.5 ER, 50, 75, 75 ER, 100, 150 ER, 225 ER	37.5–300 mg	Predominant action on serotonin
Milnacipran	Savella	12.5, 25, 50, 100 mg	12.5–100 mg bid	Predominant action on norepinephrine

yet to be done. Other pain conditions have shown some greater response to SSRIs, particularly somatization disorders, but that is not necessarily applicable to the refractory headache population. However, their high degree of tolerability may suggest that there is a role for their use, particularly among individuals who have shown difficulty with tolerating other headache preventive treatment. Even if the efficacy is low, they may be candidates for use in some individuals who require alternative treatments. However, their role in prevention of migraine, or RM, may be quite limited.

There are currently three serotonin norepinephrine reuptake inhibitors on the market (desvenlafaxine, duloxetine, and venlafaxine) and one new norepinephrine serotonin reuptake inhibitor (milnacipran.) These are differentiated by the predominant effect on a specific neurotransmitter: the first three mostly affect serotonin, and milnacipran predominantly affects norepinephrine. These differ from the SSRIs by having an affinity for norepinephrine receptors.

Although these drugs were initially developed for the treatment of major depression, they have been found to be effective for other conditions as well. Venlafaxine has been demonstrated to help with social anxiety disorder, panic disorder, and generalized anxiety disorder. Duloxetine and milnacipran have also received FDA approval for the treatment of fibromyalgia.

To date, the only studies of the SNRIs with regard to headache have involved the use of the phenyl ethylamine venlafaxine. In one crossover, blinded comparison to amitriptyline study, venlafaxine demonstrated equivalency of effect over a 12-week period and separation from placebo.[29] More patients discontinued amitriptyline than venlafaxine, predominantly because of hypersomnia, concentration difficulties, and orthostatic hypotension. In another study of migraine, venlafaxine was compared to placebo in 60 patients over a 2-month period. Of patients who received 75 mg, 80% evaluated the effect as good or very good, and of those patients who received 150 mg, 88% evaluated the effect as good or very good.[30]

Table 11-4 Monoamine Oxidase Inhibitors (MAOIs)

Generic Name	Trade Name	Available Dose Size	Reported Doses	Notes
Isocarboxazid	Marplan	10 mg	10–30 mg bid	
Phenelzine	Nardil	15 mg	15–30 mg tid	Significant side effects,
Selegiline Transdermal	Emsam	6, 9, 12 mg patch	6–12 mg daily	interactions, and medicine and food restriction
Tranylcypromine	Parnate	10 mg	10–20 mg tid	

These preliminary results suggest that further research should be done with this class of drugs for RM prophylaxis. Because they have a novel form of action, it is very possible that they may help those patients who have been refractory to other, more generally accepted, treatments.

MAOIs are older antidepressants whose use has been largely supplanted by the SSRIs and SNRIs owing to their high rate of side effects and interactions with other medicines and foods. They include the nonselective MAO-A and MAO-B hydrazines and nonhydrazines, and selective MAO-A and MAO-B inhibitors. The more recent development of selective inhibitors has brought these medications back into common usage.

The most common side effect of the MAOIs is orthostatic hypotension. However, the most concerning side effect is the interaction with tyramine-containing compounds (the so-called "Cheese reaction.") This can lead to an acute serotonin syndrome and a related hypertensive crisis. Because the earlier MAOIs were irreversible, their effects could continue weeks after the drug were discontinued. Patients who are on these medications have a long list of foods and drugs that they need to avoid. In truth, such a strict diet is difficult to accomplish. On the positive side, those dietary restrictions may have a positive effect on headache frequency.

The MAOIs have not been extensively studied with regard to their capacity to reduce headache or migraine frequency. There is some historical evidence for the use of phenelzine, tranylcypromine, and selegiline, but no extensive double-blinded placebo controlled studies to date.[31] Given that these drugs are often reserved for a refractory depressed population, consideration could be made for their use in a refractory headache population as well. The lack of response to other treatments suggests that these patients may need to look toward these otherwise nonpreferable agents.

There are a number of other antidepressants that do not easily fit into the other classifications. They vary in their mechanisms of actions, dosages, and side effects. Some of them have limited use as antidepressants owing to side effects (particularly sedation) but have been used for other purposes (e.g., the use of trazodone for insomnia.) There are limited data on their use for

Table 11-5 Other Antidepressants

Generic Name	Trade Name	Available Dose Size	Reported Doses	Notes
Bupropion HBr	Aplenzin	348, 522 ER	348–522 mg	
Bupropion HCl	Wellbutrin, SR, XL Budeprion SR, XL	75, 100, 100 ER, 150 ER, 200 ER (12 hour) 150 ER, 300 ER (24 hour)	75–450 mg	Norepinephrine dopamine reuptake inhibitors
Maprotiline		25, 50, 75 mg	25–75 mg tid	Tetracyclic inhibits norepinephrine.
Mirtazapine	Remeron, Remeron SolTab	15, 30, 45 mg	15–45 mg qhs	Tetracyclicantagonizes 5-HT_2 and alpha2-adrenergic
Nefazodone	Serzone	50, 100, 150, 200, 250 mg	50–300 mg bid	Inhibits norepinephrine and serotonin and antagonizes 5-HT_2
Trazodone		50, 100, 150, 300 mg	25–200 mg tid	Inhibits serotonin reuptake

headache disorders, but some have shown some promise. Mirtazapine has been effective in low doses for the treatment of migraine, but the data are mostly from individual case reports.[32] In addition, there is some data for its use in chronic tension type headache.[33] However, this work is very preliminary and limited by size of the studies. In addition, one study found that trazodone may be effective for headaches with features of both tension-type headaches and migraine.[34] There is also some suggestion of the utility of nefazodone.[35]

Some of these medications may be utilized as adjunct treatments in refractory headache. Trazodone, for example, may have benefit in patients who suffer from comorbid insomnia complicating their refractory headaches. Interestingly, one of the breakdown products of trazodone is meta-chlorophenylpiperazine (mCPP), which is a psychoactive drug that is known to induce headaches in humans. Up to 10% of people who are exposed to mCPP will develop a migraine headache. However, it is unknown if trazodone has a similar rate of headache-inducing effect.

Given the relative efficacies of the antidepressants and their different adverse event profiles, one can make an argument for the use of several different medications in patients with refractory headaches. However, effectiveness must be validated in future stringent studies. Antidepressants may be effective in headache prevention or on comorbid conditions but their side effects must be considered when prescribing.

Mood Stabilizers

Another common disease in the general population is bipolar illness. The estimated prevalence of bipolar I disorder, defined by the individual having at least one manic episode is estimated to be 0.4% and 1.6%.[36] The estimated prevalence of bipolar II disorder, defined by the individual having at least one hypomanic episode is 0.5%. However, the 1- year prevalence of all bipolar illness may be as high as 3.3%.[37] The incidence of diagnoses of these conditions may have increased over the last two decades as more people have been prescribed antidepressant medications and had an event triggered iatrogenically (sometimes referred to as bipolar III disorder.) In addition, bipolar disorder is often under diagnosed, as hypomanic episodes are sometimes perceived as an environmental advantage and come to treatment only during the depressed phase of the illness.

In the migraine population, the 1-year prevalence of bipolar disease may be as high as 8.8%.[38] Breslau reported that the adjusted odds ratio for lifetime risk of bipolar I disorder in migraine without aura was 2.4 and for migraine with aura was 7.3.[39] In addition, she noted the adjusted odds ratio for lifetime risk of bipolar II disorder in migraine without aura was 2.5 and 5.2 for migraine with aura.[39] The rates of bipolar illness in RM groups have yet to be analyzed, but rates are likely to be at least equal to the rates in a general migraine population. Clearly, the rate of bipolar disorder in migraine alone suggests a large number of people that need to be pharmacologically treated for both conditions.

The most common historical treatments for bipolar illness have included lithium and various antiepileptic medications. Several antidopaminergic agents have also been demonstrated to be effective in the acute phase. Of these medications, lithium has the longest history of use, stemming from the 19th century use of "lithiated" beverages used to treat gout and as nerve tonics. Valproic acid was initially utilized for seizure control, but was found to have utility for both migraine prevention and bipolar illness. Other antiepileptic treatments, including carbamazepine and lamotrigine, were also found to be effective. However, it is worth mentioning that many other antiepileptics have been tested with minimal results in bipolar illness, so one cannot assume a class effect.

Lithium is an ionic salt which was noted to have significant effect on bipolar disorder in the early 1950s, and has also been demonstrated to be effective in other cyclic psychiatric conditions. In addition, evidence has demonstrated its use as an adjunct treatment to antidepressants in refractory major depression. It has become standard of care in treating bipolar disorder. No other treatment to date has been demonstrated to be more effective. However, it does have significant side effects, and tolerability can be problematic, limiting the use of this medication.

Because of its efficacy in a psychiatric population, lithium has also been tested in the treatment of headache. To date, no studies have convincingly demonstrated effect in the treatment of migraine or tension type headache, but lithium has been found to be effective in the treatment of cluster headache.[40] Ekbom used lithium in the treatment of chronic cluster headache, showing moderate efficacy in causing partial remission.[41] It has been used in other trigeminal autonomic cephalalgias with varying degree of success.[42]

With regard to refractory headaches, lithium should be considered, particularly in cases where autonomic symptoms are present. However, there are no current good double blinded studies of its use in the refractory population. Its effect on bipolar disorder may help outcomes in patients with comorbid headache and psychiatric illness, but this still needs to be convincingly demonstrated.

Lithium has many potential side effects on almost every organ system. Common side effects include tremor, slurred speech, blurred vision, nausea, weakness, thirst, anorexia, and diarrhea. In patients with toxic levels, confusion, ataxia, tremor, nystagmus, extra pyramidal signs (EPS) and ultimately seizure and death can result. Longer term use can lead to hypothyroidism, polyuria, abnormal renal function, and polymorphonuclear leukocytosis. Lithium also interacts directly with a host of other medications including nonsteroidal anti-inflammatory drugs (NSAIDs), carbamazepine, and diuretics, and patients should be closely monitored.

Valproic acid is an interesting drug, with effects at many different sites. It increases γ-aminobutyric acid (GABA) levels, enhances postsynaptic response to GABA, causing neuronal hyperpolarization and lowering the level of serotonin in the dorsal raphe nuclei. It appears to decrease aberrant neuronal firing and increases the seizure threshold. The mechanism by which this appears to help bipolar disorder is unclear, but valproic acid has consistently shown itself to be effective not only in the acute treatment of bipolar disorder, but also in maintenance therapy.

With regard to control of migraine, both sodium valproate and divalproex sodium has demonstrated efficacy.[43] The evidence includes at least two placebo controlled studies for each of the drugs.[44] However, little evidence exists that shows that these medications are any more effective than other migraine prophylaxis such as beta blockers. The extended release form of divalproex sodium also appears to have preventive efficacy.[45]

Regardless of the form utilized, valproate appears to have fairly frequent adverse events including nausea, vomiting, and gastrointestinal discomfort. There is also evidence that valproate may effect liver function tests, and in relatively rare cases lead to hepatitis or pancreatitis. In some cases, hepatotoxicity can be quite far progressed before liver function tests demonstrate any significant abnormality. Other adverse reactions include weight gain, hair loss, bleeding disorders, hyperandrogenism, and polycystic ovarian syndrome. Valproate is a well documented teratogen and its use in young, fertile women needs to be closely monitored. Some physicians require fertile females to use two forms of birth control if valproate is prescribed. Neural tube defects may occur in fetuses exposed to valproate and patients should consider their use of birth control when on this medication.

Valproate also interacts with a host of medications, both directly and through its inhibitory effect on P-450. Other drugs (e.g., phenobarbital) used in combination with valproate should be monitored, as levels may be greater than when given alone. Valproate levels can be monitored and doses adjusted accordingly. Whether the "therapeutic" level for migraine and seizure prevention is the same is unknown.

Carbamazepine was found to be effective with regard to migraine prophylaxis in one placebo-controlled study,[46]; however, other studies have failed to demonstrate efficacy above placebo.[47] With regard to control of bipolar disorder, there is significantly more evidence. Several studies have demonstrated efficacy in maintaining euthymia, particularly in the face of the manic phase of illness.[48] Other studies have shown benefit particularly in patients who are rapid cyclers.[49]

The use of carbamazepine requires close monitoring. This medication can have deleterious effects upon white blood cell count, and the therapeutic range of treatment is fairly narrow. Patients require blood level monitoring, as carbamazepine can auto-induce the P450 2D6 system and may require doses adjustments.

Lamotrigine is another antiepileptic medication that has been tested in a range of psychiatric disorders, with benefit particularly in the treatment of bipolar disorder and as an adjunct in refractory depression. It is one of the few medications that seem to be effective in helping the depressed phase of bipolar illness. Its method of action appears to be by blockade of voltage-gated sodium channels causing inhibition of glutamate release, resulting in decreasing neuronal excitability.

Lamotrigine has been studied in several open-label studies as a treatment for chronic migraine. One study used it in combination treatment with some preventive effect in patients who had migraine with aura.[50] However, there was a high dropout rate due to adverse events. Another study looked at its effect on aura, and its use appears to decrease frequency and duration of the aura even in those with persistent aura.[51] Unfortunately, one fairly large placebo blind study failed to demonstrate superiority to placebo and its role remains unclear.[52]

The side effects of lamotrigine include anorexia, weakness, tremor, and cognitive changes. The drug's most significant danger is that of rash including Stevens–Johnson syndrome. Patients should report any new rash while on lamotrigine to their physician immediately.

The most recent drugs used for mood stabilization are the atypical neuroleptics or antidopaminergics. Several of them, including risperidone, olanzapine, and aripiprazole, have been approved for the acute treatment of bipolar illness, particularly during the manic phase. Most psychiatrists will utilize them for rapid stabilization and then transfer patients to other treatments for maintenance.

More will be said about these neuroleptics in the section that discusses antipsychotic medications. These atypical neuroleptics have a wide range of

Table 11-6 Mood Stabilizers

Generic Name	Trade Name	Available Dose Size	Reported Doses	Notes
Carbamazepine	Tegretol	100 CH, 200 mg 100 mg/5 mL soln	200–600 mg bid	
Divalproex Sodium	Depakote Depakote ER	125, 250, 500 mg 250, 500 mg ER	125–500 mg bid to tid	
Lamotrigine	Lamictal	25, 100, 150, 200 mg 2, 5, 25 CH	25–200 mg daily	
Lithium	Lithobid Eskalith	150, 300, 600 mg 300, 450 mg ER	300–900 mg bid	
Oxcarbazepine	Trileptal	150, 300, 600 mg 300 mg/5 mL	300–1200 mg bid	
Valproic acid	Depakene Stavzor	125, 250, 500 mg 250 mg/5 mL	250–500 mg bid to tid	

different neurotransmitter effects and they need to be considered individually. Patients who use them over extended periods are at risk for weight gain, elevated blood sugar levels, cholesterol changes, and movement disorders.

In the use of any of these agents for bipolar disease, several things should be kept in mind. Without adequate control of bipolar illness, the treatment of refractory headaches may be even more difficult. The chief reason for failure of many of these agents is patients' lack of adherence to treatment. Many patients with bipolar illness do not have insight into their condition and are often ready to discontinue usage rapidly. These drugs do have significant side effects and can make the drug intolerable to individuals. These risks need to be discussed with the patient and monitored closely, which will improve compliance and outcomes. Table 11.6 reviews through the most common mood stabilizing agents, including generic names, trade names, doses available and reported effective doses.

Anxiolytics

Anxiety disorders are among the most common psychiatric problems in the general population. In the United States, prevalence rates of generalized anxiety disorder in the general population are about 5%, social phobia 3% to 13%, panic disorder 1% to 3.5%, and obsessive–compulsive disorder about 2.5%.[53] In the specific population of patients with migraine, 1-year prevalence of generalized anxiety has been estimated to be 9.8%, and social phobia prevalence about 6.6%.[54] Dr. Breslau noted that lifetime prevalence of anxiety in migraine patients was 54% compared to a control group with 27%, generalized anxiety disorder was 10% compared to 2%, panic disorder 11% compared to 2%, and obsessive–compulsive disorder 9% compared to 2%.[55] There appears to be a bidirectional association, as migraine increases the rates of panic disorder, and panic disorder increases the risk for migraine.[56] Again, these rates of illness are in a general population with migraine, not in RM. The rates of these specific disorders in the refractory population have not yet been established and could reflect a much higher ratio of comorbid disease.

There are many options in the treatment of anxiety disorders. A number of nonpharmacological methods have been utilized including progressive relaxation training, hypnosis and autogenics, and psychotherapy. With regard to pharmacological interventions, most medications utilized are separated into benzodiazepines and nonbenzodiazepine treatments. Among the nonbenzodiazepine medications, most common are the selective serotonin reuptake inhibitors previously discussed.

Barbiturates entered the American market in 1903 and were some of the earliest regulated medications to be used for anxiety disorders. They are all derived from barbituric acid but with different substitutions at the C-5 position. However, it became quickly apparent that their use could lead to significant ill effects, including abuse, habituation, and dependence. Acute withdrawal could lead to autonomic dysfunction, seizures, and death. Besides these issues, barbiturates also bear a significant risk of respiratory depression, induction of liver enzymes, and risk of cardiac arrhythmia at high dosage. This can be particularly a problem because of the low therapeutic index of this class of drugs.[57]

Interestingly, one of the few remaining short-acting barbiturates on the market is butalbital, which is found in several different headache preparations (e.g., Fioricet, Fiorinal, Esgic, and Esgic Plus.) Butalbital has a relatively short half-life, and this may contribute to the general risk with medication overuse and rebound headaches. Some individuals with migraine and comorbid anxiety disorders may find these preparations particularly attractive not only because of the effectiveness for headache, but because they may provide some mild relief of anxiety symptoms. This may be a group at a higher risk of developing addictive or pseudo-addictive disorders with the development of tolerance, habituation, and drug-seeking behaviors. Other barbiturate anxiolytics such as butabarbital and pentobarbital are rarely used. Some physicians still may utilize anticholinergic sedating agents (hydroxyzine) or muscle relaxants (meprobamate) for limited periods of time in the management of anxiety. There is little good evidence for their prolonged use, or for their use in the management of headaches. They may be used if other treatments are not effective or tolerated, but their use is strictly limited.

In general, patients who have been on higher quantities of short-acting barbiturates, and for an extended period, often need to be detoxified of medication to break this vicious cycle. For detoxification to be successful, one may need to treat the headache pain, the withdrawal symptoms, and the underlying anxiety or depression. This contributes to the difficulty many practitioners have in managing these patients. Part of the treatment requires switching these patients to a long-acting barbiturate or benzodiazepine to prevent withdrawal symptoms including seizures. However, this treatment often requires supplementation with acute migraine medications, and with an alternate anxiolytic.

Benzodiazepines entered the market in the 1960s and were found to be moderately safer and more effective. They are a common treatment for acute anxiety, and have a role in stabilizing patients while longer-term treatments for anxiety and depression may be initiated. However, three of the benzodiazepines (i.e., diazepam, lorazepam, and alprazolam) remain among the top abused drugs in the United States and worldwide.[58]

Benzodiazepines are classified into various categories based on time to peak onset and length of action: short-acting, mid length of action, and long-acting. The average range of time to peak plasma level is 1 to 3 hours with a secondary peak between 6 and 10 hours based on hepatic recirculation. The plasma half-life ranges from 2 to 100 hours (up to 200 hours in patients with liver disease.) Some individuals prefer a rapid time to peak effect owing to either rapid relief of anxiety or a pleasurable effect. However, a common misperception is that benzodiazepines with a longer time to peak effect are less likely to be abused. In fact, many drug abusers will seek to turn extended-release preparations into immediate release preparations in order to achieve high blood levels quickly by crushing pills to disrupt the slow release matrix. Their common site of action is on the GABA-A receptor complex. This results in their sedative hypnotic effect. They have been used not just for the treatment of anxiety, but also for maintenance of sleep, panic disorder, obsessive–compulsive disorder, akathisia, phobias, and agitation related to bipolar disorder. In Table 11.7 we have included the most common benzodiazepines and provided information as to the generic name, trade name, doses available, reported effective doses and classification by length of action

Unfortunately, there is a dearth of information on the effect that benzodiazepines have on headache. Although headache is listed as a potential side effect on nearly all of these medications, there are very little data as to whether they contribute to, cause, or are effective for treating migraine or intractable headaches.[59] However, the incidence of anxiety disorders is increased in migraine and chronic daily headache. These medications can be useful in controlling these comorbid disorders that may be complicating the underlying illness. Benzodiazepines are commonly accepted as effective in controlling anxiety in migraine patients.

The nonbenzodiazepine anxiolytics are predominantly made up of barbiturates and selective serotonin reuptake inhibitors (discussed earlier in this chapter.) However, there are other drugs in this category including buspirone. Table 11.8 includes the non benzodiazepine anxiolytics and provides details regarding generic name, trade names, available doses and reported effective doses. Buspirone is an azaspirone and does not have sedative, hypnotic, muscle relaxant, or anticonvulsant effects. It appears to act predominantly as a partial agonist at the 5-HT_{1A} receptor, with some effects at 5-HT_{2A} and as a mixed agonist antagonist at dopamine type 2 receptors The full psychotropic effect requires several weeks of treatment, suggesting that its anxiolytic effect

Table 11-7 Benzodiazepines

Generic Name	Trade Name	Available Dose Size	Reported Doses	Length of Action
Alprazolam	Niravam, Xanax, Xanax XR	0.25, 0.5, 1, 2 ODT, 0.5, 1, 2, 3ER, 1 mg/mL soln	0.25 bid–2 mg tid	
Midazolam	Versed	2 mg/mL syrup; IM; IV	1 mg IV q2–3 min	Short acting and rapid onset
Oxazepam	10, 15, 30 mg	10–30 mg tid		
Triazolam	Halcion	0.125, 0.25 mg	0.125–0.5 mg qhs	
Estazolam		1, 2 mg	0.5–2 mg qhs	
Lorazepam	Ativan	0.5, 1, 2 mg 2 mg/mL soln IV, IM	0.5 daily–3 mg tid	Mid length of action
Temazepam	Restoril	7.5, 15, 22.5, 30 mg	7.5–30 mg qhs	
Chlordiazepoxide	Librium	5, 10, 25 mg	5–25 mg qid	
Clonazepam	Klonopin, Klonopin Wafer	0.5, 1, 2 mg; 0.125, 0.25, 0.5, 1, 2 ODT	0.125–6 mg tid	Long length of action
Clorazepate	Tranxene SD, TranxeneT-tab	3.75, 7.5, 15 mg	3.75–20 mg tid	
Diazepam	Valium	2, 5, 10 mg 5 mg/5 mL soln 5 mg/mL nasal IM, IV	2–10 mg bid– qid	
Flurazepam	Dalmane	15, 30 mg	15–30 mg	

Table 11-8 Nonbenzodiazepine Anxiolytics

Generic Name	Trade Name	Available Dose Size	Reported Doses	Notes
Buspirone	Buspar	5, 7.5, 10, 15, 30 mg	7.5–30 mg bid	
Butabarbital	Butisol	30, 50 mg30 mg/5 mL	15–30 mg bid–tid	
Hydroxyzine	Atarax	10, 25, 50, 100 mg 10 mg/5 mL soln	50–100 mg q6h	
Meprobamate		200, 400 mg	400 mg tid– qid	
Pentobarbital	Nembutal	IM, IV	150–200 mg	

may work through modifying receptor expression. Buspirone has side effects of nausea, dizziness, occasional insomnia, and headache. Although, it does not appear to have the same abuse potential as the barbiturates or benzodiazepines, many psychiatrists are unimpressed with its general result on anxiety. With regard to headache, there is some small open label evidence for its use in migraine and in chronic tension type headache.[60] The current studies are limited and further trials should be done, particularly with regard to RM.

Antipsychotics

The antipsychotic medications, or neuroleptics, were predominantly derived from phenothiazine compounds that were used as synthetic dyes in Europe. Their general action is "neurolepsis" or the suppression of spontaneous complex behaviors, vigilance, aggression, impulsivity, and overactive response to stimuli. In addition, they optimally maintain intellect, coordination, and speech and have a minimal effect on other dopaminergic pathways.

Promethazine was first conceived in the 1930s, but failed to demonstrate adequate effectiveness in treating agitation. However, its antiemetic effect was significant and it continues to be used for the control of nausea. In addition, it has been used to potentiate the effect of other anesthetics. In 1949, chlorpromazine was developed to augment anesthesia. Reserpine was developed in the 1950s and demonstrated some moderate antipsychotic effects. Chlorpromazine, a derivative of reserpine, was further tested for its ability to cause hypothermic shock in humans because it lowered the core temperature of laboratory rats. It did not lower human core temperature, but it did have a positive effect on decreasing psychotic behaviors. In 1958, the first butyrophenone haloperidol was developed, leading to a host of other '"typical" neuroleptics being developed throughout the 1960s and 1970s.

In the 1980s clozapine, the first of the "atypical" neuroleptics, was developed. It differed from the typical neuroleptics in that it was a dibenzapine and had a low affinity for dopamine receptors (being somewhat D1 selective) as well as having 5-HT$_2$, muscarinic, α-adrenergic, and H1 effects. The other atypical neuroleptics followed and showed a decrease in the side effects of extrapyramidal symptoms (EPS), little effect on prolactin levels, and a greater effect on negative symptoms of schizophrenia. The 21st century has seen the introduction of the first "third–generation" neuroleptic, aripiprazole, which has a mixed agonist antagonist effect.

The total group of neuroleptics breaks down to several subclasses. Table 11.9 provides information on first, second and third generation neuroleptics including generic names, trade names, doses available and reported effective doses. There are the phenothiazenes, which split into aliphatics (such as chlorpromazine and promethazine), piperazines (including fluphenazine, perphenazine, trifluoperazine, and prochlorperazine), and piperidines (including mesoridazine and thioridazine.) There are thioxanthenes such as thiothixene, and other heterocyclics including dibenzapines (e.g., clozapine, loxapine), butyrophenones (e.g., haloperidol, droperidol), indoles (e.g., molindone, ziprasidone), benzamides, quinolones, thienobenzodiazepines, dibenzothiazepines, benzisoxazoles, and others.

Table 11-9 First- and Second-Generation Antipsychotics

First-Generation Antipsychotics

Generic Name	Trade Name	Available Dose Size	Reported Doses	Notes
Chlorpromazine	Thorazine	10, 25, 50, 100, 200 mgIM, IV	10–250 mg tid–qid	
Fluphenazine	Prolixin	1, 2.5, 5, 10 mg 2.5/5 mL elixir	1–10 mg qid	
Haloperidol	Haldol	0.5, 1, 2, 5, 10, 20 mg	0.5–5 mg tid reports up to 100 mg/day	
Loxapine	Loxitane	5, 10, 25, 50 mg	10–50 mg bid	
Molindone	Moban	5, 10, 25, 50, 100 mg	5–50 mg tid to qid	
Perphenazine	Trilafon	2, 4, 8, 16 mg	4–16 mg bid to qid	
Pimozide	Orap	1, 2 mg	1–2 mg daily to bid	
Prochlorperazine	Compazine	5, 10 mg	5–10 mg q6–8h	
Thioridazine	Mellaril	10, 15, 25, 50, 100, 150, 200 mg 30; 100 mg/mL	50–200 mg bid to qid(max 800 mg)	
Thiothixene	Navane	1, 2, 5, 10, 20 mg	2–20 mg tid	
Trifluoperazine	Stelazine	1, 2, 5, 10 mg	1–20 mg bid	

Second-Generation Antipsychotics

Generic Name	Trade Name	Available Dose Size	Reported Doses	Notes
Aripiprazole	Abilify	2, 5, 10, 15, 20, 30 mg 1 mg/mL IM	2–30 mg daily	D2, 5-HT_{1A} agonist;5-HT_{2A} antagonist
Clozapine	Clozaril FazaClo ODT	12.5, 25, 50, 100, 200 mg	12.5–300 mg bid(max 900 mg/day)	Risk of agranulocytosis
Olanzapine	Zyprexa Zyprexa Zydis	2.5, 5, 7.5, 10, 15, 20 mg	2.5–20 mg daily	
Paliperidone	Invega	3, 6, 9 mg ER	3–12 mg daily	
Quetiapine	Seroquel Seroquel XR	25, 50, 100, 200, 300, 400 mg 25, 50, 100, 200, 300, 400 mg ER	25–300 mg tid(max 800 mg/day)	
Risperidone	Risperdal	0.25, 0.5, 1, 2, 3, 4 mg 1 mg/mL	0.25–4 mg bid(max 16 mg/day)	
Ziprasidone	Geodon	20, 40, 60, 80 mg	20–80 mg bid	

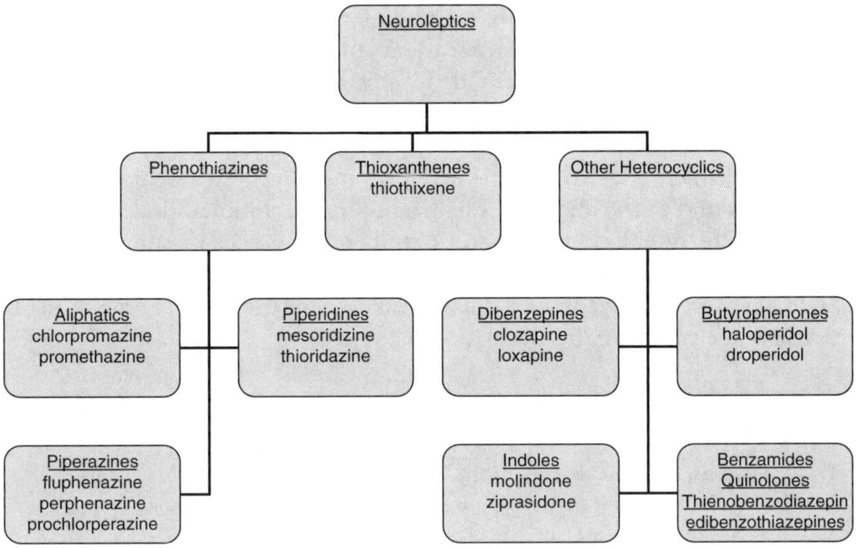

Figure 11-1 Neuroleptics

The role of dopamine in migraine has been speculated about since 1977. It has been noted that stimulation of dopamine produces many effects similar to the migraine prodrome, including yawning, mood changes, nausea and vomiting, gastrokinetic changes, and hypotensive autonomic changes.[61] The dopamine receptor is heterogeneous and consists of two general families of receptors: D1-like (including D1 and D5) and D2-like (including D2, D3, and D4). D1-like receptors stimulate adenylyl cyclase whereas D2-like inhibits adenyl cyclase. Whereas most receptors are central, D1 and D2 are also present peripherally. There are four major dopaminergic pathways including the tuberoinfundibular pathway (hypothalamus to the anterior pituitary involved in prolactin release), nigrostriatal pathway (substantia nigra to the striatum involved in movement smoothing), mesocortical pathway (ventral tegmentum to the limbic cortex involved in cognition), and mesolimbic pathway (tegmentum to nucleus accumbens involved in perception.)

The neuroleptics also have a diverse effect on a range of other neurochemical messengers including serotonin, epinephrine and norepinephrine, acetylcholine, and histamine. Some of these effects account for their particular side effects. These include hyperprolactinemia, dry mouth and eyes, hypotension, weight gain, metabolic syndrome, sedation, QTc prolongation and risk of sudden death, lowered seizure threshold, and extrapyramidal movement disorders including tardive dyskinesia.[62]

There is evidence of use of some of the neuroleptics for treatment of other conditions besides psychosis. Pimozide is a classic treatment for Tourette's syndrome, and some of the second- generation drugs have been approved for treatment of the acute manic phase of bipolar disease. Although none of the neuroleptics have been approved for the treatment of migraine, several studies have looked at this question. Evidence exists for the use of chlorpromazine, prochlorperazine, haloperidol, droperidol, and metoclopramide in migraine.[63–66] Limited evidence exists for olanzapine, quetiapine, ziprasidone, and aripiprazole.[67–70] Haloperidol prevented migraine in two small open studies in 1995 and 2004, and in a small randomized double-blinded study in 2006.[71–73] One double-blind crossover study of fluphenazine showed benefit with tension-type headache.[74] None of these studies meet Level 1 evidence, and further research needs to be done to validate the use of these potent medications in the refractory headache population.

Dopamine Receptors

D1: Thalamus, superior chiasmatic nucleus, supraoptic nucleus, arterial walls
D2: Periaqueductal Gray, hypothalamus, raphe nuclei, basal ganglia, solitary nucleus, dorsal motor vagal nucleus, presynaptic sympathetics
D3: Area postrema, brain stem
D4: Brain stem
D5: Limbic regions, basal ganglia

Attention–Deficit/Hyperactivity Disorder

Very little has been written about the use of stimulant and nonstimulant medications for attention-deficit disorder and their effect on migraine. Although all of these drugs have headache listed as a side effect, there is no distinction as to whether this side effect is medication induced or acts as a trigger for migraine episodes. Table 11.10 provides information on the medications used for attention deficit disorder including generic names, trade names, available dosing strengths, and reported effective doses.

Some physicians have used these medications to compensate for the cognitive impairments that result from other medications. This use lacks evidence and is off label, but is an area where further research is required. In addition, some of these medications can have the side effects of insomnia and anorexia, both of which can be triggers for migraines. These medications should be used with caution, particularly when mixed with other psychiatric medications.

In conclusion, many classes of psychopharmacological agents are used in the management of refractory headaches, both for the treatment of the headache disorder and for the treatment of comorbid psychiatric disorders. The rates of Axis I psychiatric disorders such as major depression, dysthymia, bipolar I and II, generalized anxiety disorder, social phobia, and obsessive–compulsive disorder are higher among patients with migraine and RM. These comorbidities complicate medical care and require individualized assessment

Table 11-10 Stimulants and Nonstimulants

Generic Name	Trade Name	Available Dose Size	Reported Doses	Notes
Amphetamine/ Dextroamphetamine	Adderall Adderall XR	5, 7.5, 10, 12.5, 15, 20, 30; 5, 10, 15,20, 25, 30 ER	5–60 mg qd–bid	
Atomoxetine	Strattera	10, 18, 25, 40, 60, 80, 100	10–100 mg daily	
Dextroamphetamine	Dexedrine Procentra	5, 10, 15 mg ER	5–60 mg daily	
Dexmethylphenidate	Focalin Focalin XR	2.5, 5, 10 mg; 5, 10, 15, 20 ER	2.5–10 mg daily–bid	
Lisdexamfetamine	Vyvanse	20, 30, 40, 50, 60, 70 mg	20–70 mg daily	
Methylphenidate	Ritalin (LA, SR) Metadate (CD, ER) Methylin (ER) Daytrana	2.5, 5, 10, 20 18, 27, 36, 54 ER	2.5–15 mg tid	

and management. An understanding of psychopharmacological agents is essential, as their actions can be beneficial, but their side effects and interactions may be devastating. Whether one measures outcomes by following pain scores or by measuring functionality, the final goal is the same: doing the best for our patients.

References

1. Schulman EA, Lake AE 3rd, Goadsby PJ, Peterlin BL, Siegel SE, Markley HG, Lipton RB. Defining refractory migraine and refractory chronic migraine: proposed criteria from the Refractory Headache Special Interest Section of the American Headache Society. *Headache.* 2008; 48(6):778–782.
2. Sheftell FD. Understanding the headache patient with complex comorbidities: a headache specialist's perspective. *Headache.* 2006;46(Suppl. 3):S165–S167.
3. Baskin SB, Lipchik GL, Smitherman TA. Mood and anxiety disorders in chronic headache. *Headache.* 2006;46(Suppl. 3):S76–S87.
4. Hamelsky SW, Lipton RB. Psychiatric comorbidity of migraine. *Headache.* 2006;46:1327–1333.
5. Lipchik GL, Penzian DB. Psychiatric comorbidities in patients with headaches. *Semin Pain Med.* 2004;2:93–105.
6. Breslau N, Davis GC, Andreski P. Migraine, psychiatric disorders, and suicide attempts: an epidemiologic study of young adults. *Psychiatry Res.* 1991;37:11–23.
7. Lipton RB, Diamond S, Reed M, Diamond ML, Stewart WF. Migraine diagnosis and treatment: results from the American Migraine Study II. *Headache.* 2001;41:638–645.

8. Silberstein S, Lipton R, Dodick D. *Wolff's Headache and Other Head Pain*, 8th ed. New York: Oxford University Press;2007:95–120.
9. Lake A III, Lipchik D, Penzian D, Rains J, Saper J, Lipton R. Psychiatric comorbidity with chronic daily headache: evidence based clinical implications—introduction to the supplement. *Headache.* 2006;46(Suppl. 3): S73–S75.
10. Hamelsky SW, Lipton RB. Psychiatric comorbidity of migraine. *Headache.* 2006;46:1327–1333.
11. Lipton RB, Bigal ME, Diamond M, Freitag F, Reed ML, Stewart WF. AMPP Advisory Group. Migraine prevalence, disease burden, and the need for preventive therapy. *Neurology.* 2007;68:343–349.
12. Huffman JC, Stern TA. Neuropsychiatric consequences of cardiovascular medications. *Dialogues Clin Neurosci.* 2007;9:29–45.
13. Evans R. FDA Alert on serotonin syndrome with combined use of SSRI's and SNRI's and triptans: an analysis of the 29 case reports. *Med Gen Med.* 2007;9:48.
14. Kessler R, McGonagle K, Zhao S, et al. Lifetime and 12-month prevalence of DSM-III-R psychiatric disorders in the United States: results from the National Comorbidity Survey. *Arch Gen Psychiatry.* 1994;51(1):8–19.
15. Merikangas KR, Stevens DE. Comorbidity of migraine and psychiatric disorders. *Neurol Clin.* 1997;15:115–123.
16. Breslau N. Psychiatric comorbidity in migraine. *Cephalalgia.* 1998;18 (Suppl 22):56–61.
17. Swartz KL, Pratt LA, Armenian HK, Lee LC, Eaton WW. Mental disorders and the incidence of migraine headaches in a community sample: results from the Baltimore Epidemiologic Catchment area follow-up study. *Arch Gen Psychiatry.* 2000;57:945–950.
18. Breslau N, Davis GC, Andreski P. Migraine, psychiatric disorders, and suicide attempts: an epidemiologic study of young adults. *Psychiatry Res.* 1991;37:11–23.
19. Patel NV, Bigal ME, Kolodner KB, et al. Prevalence and impact of migraine and probable migraine in a health plan. *Neurology.* 2004;63:1432–1438.
20. Breslau N, Lipton RB, Stewart WF, et al. Comorbidity of migraine and depression: investigating potential etiology and prognosis. *Neurology.* 2003;60:1308–1312.
21. Zwart JA, Dyb G, Hagen K, et al. Depression and anxiety disorders associated with headache frequency. The Nord-Trondelag Health Study. *Eur J Neurol.* 2003;10:147–152.
22. Melfi C, Chawla A, Croghan T, Hanna M, Kennedy S, Sredl K. The effects of adherence to antidepressant treatment guidelines on relapse and recurrence of depression. *Arch Gen Psychiatry.* 1998;55:1128–1132.
23. Ziegler DK, Hurwitz A, Hassanein RS, Kodanaz HA, Preskom SH, Mason J. Migraine prophylaxis. A comparison of propranolol and amitryptyline. *Arch Neurol.* 1987;44:486–489.
24. Krymchantowski AV, Silva MT, Barbosa JS, Alves LA. Amitriptyline versus amitriptyline combined with fluoxetine in the preventative treatment of transformed migraine: a double-blind study. *Headache.* 2002;42:510–514.
25. Martucci N, Manna V, Agnoli A. Antidepressant drugs and migraine. *Cephalalgia.* 1985;5(Suppl. 2):225–228.

26. Song F, Freemantle N, Sheldon T A, House A, Watson P, Long A, Mason J. Selective serotonin reuptake inhibitors: meta-analysis of efficacy and acceptability. *BMJ.* 1993;306:683–687.
27. Barbui C, Campomori A, D'Avanzo B, Negri E, Garattini S. Antidepressant drug use in Italy since the introduction of SSRIs: national trends, regional differences and impact on suicide rates. *Social Psychiatry and Psychiatric Epidemiol.* 1999;34:152–156.
28. Saper JR, Silberstein SD, Lake AE III, Winters ME. Double-blind trial of fluoxetine: chronic daily headache and migraine. *Headache.* 1994;34: 497–502.
29. Bulut S, Berilgen MS, Baran A, Tekatas A, Atmaca M, Mungen B. Venlafaxine versus amitriptyline in the prophylactic treatment of migraine: randomized, double-blind, crossover study. *Clin Neurol Neurosurg.* 2004;107:44–48.
30. Ozyalcin SN, Talu GK, Kiziltan E, Yucel B, Ertas M, Disci R. The efficacy and safety of venlafaxine in the prophylaxis of migraine. *Headache.* 2005;45:144–152.
31. Punay NC, Couch JR. Antidepressants in the treatment of migraine headache. *Curr Pain Headache Rep.* 2003;7:51–54.
32. Levy E, Margolese HC. Migraine headache prophylaxis and treatment with low-dose mirtazapine. *Int Clin Psychopharmacol.* 2003;18:301–303.
33. Bendtsen L, Jensen R. Mirtazapine is effective in the prophylactic treatment of chronic tension-type headache *Neurology.* 2004;62:1706–1711.
34. Pies R. Trazodone and intractable headaches. *J Clin Psychiatry.* 1983;44(8):317.
35. Saper J, Lake A, Tepper S. Nefazodone for chronic daily headache prophylaxis: an open-label study. *Headache.* 2001;41(5):465–474.
36. Kessler R, McGonagle K, Zhao S, et al. Lifetime and 12-month prevalence of DSM-III-R psychiatric disorders in the United States: results from the National Comorbidity Survey. *Arch Gen Psychiatry.* 1994;51(1):8–19.
37. Kessler R, McGonagle K, Zhao S, et al. Lifetime and 12-month prevalence of DSM-III-R psychiatric disorders in the United States: results from the National Comorbidity Survey. *Arch Gen Psychiatry.* 1994;51(1):8–19.
38. Radat F, Swendsen J. Psychiatric comorbidity in migraine: a review. *Cephalalgia.* 2004;25:165–178.
39. Breslau N. Psychiatric comorbidity in migraine. *Cephalalgia.* 1998;18 (Suppl 22):56–61.
40. Peatfield RC. Lithium in migraine and cluster headache: a review. *J R Soc Med.* 1981; 74(6):432–436.
41. Ekbom K. Lithium for cluster headache: review of the literature and preliminary results of long-term treatment. *Headache.* 1981;21:132–139.
42. Cohen A, Matharu, M, Goadsby P. Trigeminal autonomic cephalalgias: current and future treatments. *Headache.* 2007;47(6):969–980.
43. Hering R, Kuritzky A. Sodium valproate in the prophylactic treatment of migraine: a double blind study versus placebo. *Cephalalgia.* 1992;12:81–84.
44. Yoon MS, Savidou I, Diener HC, Limmroth V. Evidence-based medicine in migraine prevention. *Expert Rev Neurother.* 2005;5(3):333–341.
45. Freitag FG, Collins SD, Carlson HA, et al.; Depakote ER Migraine Study Group. A randomized trial of divalproex sodium extended-release tablets in migraine prophylaxis. *Neurology.* 2002;58(11):1652–1659.

46. Rompel H, Bauermeister PW. Aetiology of migraine and prevention with carbamazepine (Tegretol): results of a double-blind, cross-over study. *S Afr Med J.* 1970;44(4):75–80.
47. Silberstein S, Lipton R, Dodick D. *Wolff's Headache and Other Head Pain*, 8th ed. New York: Oxford University Press; 2007:95–120.
48. Ceron-Litvoc D, Soares BG, Geddes J, Litvoc J, de Lima MS. Comparison of carbamazepine and lithium in treatment of bipolar disorder a systematic review of randomized controlled trials. *Hum Psychopharmacol.* 2009;24(1): 19–28.
49. Stoner SC, Nelson LA, Lea JW, Marken PA, Sommi RW, Dahmen MM. Historical review of carbamazepine for the treatment of bipolar disorder. *Pharmacotherapy.* 2007;27(1):68–88.
50. Lampl C, Katsarava Z, Diener HC, Limmroth V. Lamotrigine reduces migraine aura and migraine attacks in patients with migraine with aura. *J Neurol Neurosurg Psychiatry.* 2005;76:1730–1732.
51. Chen WT, Fuh JL, Lu SR, Wang SJ. Persistent migrainous visual phenomena might be responsive to lamotrigine. *Headache.* 2001;41(8):823–825.
52. Steiner TJ, Findley LJ, Yuen AW. Lamotrigine versus placebo in the prophylaxis of migraine with and without aura. *Cephalalgia.* 1997;17(2): 109–112.
53. Kessler R, McGonagle K, Zhao S, et al. Lifetime and 12-month prevalence of DSM-III-R psychiatric disorders in the United States: results from the National Comorbidity Survey. *Arch Gen Psychiatry.* 1994;51(1):8–19.
54. Baskin SB, Lipchik GL, Smitherman TA. Mood and anxiety disorders in chronic headache. *Headache.* 2006;46(Suppl. 3):S76–S87.
55. Breslau N. Psychiatric comorbidity in migraine. *Cephalalgia.* 1998;18(Suppl 22): 56–61.
56. Guidetti V, Galli F, Fabrizi P, et al. Headache and psychiatric comorbidity: clinical aspects and outcome in a 8-year follow-up study. *Cephalalgia.* 1998; 18:455–462.
57. Bigal ME, Serrano D, Buse D, Scher A, Stewart WF, Lipton RB. Acute migraine medications and evolution from episodic to chronic migraine: a longitudinal population-based study. *Headache.* 2008;48(8):1157–1168.
58. Christensen R, Garces L, The growing abuse of commonly prescribed psychiatric medications. *Am J Emerg Med.* 2006;24(1): 137–138.
59. Covelli V, Maffione AB, Nacci C, Tatò E, Jirillo E. Stress, neuropsychiatric disorders and immunological effects exerted by benzodiazepines. *Immunopharmacol Immunotoxicol.* 1998;20(2):199–209.
60. Lee S, Park J, Kim M. Efficacy of the 5-HT_{1A} agonist, buspirone hydrochloride, in migraineurs with anxiety: a randomized, prospective, parallel group, double-blind, placebo-controlled study. *Headache.* 2005;45: 1004–1011.
61. Fernandez F, Colson N, Quinlan S, MacMillan J, Lea RA, Griffiths LR. Association between migraine and a functional polymorphism at the dopamine beta-hydroxylase locus. *Neurogenetics.* 2009;10(3):199–208. Epub 2009 Feb 14.
62. Edlinger M, Hofer A, Rettenbacher MA, et al. Factors influencing the choice of new generation antipsychotic medication in the treatment of patients with schizophrenia. *Schizophr Res.* 2009;113(2-3):246–251.

63. Miller MA, Levsky ME, Enslow W, Rosin A. Randomized evaluation of octreotide vs prochlorperazine for ED treatment of migraine headache. *Am J Emerg Med.* 2009;27(2):160–164.
64. Honkaniemi J, Liimatainen S, Rainesalo S, Sulavuori S. Haloperidol in the acute treatment of migraine: a randomized, double-blind, placebo-controlled study. *Headache.* 2006;46(5):781–787.
65. Silberstein SD, Young WB, Mendizabal JE, Rothrock JF, Alam AS. Acute migraine treatment with droperidol: a randomized, double-blind, placebo-controlled trial. *Neurology.* 2003;60(2):315–321.
66. Griffith JD, Mycyk MB, Kyriacou DN. Metoclopramide versus hydromorphone for the emergency department treatment of migraine headache. *J Pain.* 2008;9(1):88–94. Epub 2007 Nov 5.
67. Silberstein SD, Peres MF, Hopkins M, Schecter AL, Young W, Rozen T. Olanzapine in the treatment of refractory migraine and chronic daily headache. *Headache.* 2002;42:515–518.
68. Krymchantowski AV, Jevoux C. Questiapine for the prevention of migraine refractory to the combination of atenolol + nortriptyline + flunarizine: an open pilot study. *Arq Neuropsiquiatr.* 2008;66(3B):615–618.
69. Boeker T. Ziprasidone and migraine headache. *Am J Psychiatry.* 2002;159(8): 1435–1436.
70. LaPorta LD. Relief from migraine headache with aripiprazole treatment. *Headache.* 2007;47(6):922–926.
71. Fisher H. A new approach to emergency department therapy of migraine headache with intravenous haloperidol: a case series. *J Emerg Med.* 1995;13(1):119–122.
72. Monzillo PH, Nemoto PH, Costa AR, Sanvito WL. [Acute treatment of migraine in emergency room: comparative study between dexamethasone and haloperidol. *Preliminary results] Arq Neuropsiquiatr.* 2004;62(2B):513–518. Epub 2004 Jul 20.
73. Honkaniemi J, Liimatainen S, Rainesalo S, Sulavuori S. Haloperidol in the acute treatment of migraine: a randomized, double-blind, placebo-controlled study. *Headache.* 2006;46(5):781–787.
74. Hakkarainen H. Fluphenazine for tension headache; double-blind study. *Headache.* 1977;17(5):216–218.

12

Psychological Aspects of Refractory Migraine Management

Alvin E. Lake III, PhD, BCIAC-SF

It was the best of times.
It was the worst of times.
It was the age of triptans and extended release opioids.
It was the age of medication overuse and dependency.
It was the epoch of anticonvulsants and botulinum toxin.
It was the epoch of adverse effects and limited efficacy.
It was the era of behavioral therapy and nonpharmacology.
It was the era of passivity and noncompliance.
It was the season to function heroically.
It was the season of disability.
It was the spring of hope.
It was the winter of psychiatric comorbidity and traumatic life events.

—(With appreciation to Charles Dickens, Tale of Two Cities)

Introduction

One of the ironies of headache management in the current era is that the emergence of effective therapies for the control of migraine has widened the gap between treatment-responsive and treatment-refractory headache sufferers. Factors contributing to refractory migraine (RM) need to be identified, with the hope of devising therapies that reduce the suffering of those whose headaches fail to respond to established conventional treatment. Patients deserve and appreciate our compassion and empathy. Many have endured well-meaning or frustrated suggestions from family, friends, employers—even physicians—that their own inadequacies lie at the route of their problems, that they are the cause of their own suffering: "Just relax, you worry too much," "Your headaches are a symptom of your depression—get that under control and you'll feel better," "You're too stressed—quit your job, straighten out your marriage, get control of your kids," "You should get rid of all your drugs, they're just making you worse."

Effective management of RM requires sailing a course through the straits between *empathy for the patient's suffering* on one side of the ship, with *identification of behavioral factors that may contribute to headache activity (without blaming the patient)* on the other—the Scylla and Charybdis through which both Odysseus and the contemporary headache physician must navigate to reach home successfully. The following observations and treatment suggestions are based on the emerging migraine and general pain literature, as well as clinical experience over the past 30 years in a multidisciplinary tertiary care setting. This chapter highlights seven selected areas of behavioral inquiry and intervention in treating patients with RM:

1. Appropriate goal-setting
2. Biofeedback and relaxation training
3. Cognitive–behavioral therapy
4. Coping styles—dysfunctional versus adaptive
5. Life events, trauma, and histories of abuse
6. Behavioral factors underlying medication overuse
7. Family interaction related to headache

This is not intended to be an exhaustive review of the behavioral literature in headache treatment. Other, equally important psychological topics are addressed in chapters on psychiatric comorbidity, nonpharmacological and physical treatments, fostering adherence and the therapeutic relationship, managing disability issues, management of other refractory headache disorders (e.g., chronic tension-type headache), and inpatient strategies.

Discussion of Treatment Goals: Pain Reduction versus Pain Management

The primary goal of most headache sufferers is pain reduction (acute relief, sustained relief, and prevention), along with control of pain-associated symptoms (e.g., nausea, excessive sensitivity to light and sound, dizziness in some cases).[1] These primary goals have eluded the grasp of the patient with RM. A history of ineffective treatments can condition negative expectations about any potential benefit from future therapies—expectations that can further reduce the likelihood of pain relief from new approaches.[2]

Some patients come to treatment with overblown expectations—"Maybe this time my headaches will be cured!"—that can lead to an increased sense of demoralization when the goal is not reached, or not reached in as timely manner as the patient believes should be the case. While positive expectations may improve treatment success, *unrealistic* expectations can breed disappointment down the road. Studies of the placebo analgesic response often rely on the communication of what might be called "cautious optimism"—the *possibility* of pain reduction ("You will receive a treatment that has been shown to be effective in a number of studies")[3] rather than attempting to communicate an *absolute certainty of success* ("This will definitely reduce your pain"). The treatment experience of some patients with RM can be analogous to riding a roller-coaster with more disappointments than thrills—a series of rising hopes and expectations followed by descents that return the patient to the starting position, when treatments prove ineffective or trigger intolerable adverse effects.

The first step in the behavioral management of RM is an explicit discussion of goals and reasonable expectations before starting treatment, beginning with an inquiry into the patient's thoughts—*the unexpressed attitude is the most difficult attitude to change.* In our setting, patients are requested to write their goals down before seeing the doctor, which offers an opportunity to clarify what may or may not be possible.

It is important to broaden the patient's perceptions of treatment goals from a narrow focus on *pain and symptom reduction* to a more wide angle lens that includes *pain management*—defined as reducing pain-related distress (including comorbid pain-related depression or anxiety) for the patient and family, along with increased functioning and quality of life—even when pain reduction is difficult to achieve. I often tell patients that there is reason for considerable optimism about improved control over pain, reduced distress, and improved function, but that "cure"—in the sense of no headaches, never again—is not the expected outcome. We also encourage patients to discuss realistic (cautiously optimistic) treatment goals with family members and employers. Some of our patients who achieve meaningful but limited success in our inpatient program become more stressed as discharge approaches, and they fear they are not reaching the expectations of family members and employers.

In addition to pain relief, most headache patients also express interest in a diagnosis and explanation of the factors contributing to their headaches.[1] Cognitive understanding of headache mechanisms can help impart a sense of control. The implicit goal is to assist the patient who has failed to improve from previous therapies to shift from an external locus of control with a sense of helplessness, to an internal locus of control[4] and a sense of self-efficacy[5,6]—the belief that "I can take action that will reduce my distress and improve my ability to function." Beliefs about pain have significant physiological consequences.[7] A series of small treatment successes (rather than giant leaps) can condition positive expectations, with increasingly potent benefits over time.[2,8,9]

Biofeedback and Relaxation Training

The proposed definition of RM[10,11] discussed in Chapter 2 implies a two-step approach to treatment: (1) initial use of established treatments (the basics) that merit application before a headache is deemed "refractory," and should be revisited if those treatments have not been given an adequate trial, followed by (2) referral of appropriate patients for advanced, specialized treatment, including the creative application of treatment approaches that may not yet have been fully validated if the basics have not yielded sufficient benefit. Although the definition requires modification of triggers and lifestyle factors, the proposed definition of "refractory" is primarily based on lack of success or adverse effects to specific classes of acute and preventive medications.

The multiple authors of the proposed definition (including myself) struggled with whether to include biofeedback and cognitive behavioral therapy as "treatments with established efficacy." The decision to omit them was based on our concern about the lack of ready access to these treatments for many patients in primary care settings, and was not intended to relegate these approaches to a secondary status. More than a decade ago, the U.S. Headache Consortium (consisting of the American Headache Society and six other medical societies) reviewed the available evidence and put forward an evidence-based treatment guideline with the following recommendations related to behavioral medicine:[12]

1. Relaxation training, thermal biofeedback combined with relaxation training, electromyographic (EMG) biofeedback, and cognitive–behavioral therapy may be considered treatment options for the prevention of migraine (Grade A evidence).
2. Behavioral therapy may be combined with preventive drug therapy to achieve added clinical improvement for migraine (Grade B evidence).

Continuing meta-analytic reviews of multiple studies have confirmed that behavioral headache interventions are effective primary treatments for migraine and tension-type headache. The most recent review of biofeedback for migraine at the time of this writing was by Nestoriuc and Martin (2007),[13] who found 88 studies, 55 of which were rigorous enough to meet their inclusion criteria, including randomized controlled trials as well as pre–post trials. Biofeedback was more effective than control conditions, with a medium effect size ($d = 0.58$, 95% CI = 0.52, 0.64) for all biofeedback interventions, and remained stable over an average follow-up phase of 17 months. The strongest evidence for improvement was for reduced frequency of migraine attacks and perceived self-efficacy (the person's belief that he or she can exert control over headache). An intent-to-treat analysis revealed stable treatment effects, even when dropouts were considered as nonresponders.

This review included three primary types of biofeedback for migraine: peripheral skin temperature feedback (hand warming—a measure of reduced noradrenergic outflow), surface EMG feedback from facial and neck muscles, and blood-volume-pulse feedback from the temporal artery (using photoplethysmography). Blood-volume-pulse feedback yielded higher effect sizes than peripheral skin temperature or EMG feedback, but is not widely available in most clinical biofeedback settings. Moderator analyses revealed biofeedback in combination with home training (e.g., finger thermometers, such as inexpensive alcohol thermometers or relatively inexpensive electronic digital thermometers capable of displaying 0.1 degree changes in temperature) to be more effective than therapies without home training.

Not all types of biofeedback are equally effective. For example, neurofeedback is a novel type of electroencephalographic (EEG) biofeedback now available in some communities, often marketed as a state-of-the-art tool that allows the brain to reorganize itself. Although it has shown promise in the management of certain conditions such as attention-deficit/hyperactivity disorder,[14] there are very few published reports in the medical literature of its successful use in the treatment of headache. In contrast to conventional biofeedback that can often be learned within a few sessions with structured therapy manuals, neurofeedback typically requires a large number of sessions occurring several times a week, making it one of the more expensive and least validated of the biofeedback modalities when applied to migraine. At the time of this writing, only a handful of studies surfaced in an online survey of articles through pubmed MEDLINE for "neurofeedback" or "EEG biofeedback" in conjunction with "migraine," "headache," or "pain," with minimal data from uncontrolled studies with a very small number of patients.

Kropp, Siniatchkin, and Gerber have proposed an "empirically based" neurofeedback approach that utilizes feedback of slow cortical potentials with pronounced negativity that have been empirically shown to precede migraine attacks, sometimes by several days.[15] The results of their pilot research appear promising, but have limited clinical availability at this time. However, this specific type of neurofeedback differs from what is typically used by neurofeedback practitioners for other conditions.

The physician's role in biofeedback and relaxation training can be critical to its success. Patients may need an appropriate referral. The physician needs to inquire about the patient's progress, reinforce adherence to relaxation training and home practice, and provide compassionate confrontation on the need to increase adherence in noncompliant patients. Physicians can also direct motivated patients to self-help sources, including relaxation CDs and self-help books—Research Press is one excellent resource. Perhaps most importantly, physicians, nurses, and other health professionals can provide education on the *importance* of attending to behavioral factors in headache management.

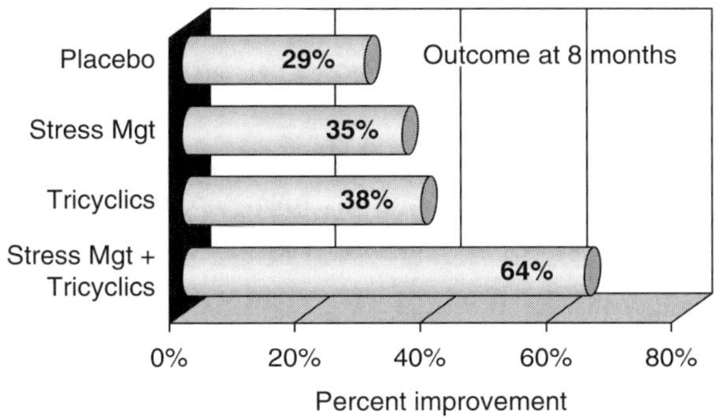

Figure 12-1 Stress management and tricyclics for chronic tension-type headache. From Holroyd, O'Donnell, Stensland et al, 2001[16]

Cognitive–Behavioral Therapy

Biofeedback and relaxation therapy is often combined with cognitive–behavioral therapy (CBT), a therapeutic modality that has shown significant benefit in the treatment of various psychiatric conditions that are common comorbid conditions with migraine, including anxiety,[16] obsessive–compulsive,[17] depressive,[18] and personality disorders.[19] CBT in combination with antidepressant and antianxiety medications appears particularly fruitful in preventing relapse when compared to psychotropic medication alone.[20] The combination of relaxation skills with CBT is sometimes referred to as "stress management training," and has been shown to add significantly to the benefit from tricyclic drug therapy for chronic tension-type headache, as illustrated in Figure 12.1.[21] See the chapter on other headache disorders by Jensen and Olesen for more detailed discussion of this study.

In brief, CBT incorporates a range of coping skills, including the recognition and correction of distortions in thinking such as categorizing stressors in "all or nothing" terms, overgeneralization, bias toward negative predictions of the future, and excessive self-blame. Patients are encouraged to become objective, dispassionate observers of their own thoughts rather than becoming "hooked" and active participants in counterproductive thinking. For example, patients can learn to address negative thoughts about headache or stressors in diverse ways:

- Confronting distorted negative thinking with logical self-talk
- Framing thoughts about stressors by devoting attention in limited periods of time (the "10-minute rule") and specific settings (a chair in the study, not the dinner table or when trying to sleep), followed with an appointment to return to it at a later time with reminders to "stop" if thoughts intrude before the appointment, or

- Mindfulness—allowing stressful thoughts to pass in and pass on, like watching a leaf fall from a tree to a floating stream, then drifting out of sight.

CBT also may incorporate elements of assertiveness training, with encouragement to confront stressful situations in an *appropriate* way rather than retreat and avoid, as in the following case example:

Case Example 1 : Self-efficacy

A woman in her 40s with continuous daily pain also experienced periodic acute migraines, some of them triggered by marital arguments. Her typical coping style was to escalate the argument, aggressively defend herself, then retire to her room and brood—"How can he keep doing this to me?"—convinced that she would have an inevitable, incapacitating headache the next day. Therapeutic discussion focused on the potential for her to control her emotional responses and prevent similar stress-related migraines, even if her husband persisted in provoking her.

She was successful at relaxation and biofeedback in the office, and began to believe that headache prevention was within her capability. The next time an argument emerged, she elected to stop the escalation, told her husband she was going to take a drive, turned on a classical music station on the car stereo, and told herself "I may not be able to control my husband's behavior, but I don't have to give him the keys to my emotions." She tried to look at the humor in the situation, as if she were watching a dark situation comedy. She maintained a sense of optimism that although she had been emotionally upset, she had succeeded in calming herself.

She expressed particular delight that there was no increase in headache activity the next day, for the first time after one of these fights. Of particular interest from a self-efficacy perspective is the observation that she did not employ the specific relaxation techniques she had practiced in the office, but creatively applied a number of different distraction and self-talk approaches that were already in her capability—the difference was a cognitive shift in her approach to the stressor, motivated by the belief that she could take control of her own emotional responding.

Coping Styles: Dysfunctional versus Adaptive

As headaches become more frequent, the headache itself often emerges as the primary stressor faced by the patient. A coping *style* is marked by a pervasive *pattern* of responding to pain, stressors, and/or affective distress. Attention, expectation, and beliefs about pain have physiological consequences. Although much of the work on the pathophysiology of migraine has focused on brain stem and neurovascular factors, "top-down" control or facilitation of pain processing is an important aspect of pain modulation, and may be central to understanding some cases of RM.[22]

Optimal Coping Requires Balance—Dysfunctional Coping Is Marked by Extremes

Functional coping styles rely on flexibility and balance, with a willingness to directly confront the experience of pain in a calm and intentional way. Adaptive coping is associated with enhanced treatment outcomes and a sense of self-efficacy—the individual's belief in the ability to control the headache, control emotional reactivity to pain, and/or achieve functional goals in the presence of pain. Dysfunctional coping is often marked by extremes: *excessive negative attention* to pain on the one hand, versus *failure to attend* to cues of impending or increasing pain severity of insufficient recognition or expression of negative affect. Optimal coping involves *balance* between these extremes.

Table 12.1 summarizes the need for balance in the application of relaxation versus distraction techniques. In clinical practice, some patients report becoming more aware of their pain when they attempt to relax, and do much better with distraction techniques, which can range from imagery (even active imagery, like watching a hockey game or redecorating their home), to crossword puzzles, to Sudoku, to drawing, listening to music (even hard rock in some cases), or talking with others about non–pain-related topics. But distraction can have a down side. For example, some patients note that they may block their awareness of migraine when deeply involved in their work, only to experience an intense escalation of pain with the let-down at the end of the work day. Exclusive reliance on distraction may block the patient's awareness of muscle tension and stress-related physiological arousal that continue to drive the headache.

The key to optimal coping is often learning how to balance these two approaches, shifting attention from one to the other depending on the situation and current level of pain. When patients are wired to biofeedback

Table 12-1 Relaxation vs. Distraction: Need for Balance

Relaxation	Distraction
Benefits	**Benefits**
Reduce arousal.	Reduce pain awareness.
Reduce anxiety and distress.	Activate brain stem mechanisms to block conscious awareness of nociception.
Prevent stress-related pain.	
Liabilities	**Liabilities**
Focus on body can enhance pain awareness.	Focus away from body can increase arousal, muscle tension.

Table 12-2 Two Extremes of Dysfunctional Coping

Sensitizing	Minimizing
Hypervigilance	**Alexithymia**
Attention to pain and changes in pain	(no words for feelings)
Catastrophizing	**Denial and Stoicism**
Rumination	Dissimulation
Magnification	
Helplessness	
Hyperempathy	**Suppression**
Excessive concern for others' pain	Distraction while maintaining high, unexpressed, or unacknowledged physiological arousal

machines, increases in physiological arousal can be easily observed and rectified when the patient is instructed to redirect attention to relaxing their neck or jaw, for example. Just as a golfer carries a bag of different clubs, each with its own advantage depending on the lay of the ball, the headache sufferer can benefit from a "bag" of coping techniques from both the relaxation and distraction ends of the spectrum, each with their advantages depending on the level of pain and the situation.

Dysfunctional coping be classified as excessively *sensitizing* or *minimizing*, as depicted in Table 12.2.

Hypervigilance

When individuals focus attention on the unpleasantness ("hurt") of painful sensations associated with nociceptive input, there is an increase in reported pain intensity, correlated with changes in the neural pain matrix from the midbrain through cortical regions, revealed through functional magnetic imaging (fMRI). In contrast, when the same subjects distract themselves from nociceptive input—whether through their own internal strategies, attention to more complex environmental tasks, or refocusing attention in a neutral way on the location of sensation rather than the associated discomfort—then pain intensity declines, with corresponding changes in the pain matrix.[23–26] Attention to pain speeds the processing of nociceptive stimuli.[27]

Some patients (and their families) maintain a frequent but ultimately dysfunctional cognitive search for any signal of an impending change in pain, analogous to instructions to focus on pain in the fMRI studies noted earlier. High levels of vigilance for pain are associated with heightened pain severity and pain-related fear.[28] For patients with episodic migraine, the headache diary can be an indispensable tool for uncovering triggering factors and monitoring treatment effectiveness. However, for RM patients with continuous pain—particularly those with high levels of pain intensity that vary little over time—maintaining a detailed headache diary over time can be counter-therapeutic, contributing to pain-related distress by requiring continued attention to pain. In contrast, diaries that focus on positive changes—goals accomplished, successful reductions in distress from relaxation techniques—can serve as distraction devices and help reinforce movement toward behavioral goals.

Catastrophizing

Catastrophizing goes beyond vigilance for pain to exaggerated negative cognitions about the actual or anticipated experience of pain. Clinical examples include thoughts such as "I can't stand this...this is killing me...my life is over...there is nothing I can do...I'll never get better." Factor analyses of the Pain Catastrophizing Scale have identified 3 independent factors in catastrophizing: rumination, magnification, and helplessness.[29] Pain catastrophizing is associated with increased activity in brain areas related to anticipation of pain, attention to pain, emotional aspects of pain, and motor control, with consequent influences on pain perception.[30]

In a nonclinical sample of 1018 subjects, higher scores on the Pain Catastrophizing Scale predicted the presence of weekly headache.[31] Within an otherwise healthy population of headache sufferers, higher levels of pain catastrophizing are associated with higher levels of depressive symptoms, greater headache pain, and more pain-related interference in functioning.[32] In a study of episodic migraine ($n = 1127$) and chronic daily headache with migrainous features ($n = 407$), reliance on catastrophizing and pain avoidance as coping strategies was predictive of headache chronicity; other predictors included psychological distress, an external locus of control, and the perceived headache impact.[33] For 232 frequent migraine sufferers, catastrophizing predicted impairment across five measures of functioning and quality of life—including a daily diary of the level of migraine-related disability—independent of migraine characteristics and other demographic and psychological variables.[34]

If not addressed, catastrophizing can play an important role in treatment failure. The strongest predictors of nonresponse to acute pharmacological therapy for migraine in a study of 1443 treated patients were psychological variables, including elevated scores on a measure of catastrophizing, suggesting that behavioral modification of coping strategies might improve outcome for pharmacological treatment.[35] Headache sufferers can learn to reduce catastrophizing, with associated reductions in anxiety and enhanced self-efficacy. In a randomized controlled trial, CBT targeting reduction of catastrophizing for chronic headache pain, half of the participants also experienced clinically meaningful reductions in headache indicators.[36]

Case Example 2 : Hypervigilance and Catastrophizing.

A woman in her mid-30s whom I had seen for several sessions was seated in the "dark room" (a separate waiting room left relatively dark and quiet for patients with light and sound sensitivity) when I went to get her for her appointment. In my office she reported a particularly severe headache that

(continued)

had not responded to her acute medication, and had almost considered cancelling her appointment. Since her compliance with home relaxation training had been minimal—despite my best efforts at facilitating adherence (see the chapter by Cady and others in this book)—I engaged her in a conversation about her pre-teen daughter, activities they enjoyed together, their summer vacation, and plans for the school year. She became more animated during the discussion, and after about 30 minutes she said her headaches had remitted to a moderate level. She reported a flash of insight—as she was retreating from pain, focusing on how severe it was, catastrophizing in the darkness, the pain remained up front and center; as she became involved in distraction and focusing on pleasurable activities, the pain actually lessened. We discussed how she could apply this concept at home, for example, playing cards or simple games with her daughter rather than retreating to her darkened bedroom.

Hyperempathy: Excessive Concern for the Pain of Others

Recent neuroimaging studies have shown that the neural substrates evoked in viewing others in painful circumstances (empathy for pain) share commonalities with the pain matrix activated by direct nociceptive stimulation.[37–40] In their article titled "Empathy hurts: compassion for another increases both sensory and affective components of pain perception," Loggia et al. were able to manipulate experimentally the level of empathy subjects felt for an actor, and then exposed the participants to heat stimuli of varying intensities while viewing the actor being exposed to similar stimuli. Subjects in the "high empathy" group rated the directly experienced noxious stimuli as both more intense and unpleasant than those in the "low empathy" group.[39] "Dispositional empathy" is significantly related to the level of parental distress and concern reported by parents when asked to imagine their child in several painful and stressful situations, further compounded by the degree of catastrophizing, and may lead to excessive reinforcement of pain behavior.[41]

Although hyperempathy has not been studied systematically in headache patients, in clinical practice some patients with RM are consumed by the physical or emotional pain of their parents or children, and can become swept up in the pain of others. Based on the evolving neuroimaging literature on empathy for others' pain, it appears plausible that this excessive level of concern can contribute to treatment intractability, and needs to be addressed.

Case Example 3 : Hyperempathy for a Significant Other's Pain

A high-school–age young man had failed to show any significant improvement in headache despite two admissions to our inpatient unit, multiple trials of prophylactic medications, and extensive practice of biofeedback and relaxation skills. Despite the continuous high level of pain, he maintained school attendance, had excellent grades, and planned a career in environmental law. He had a particularly close but supportive and non-controlling relationship with his mother, who had multiple pain problems of her own, and often accompanied him to his appointments.

It was only on detailed inquiry that he described his tendency to over-empathize with his mother's problems, consistent with what drove his interest in law—a desire to help others and contribute to a better world. This opened the door for a discussion of the difficulties posed by hyperempathy—that *feeling* another's pain can actually be an impediment. He did not feel responsible for his mother's medical problems, but reported feeling guilty if he directed attention elsewhere and did not remain mindful of them. We then discussed a number of coping and distancing techniques, including the use of self-talk to remind himself that distancing himself from feeling her hurt could actually allow him to feel better and more functional, just as a surgeon needs to remain focused on the task at hand rather than feeling his patient's discomfort and anxiety. He understood the concept, applied the approach, was able to graduate and go on to college away from home, with a gradual reduction in the severity of his headaches over time although they remained continuously present.

Alexithymia

Literally defined as "without words for feelings," alexithymia refers to significant difficulty in identifying feelings, differentiating emotional from physical states, and difficulty perceiving emotions in others, in stark contrast to the hypervigilant, catastrophizing, hyperempathic end of the spectrum of coping styles. Examples from clinical practice include those with intractable headache and significant functional impairment who deny even normal levels of frustration, report never feeling angry, and have the "perfect" marriage or family. Patients with alexithymia may score "zero" on depression or anxiety scales, well below the mean scores of nondepressed and nonanxious patients who report normal affect. Inquiry about the emotional impact of frequent, severe pain may lead to brief answers without elaboration—"it just hurts."

Although alexithymia has not yet been systematically studied in headache patients, the failure to recognize or differentiate emotional distress from pain is associated with increased difficulty in managing other chronic pain disorders. Large workplace samples[42] and epidemiological studies[43] have found significant associations between alexithymia and temporomandibular (TMD) symptoms, including the frequency of neck pain, head pain, tender teeth, overall pain symptoms, and painless TMD-related symptoms;[42] as well as facial pain, orolingual and dental pain, and difficulties in mouth opening.[43] In a study of adolescents with somatoform pain disorder, 59% had significant elements of alexithymia in contrast to only 1% of control subjects.[44] Low back pain is an occupational risk for San Francisco transit officers, reported by 31%.

Those who scored in the upper quartile of an alexithymia scale had an adjusted odds ratio (OR) of 2.00 for low back pain, an association that was significantly stronger for women (OR = 4.35) than men (OR = 1.83). The strongest association with low back pain was the factor "difficulty expressing feelings" (OR = 2.23).[45] In a study of chronic myofacial pain, alexithymia correlated positively with the affective (unpleasantness) component of pain, independent of self-efficacy or catastrophizing.[46]

Denial

Where alexithymia is generally understood to reflect a deficit in understanding and identifying emotional responding, denial is an active process, and can occur in patients who are capable of describing a wide range of feelings. Dysfunctional denial is marked by incongruity, either between a person's statements and behavior (e.g., loud voice and clenched fists while denying anger, lying about medication use) or between behavior and events (the father who calmly reads his paper during an explosive interaction between the son and mother; the wife who acts as if everything were normal when her spouse becomes increasingly intoxicated, loud, and inappropriate). Denial is often a significant issue in complex cases of medication overuse headache, where patients may lie about use, and dissimulate about the use of opioids to control negative affect, denying much distress in general.[47] The extent to which a patient relies on denial may not become clear until the patient has been in treatment for a period of time, or observed in a 24-hour milieu such as an inpatient unit. Denial is a "red flag" for trouble ahead. Denial has received little recent attention in the pain literature, although a recent phenomenological study of individuals with long-standing musculoskeletal pain has identified denial as one of four distinct coping styles, with acceptance at the other end of the spectrum[48] (see discussion of acceptance later).

Suppression of Anger and Negative Affect

The conscious suppression of negative emotions also differs from alexithymia, which appears to represent a deficit in the awareness and identification of emotions. Most work in this area has focused on anger. Several independent studies have consistently noted that suppressing anger by holding it in (anger-in) differentiates headache patients from non-headache controls, including unspecified headache,[49] tension-type headache,[50–52] and migraine.[52] Nicholson used statistical methods to control for the presence of depression and anxiety in a large-scale study of differences in anger expression between 171 individuals with nonspecified headache and 251 sex-matched controls. Those in the headache group had significantly higher levels of anger-in after controlling for depression and anxiety. In this study, it was the *coping style* of holding anger in that was strongest predictor of headache status, not the tendency to anger easily—trait anger was not a significant predictor of headache.[49] However, Perozzo et al. found not only an impairment in anger control, but also a higher level of angry temperament and angry reaction in both migraine and chronic tension-type headache than in headache-free subjects, and also suggested a connection between anger and the duration of headache experience.[53] Both anger and coping style were predictive of headache activity in a daily diary over the 2 weeks after the anger assessment for both migraine and chronic tension-type headache.[52]

Most of the research on anger suppression and pain is based on psychometric tests and correlational designs, and subject to criticism on that basis. In an alternative in vivo research design, Burns et al. were able to induce anger by use of a confederate who harassed their research subjects during completion of a computer maze task. Chronic low back pain patients who were instructed to suppress their expression of anger during this provocation reported more internally experienced anger and greater pain intensity during a subsequent structured task, and showed more pain behavior than those who were not so instructed.[54] Burns suggests that suppressing anger may ironically increase feelings of anger and sustain anger over time, leading to an exacerbation of experienced and expressed pain down the road. In a previous study of the relationship among anger management style, emotional suppression, and responses to experimentally induced pain (cold pressor test) in healthy subjects, subjects who scored high on measures of typically expressing anger (anger-out), who then suppressed negative emotions, were the most vulnerable to the pain-augmenting impact of anger-suppression.[55] Burns recently reviewed the evidence from several other studies that provide further support for the finding that suppressing anger expression during a provocative event may increase pain at a later point in time.[56]

Anger control includes aspects of both sensitizing and minimizing response styles, reflected in Burns' discussion of the "ironic process model"—the attempt to suppress anger when provoked (minimizing anger in the interpersonal relationship) can keep it smoldering under the surface (sensitizing).[56] For non-headache pain disorders, both anger-in and anger-out are associated with elevated chronic pain intensity across a diverse range of non-headache pain disorders.[57]

If suppressing appropriate anger is associated with augmentation of pain, what is the evidence that appropriate expression of anger has a salutatory effect for pain patients? Graham et al. randomly assigned patients at an outpatient chronic pain treatment center to two different letter-writing tasks: (1) constructive expression of anger about real-life events or (2) writing about goals in a nonemotional way. Over a 9-week period, participants in the anger-expression group ($n = 51$) experienced greater improvement in control over pain and depressed mood, and marginally greater improvement in pain severity than the control group ($n = 51$). Mediators of improvement included the degree of expressed anger. The extent to which the patients were able to speculate and express insight into the circumstances that precipitated their anger had a mediating effect on mood improvement.[58]

Although more research is necessary, these preliminary findings suggest that appropriately expressing anger—even at a later point in time about meaningful past events, and in a manner that may not directly be communicated to the individual involved in the anger provocation—may be helpful for chronic pain sufferers. Neuroimaging data reveal overlapping circuits underlying regulation of both pain and anger.[59] The association between anger-out expression and chronic pain intensity is at least partially mediated by endogenous opioid dysfunction.[60]

Proactive versus Reactive Coping

The most effective stress management strategy is to plan in advance how to address a situation, rather than attempting to manage the pain only when it reaches a severe level. This concept has equal applicability to the use of abortive medication (e.g., triptans) at the onset of headache, as it does to the use of behavioral methods.

Case Example 4 : Proactive Coping

A woman in her late 50s experienced a severe migraine at the end of her weekly phone calls to her elderly "controlling" mother. Despite excellent biofeedback skills and a consistent pattern of home practice, her migraine failed to respond to her efforts to relax once the call was over. Until she discussed it in therapy, it had not occurred to her to relax herself deeply *before* placing the call, while setting a mental goal to remain calm regardless of anything her mother said to her. When she began consistent use of that strategy, along with the thought "I may not be able to control my mother's behavior, but I don't have to allow her to control my emotions," she found she was able to complete the call with no escalation of headache. She also noted a few weeks later that "my mother is becoming a much nicer person." Her own emotional reactions to her mother's behavior had served to escalate an unpleasant interaction. When she no longer responded with nonverbal signs of irritation in response to perceived provocative comments, the calls evolved to a pattern of more pleasant interactions.

Proactive planning can increase functioning. For example, rather than decide at the last minute to avoid a family gathering due to a severe headache, or to go and suffer with the risk of creating a dramatic event if the pain gets out of hand, the patient can develop an "escape plan" in advance, including staying for a shortened time (pacing), how to signal her desire to leave when at the event, how to communicate her needs to the host or hostess, and how to get back home. The concept is to avoid a "black or white, either-or" approach to events, and to set behavioral goals to increase function rather than rely on avoidance and withdrawal.

Acceptance

Acceptance can be defined as the willingness to have pain and other uncomfortable private experiences—without taking action to control or eliminate them—as opposed to maintaining exclusive focus on pain reduction as the only acceptable outcome. In most cases, headache disorders are chronic conditions that can be managed and ameliorated, but not "cured" in the sense of total remission. The goals of behavioral interventions are not limited to reductions in the frequency and severity of headache, but also include less affective distress, or what might be referred to as increased "pain tolerance."[61] Some patients with severe forms of chronic daily headache initially reject behavioral interventions due to preconceived attitudes that pain reduction is the only acceptable outcome, reflected in comments such as "It doesn't 'work' if it doesn't take my pain away;" "I need pain control, not 'pain management;" or "I am not going to live my life like this."

Acceptance and Commitment Therapy (ACT) includes a commitment to engage in activities and set achievable goals regardless of pain, and to observe negative pain-related sensations and thoughts in a neutral or "mindful" way, rather than reacting emotionally to them.[62] Chronic pain patients who score high on measures of pain acceptance appear to be less detrimentally affected by catastrophizing.[63] In a review of 15 laboratory and clinical studies of pain, McCracken found that acceptance predicts positive outcomes, including lower pain intensity, less pain-related anxiety and avoidance, less depression, less functional impairment, more daily uptime, and better work status.[64] In a study of 252 consecutive patients who completed treatment on an interdisciplinary pain treatment unit, increasing acceptance and decreasing catastrophizing both accounted for significant variance in functional improvement, independent of and larger than the variance accounted for by change in pain intensity.[65] From survey research of a sample of 501 chronic pain patients, Viane et al. found that those scoring higher on a measure of pain acceptance reported giving less attention to pain. In a prospective diary study reported in the same article, patients with chronic pain kept records of pain intensity, the degree of attention to pain, and characteristics of goal-oriented behavior eight times a day. Higher levels of pain acceptance were associated with less attention to pain, more engagement with daily activities, greater motivation to complete activities, and increased efficacy in performing daily activities.[66]

In her book *The Body Broken*, Lynne Greenberg (associate professor of English at Hunter College) chronicles the onset of intractable, continuous head and neck pain 22 years after a serious motor vehicle accident that almost took her life.[67] The second half of the book discusses her treatment in a multidisciplinary inpatient headache program with outpatient follow-up. After learning that her cervical fusion after the accident rendered the pain-relevant nerves almost inaccessible for any anesthesiological intervention, she wrote the following in a chapter titled "Acceptance":

> One could no longer say with certainty that my condition had a surefire cure. No longer could I continue looking for the next

> doctor, the next procedure, the next drug to cure me....So I found myself in a new place. It was one of *acceptance* [italics added], a giving in, a letting go, accompanied by a firm faith in endurance....I could no longer stand the constant focus on getting better....Instead of focusing on a cure, I would place my energy into healing—in all its varied forms. I would practice calm. I would search for inner resolve....I might have chosen resignation, but in the interests of goodwill, of free will, of good coming of my will, I willed myself to choose acceptance instead. (pp 156–157)[67]

There is preliminary evidence of ACT efficacy for a variety of conditions in addition to chronic pain, including anxiety disorders, depression, trichotillomania, psychosis, drug abuse, and the management of epilepsy and diabetes,[62] suggesting a potentially fruitful area for future headache research.

Life Events, Trauma, and Histories of Abuse

Major Life Changes Within the Past Year

Significant life events and stressors in the preceding year are a risk factor for both the emergence of primary headache (see Fig. 12.2),[68] and the transformation of episodic migraine to chronic daily headache.[69] So-called "exit events"—deaths, separations, losses—appear to take the greatest toll.[68,69] The persistence of headache appears more related to the perceived frequency of daily hassles in a person's life.[70]

Sexual, Physical, and Emotional Abuse

Past traumatic events can influence how a person views subsequent situations that might appear to be of much less objective significance. In a study of 949 women with migraine from six specialty headache clinics, who completed

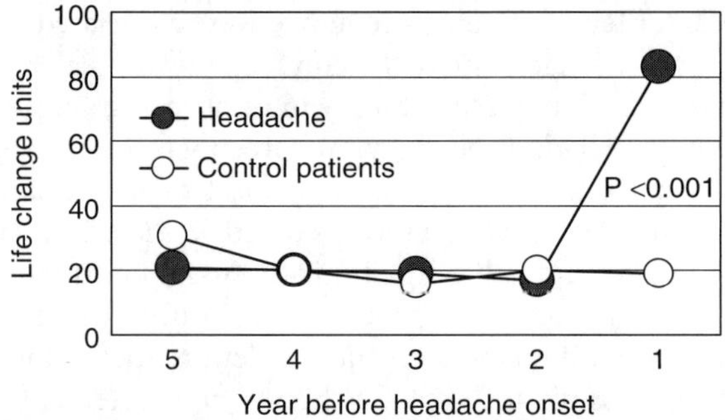

Figure 12-2 Major life changes in the years before headache onset.
From De Benedittis, Lorenzetti, & Pieri, 1990[64]

Table 12-3 Relationship of Childhood Abuse to Major Depression in Migraine Patients

Migraineurs with current major depression:
• More likely to report history of physical and sexual abuse than nondepressed patients ($p < 0.001$)
• More likely to report sexual abuse before age 12, Odds Ratio = 2.30 [95% CI = 1.14–4.77]
• For abuse both before and after age 12, risk of major depression increases significantly Odds Ratio = 5.08 [95% CI = 2.15–11.99]
• More likely to report multiple types of maltreatment Odds Ratio = 2.07 [95% CI = 1.27–3.35]

From ref. 67.

a confidential questionnaire regarding childhood maltreatment, Tietjen and colleagues found a prevalence of childhood physical or sexual abuse in 38% (12% reporting both types of abuse). Histories of abuse were significantly related to comorbid depression, as shown in Table 12.3.[71]

How does this high rate of reported abuse in headache patients at specialty clinics—a nonrandom sample—compare with base rates of reported abuse in the general population? A meta-analysis of 65 epidemiological studies covering 22 countries published in 2009 by Pereda and colleagues found an international prevalence of sexual abuse as a child in 7.9% of men and 19.7% of women.[72] A geographic, randomized sample of 1442 subjects in the United States (2003) found a prevalence of childhood *sexual abuse* in 14.2% of men and 32.3% of women. Childhood *physical abuse* was more prevalent in men (22.2%) than in women (19.5%).[73] Studies in Europe find prevalence rates for sexual abuse of 6% to 36% of girls under age 16 and 1% to 15% of boys, with physical abuse prevalence ranging from 5% to 50% across both sexes.[74] The National Comorbidity Survey in the United States (population sample, $n = 5877$) found childhood sexual and physical abuse to be associated with the 1-year prevalence of serious health problems for men and women, partially mediated by the participants' psychiatric disorders.[75]

Several studies have identified a history of childhood sexual or physical abuse as a statistical risk factor for the incidence of recurrent headaches.[76–80] However, a recent meta-analysis of childhood sexual abuse and lifetime diagnosis of somatic disorders published by Paras et al. in *JAMA* (2009) found no statistically significant association between sexual abuse and a lifetime diagnosis of headache (or fibromyalgia or obesity), but did reveal abuse history as a significant risk factor for chronic nonspecific pain and pelvic pain, functional gastrointestinal disorders, and psychogenic seizures.[81] Abuse involving penetration and multiple incidents appears to be the most harmful, and the health effects associated with a history of abuse occur in men as well as women.[79] For example, when abuse involved rape, the odds ratio (OR) for the relationship with abuse and fibromyalgia in the Paras study increased from 1.61 (nonsignificant) to 3.35, although abuse including rape headache still did not emerge as a risk factor for headache disorders.[81]

From a clinical perspective, perhaps the most important question is whether a history of abuse in headache sufferers is associated with headache chronicity or intractability, rather than simply the incidence or presence of a headache disorder. In a retrospective chart review of 183 consecutive new patients at an outpatient tertiary-care headache center, Peterlin et al. found a significantly higher rate of reported abuse history in patients with chronic daily headache (40.0%) than episodic migraine (27.3%), suggesting that this may be the case.[82] Women with both migraine and major depression are more likely to report sexual abuse occurring before age 12 than those without depression, with the strongest relationship for comorbid relationship with abuse occurring both before and after age 12.[71]

One positive note is that several structured approaches to psychotherapy, including (but not limited to) exposure therapy with or without CBT, can help meliorate some of the psychological sequelae of abuse such as post-traumatic stress disorder,[79,83,84] with resultant improvement in quality of life. It appears plausible that reducing current distress related to memories of past abuse could be of significant benefit to the patient with RM. However, no study has yet shown a significant reduction in headache activity after psychotherapy directed toward managing feelings about past abuse.

Patients with RM may fail to spontaneously volunteer information about ongoing situations or past events that may play a significant role in contributing to treatment intractability. The reasons for reticence are multiple, but sometimes it can be as simple as "no one asked me." Patients in our practice complete a detailed questionnaire before the initial visit about their life experiences, beginning with straightforward information about marriage, children, occupation, education, and family of origin to more personal information about stressors including past histories of abuse or traumatic events. Responses to the questionnaire serve as points of departure for further questioning. However, even when patients leave those sections blank, it is helpful to routinely repeat the question in the interview, sometimes two or three times in different formats: "Any significant changes in your life in the past year?" "Any difficult circumstances in your life that we haven't discussed?" It is important to be direct: "This is a question I routinely ask all my patients—have you ever

Table 12-4 Suggestions for Inquiry and Discussion of Abuse in Headache Patients

- Ask clear and specific questions, but
  - Discussion of abuse can cause significant distress—assess patient's comfort level, ask permission to inquire further, offer empathy.
- Separate patient from family for in depth inquiry.
- Current abuse is greatest concern!
- Don't blame patient's headaches on abuse ("Your limbic system has been damaged.")
- Patients differ significantly in the extent to which they have emotionally processed abuse.
- Refer appropriate patients for psychotherapy.

Case Example 5 : Past Sexual Abuse and Its Current Impact

In my initial interview, one patient wrote a brief comment about having been molested by an older male cousin when she was 5 years old. The abuse was time-limited during a family vacation one summer. She never reported it to her family. When asked about the extent to which it still affected her, she tearfully said "I think about it every day." I then inquired about the extent to which she was addressing this in her ongoing psychotherapy. She replied that it never came up—"The therapist never asked me if had been abused, and now I'm embarrassed to bring it up." After taking a few moments to help her calm herself, commending her for her courage in revealing this traumatic event, she agreed to allow me to communicate this to her therapist, and assured me she would open discussion of the issue in her next scheduled session.

been physically, sexually, or emotionally mistreated?" When the question is greeted with silence, a compassionate comment ("This can be difficult to talk about…") may open the door for further discussion. Table 12.4 offers suggestions for inquiry and discussion of abuse issues.

Emotional abuse can be as devastating as physical maltreatment. Ongoing, current abuse is of even greater significance than remote histories of abuse,[85] and needs to be identified, as illustrated in Case Example 6.

Case Example 6 : Undisclosed Current Major Stressors

A woman in her mid-50s was referred to our practice by another headache specialist, having failed numerous prior treatment approaches. She requested her current husband come into the psychological interview with her, and appeared to be quite supportive. On our written questionnaire—which she had reviewed with her husband—she identified no significant stressors in her life at this time other than her disabling headache and "hyperactivity" in her preteen daughter, for which they were in family counseling. She also reported a 20-year history of physical abuse in her first marriage, with at least one episode of forced sexual activity.

In the interview, I asked again if there were any significant *current* stressors. She turned away from her husband in her chair, and looking at him out of the corner of her eye said "It's hard to live with a perfectionist." After further discussion, I asked her husband to leave the room so that I might talk with her privately. She was then able to share with me details about her husband's periodic explosions of anger at her subsequent to his traumatic brain injury several years previously, which occurred several days a month.

(continued)

It was only in the second interview several days later, when I asked again if her current husband had ever physically touched her in anger, that she tearfully confided there were two occasions: a shoving incident she discussed on the first interview, and a second incident during which he had put his hands around her neck as if to choke her. She had never discussed this with her referring neurologist, had never pursued psychotherapy despite her headache-related depression, and never attempted relaxation training despite her obvious levels of headache-related distress. Since her husband's anger was directed at her and not her daughter, it had apparently never surfaced in their family counseling either.

With her permission, I compassionately confronted her husband on the need for him to take responsibility to control his anger, while underscoring that he clearly cared about her or he would not have driven with her several hundred miles to come to this appointment. I referred her for individual cognitive–behavioral psychotherapy to deal with these issues (which were not a part of her daughter's family-focused counseling), and that he might benefit from structured help (possibly including medication) to control his anger. These types of problems are not resolved quickly or easily, but the first step to resolution is identification of the problem, followed by acceptance of responsibility to do something about it. Her headaches had actually improved significantly during several days of outpatient medical treatment. However, *maintenance* of improvement on return to her home may require continued attention to stress management.

Behavioral Factors Underlying Medication Overuse

Medication overuse headache (MOH) is not a unitary phenomenon. In cases of RM with medication overuse, behavioral issues of obsessive drug-taking may be particularly important. The proposed distinction by Saper and Lake between Simple MOH (type 1) and Complex MOH (type 2) is discussed in detail in our chapter on inpatient treatment and other sources. In brief, relatively short-term overuse of triptans or simple analgesics (type 1) may be more easily managed than overuse of opioids and butalbital over a longer time, in patients with comorbid psychiatric disorders (including personality disorders) and a history of relapse (type 2).[61,86]

Using the Mini International Neuropsychiatric Interview to determine psychiatric diagnoses, Radat et al. completed a comparative study of psychiatric comorbidity in 41 patients with episodic migraine with no history of medication overuse with 41 patients with MOH evolving from a prior history of episodic migraine.[87] As illustrated in Tables 12.4 and 12.5, they found a higher rate of psychiatric comorbidity in the MOH patients. In addition, they

Table 12-5 DSM-IV Psychiatric Disorders in MOH vs Episodic Migraine

DSM-IV Diagnosis	MOH (%)	Migraine (%)	Odds Ratio
Major depression	39	2	21.8
Panic disorder	24	2	12.1
Generalized anxiety	42	10	6.0
Social phobia	34	12	4.3
Substance disorders	44	15	7.6

n = 82 (41 MOH, 41 migraine). Headache clinic sample. Diagnosis based on Mini-International Neuropsychiatric Interview (MINI). From ref. 83.

Table 12-6 Psychiatric Disorders in MOH: Chronology of Onset

DSM-IV Diagnosis	Precedes MOH (%)	Follows (%)
First major depressive episode	76	24
Panic disorder	79	21
Generalized anxiety disorder	80	20
Social phobia	100	0
Substance disorder	89	11

N = 41 (MOH evolving from migraine). Headache clinic sample. Diagnosis and chronology of onset based on Mini International Neuropsychiatric Interview (MINI) From ref. 83.

Table 12-7 Psychiatric Disorders in Family Members of Patients with MOH

DSM-IV Diagnosis	Odds Ratio
Mood disorders	1.7
Substance disorders (alcohol or illicit drugs)	2.8

From ref. 83.

found that development of the psychiatric disorder was much more likely to *precede* than *follow* the onset of MOH. They also interviewed the family members of patients, and found that the presence of both mood and substance use disorders in family members increased the relative risk of developing MOH, suggesting the potential relevance of both genetic factors and psychosocial modeling in predisposing patients to MOH.

In a later study by Radat and colleagues, senior neurologists using a structured questionnaire interviewed 247 patients with MOH, most of whom (87%) had a prior history of primary migraine.[88] Overused drugs included triptans (46%), opioids (43%), or nonopioid analgesics (28%), with some patients overusing more than one class of medications. Based on a structured interview with senior neurologists, two-thirds of these patients met criteria for drug dependence as established by the American Psychiatric Association (DSM-IV),[89] requiring three or more of the following:

1. Tolerance
2. Withdrawal symptoms
3. Substance taken in larger amounts or longer than intended
4. Persistent desire or failed efforts to reduce substance use
5. Significant time spent in activities necessary to obtain the substance
6. Giving up important activities due to substance use
7. Substance use is continued despite knowledge of persistent or current physical or psychological problems that are likely to have been caused or exacerbated by the substance.

Risk factors for dependence were both headache-related (prior history of migraine, unilateral headaches) and behavioral (reliance on opioids, previous history of withdrawal). Cupini et al. found a significantly higher rate of subclinical obsessive–compulsive behavior in patients with medication overuse headache compared to chronic migraine without MOH, episodic migraine, and non-headache control subjects, and raise the possibility of obsessive drug-taking as a contributing factor to MOH.[90]

The importance of addressing behavioral factors in MOH is illustrated by studies of relapse rates after drug withdrawal and prophylactic pharmacotherapy. Most relapse occurs during the first year after treatment: 31% at 6 months, 41% at 1 year, and 45% at 4 years post-withdrawal.[91,92] As shown in Figure 12.3, the highest rates of relapse involved analgesics, including opioids.

The addition of behavioral therapy (biofeedback) along with withdrawal of the overused drug and prophylactic pharmacotherapy can reduce relapse rates significantly.[93–95] In addition to the lower relapse rate shown in Figure 12.4, Grazzi et al. also found a significantly lower frequency of headaches in the combined biofeedback + prophylactic medication group 4 years after drug withdrawal (11 vs. 18 days/month), with less reliance on analgesics (4 vs. 20 analgesics/month). For most patients in my experience, biofeedback may

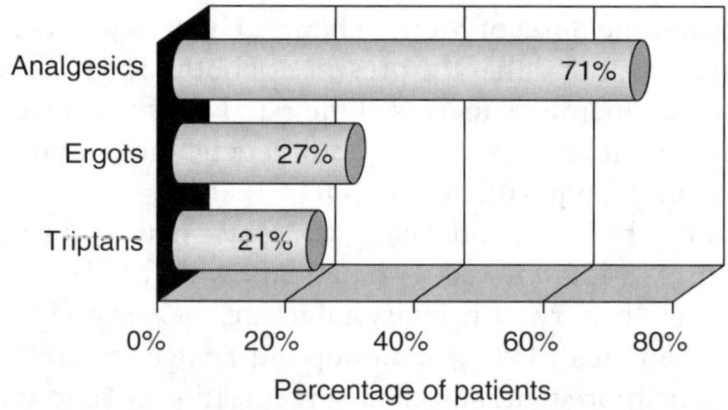

Figure 12-3 Medication overuse headache: Relapse rates 4 years after withdrawal.
From Katsarava, Muessig, Dzagnidze et al. 2005[88]

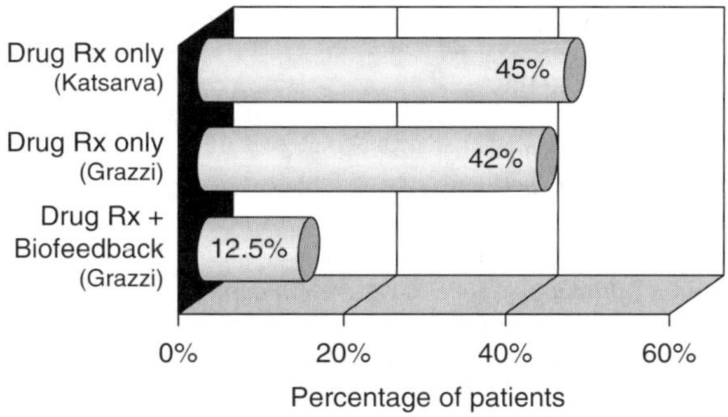

Figure 12-4 Behavioral therapy reduces medication overuse headache relapse rates 3–4 years after withdrawal.

Katsarava et al. 2005[88] (4 years post withdrawal)
Grazzi et al. 2002[90] (4 years post withdrawal)

allow the patient to abort *some* headaches, but the significant difference in the ratio of analgesics to headache days in the Grazzi study suggests that patients are learning *pain tolerance*,[96] using biofeedback skills to reduce pain-related distress rather than medicating all their headaches. Continued reliance on drugs as the only means of managing acute headache episodes puts the headache sufferer at higher risk of MOH relapse.

A small pilot study by Altieri et al. of short-term psychodynamic psychotherapy as an addition to drug withdrawal and prophylactic pharmacotherapy has also showed promise of improved outcomes in terms of headache frequency, medication use, and lower rates of relapse at 12-month follow-up.[97]

Rothrock has demonstrated the value of behavioral education in the form of a "headache school" consisting of three 90-minute structured classes taught by lay migraineurs who had all received intensive training from a senior neurologist. At 6-month follow-up, those who attended the school used significantly less abortive therapy, with less analgesic overuse than the control group. The also reported less headache days per month, experience less headache-related functional incapacitation, and made fewer headache-related calls to the clinic or unscheduled visits.[98]

Family Interaction Related to Headache

Even episodic migraine takes a significant toll on the family, with multiple adverse effects.[99–102] Families can be allies in treatment, advocating for the patient, providing supplemental information, helping the patient recall what occurred in his or her medical or psychological consultations, and providing cuing and reinforcement for adaptive coping skills. On the other hand, families can sometimes enable dysfunctional behavior, and act as angry warriors on behalf of the patient.[47] All of the preceding six issues, beginning with goal setting, take place in a family context. Pain-related behavior communicates a message that can transcend the acknowledgement of hurt. Some of the more

Table 12-8 Optimal Family Functioning in Refractory Migraine – Need for Balance

Modulate family attention to pain
• Set limited time frame for discussion of pain (the "10-minute rule")
• Center most communication on non-pain topics
Determine appropriate level of self-care
• *Provide support – avoid excessive dependency*
Set achievable functional goals, regardless of pain
• *Avoid "all or nothing" thinking – "Some is better than none"*
Plan and reinforce proactive coping
Encourage others to maintain normal activities
• *Avoid lifestyle centered around patient's limitations*

troubling aspects of pain-related family interaction are discussed in more detail in the chapter on inpatient strategies.

In our experience, patients and families often benefit from developing a proactive strategy for the discussion and management of pain. We encourage the selection of certain times of day for the report of headache to family members, including a discussion of what the patient intends to do about it (take medication, relax, keep going) and any appropriate requests of the family (keeping the sound level down a little). Appropriateness of requests for help are discussed openly and negotiated—appropriate self-care lessens excessive dependency and facilitates self-efficacy. The patient agrees to let others know when the pain improves, or keep them updated on pain status at some later point in time. Family members are encouraged to continue normal activities, rather than let the patient's pain totally dominate family functioning. These suggestions are outlined in Table 12.8.

Concluding Comments: Role of Physician, Successful Referrals

Most patients first seek help for their headaches from physicians. Physicians may need to provide the spark to ignite patient interest in self-help and behavioral issues that may be critical to effective remediation of RM, and encourage follow-through on referrals to psychologists and other behavioral health-care providers. Biofeedback and relaxation training are among the "basics" of headache management for primary migraine, and should not be ignored when a patient's headache fails to respond to standard pharmacological treatment. At times, the physician may need to schedule a special session to discuss coping styles, to encourage and reinforce self-help efforts, to ask about traumatic life events including histories of abuse, to identify behavioral factors in medication overuse headache, and/or to involve the family in a discussion of headache-related interaction.

Most patients with RM can benefit from consultation with appropriately trained psychologists, clinical social workers, or licensed counselors who have interest and training in the treatment of chronic headache. The key to a successful referral is communication—communication with the patient on the potential benefit; communication with the consultant through brief letters, copies of chart notes, or phone calls; and follow-up communication to assess patient involvement in treatment and adherence with behavioral recommendations. Successful management of RM often requires a team approach of physicians with other allied health professionals who communicate with each other and work toward a common goal.

References

1. Packard RC. What does the headache patient want? *Headache.* 1979;19(7): 370–374.
2. Colloca L, Sigaudo M, Benedetti F. The role of learning in nocebo and placebo effects. *Pain.* 2008;136(1–2):211–218.
3. Zubieta JK, Bueller JA, Jackson LR, et al. Placebo effects mediated by endogenous opioid activity on mu-opioid receptors. *J Neurosci.* 2005;25(34): 7754–7762.
4. Heath RL, Saliba M, Mahmassani O, Major SC, Khoury BA. Locus of control moderates the relationship between headache pain and depression. *J Headache Pain.* 2008;9(5):301–308.
5. Marlowe N. Self-efficacy moderates the impact of stressful events on headache. *Headache.* 1998;38(9):662–667.
6. Nestoriuc Y, Martin A, Rief W, Andrasik F. Biofeedback treatment for headache disorders: a comprehensive efficacy review. *Appl Psychophysiol Biofeedback.* 2008;33(3):125–140.
7. Wiech K, Ploner M, Tracey I. Neurocognitive aspects of pain perception. *Trends Cogn Sci.* 2008;12(8):306–313.
8. Colloca L, Tinazzi M, Recchia S, et al. Learning potentiates neurophysiological and behavioral placebo analgesic responses. *Pain.* 15 2008;139(2):306–314.
9. Zubieta JK, Stohler CS. Neurobiological mechanisms of placebo responses. *Ann N Y Acad Sci.* 2009;1156:198–210.
10. Schulman EA, Lake AE, 3rd, Goadsby PJ, et al. Defining refractory migraine and refractory chronic migraine: proposed criteria from the Refractory Headache Special Interest Section of the American Headache Society. *Headache.* 2008;48(6):778–782.
11. Schulman EA, Peterlin BL, Lake AE, 3rd, et al. Defining refractory migraine: results of the RHSIS Survey of American Headache Society members. *Headache.* 2009;49(4):509–518.
12. Campbell J, Penzien D, Wall E, et al. Evidence-based guidelines for migraine headache: behavioral and physical treatments. http://www.aan.com. 1999.
13. Nestoriuc Y, Martin A. Efficacy of biofeedback for migraine: a meta-analysis. *Pain.* 2007;128(1–2):111–127.
14. Arns M, de Ridder S, Strehl U, Breteler M, Coenen A. Efficacy of neurofeedback treatment in ADHD: the effects on inattention, impulsivity and hyperactivity: a meta-analysis. *Clin EEG Neurosci.* 2009;40(3): 180–189.
15. Kropp P, Siniatchkin M, Gerber WD. On the pathophysiology of migraine–links for "empirically based treatment" with neurofeedback. *Appl Psychophysiol Biofeedback.* 2002;27(3):203–213.

16. Ost LG. Cognitive behavior therapy for anxiety disorders: 40 years of progress. *Nord J Psychiatry.* 2008;62(Suppl 47):5–10.
17. Anholt GE, Kempe P, de Haan E, et al. Cognitive versus behavior therapy: processes of change in the treatment of obsessive-compulsive disorder. *Psychother Psychosom.* 2008;77(1):38–42.
18. Fava GA, Ruini C, Rafanelli C, Finos L, Conti S, Grandi S. Six-year outcome of cognitive behavior therapy for prevention of recurrent depression. *Am J Psychiatry.* 2004;161(10):1872–1876.
19. Leichsenring F, Leibing E. The effectiveness of psychodynamic therapy and cognitive behavior therapy in the treatment of personality disorders: a meta-analysis. *Am J Psychiatry.* 2003;160(7):1223–1232.
20. Hollon SD, Stewart MO, Strunk D. Enduring effects for cognitive behavior therapy in the treatment of depression and anxiety. *Annu Rev Psychol.* 2006; 57:285–315.
21. Holroyd KA, O'Donnell FJ, Stensland M, Lipchik GL, Cordingley GE, Carlson BW. Management of chronic tension-type headache with tricyclic antidepressant medication, stress management therapy, and their combination: a randomized controlled trial. *Jama.* 2001;285(17): 2208–2215.
22. Lake AE, 3rd. Headache as a stressor: dysfunctional versus adaptive coping styles. *Headache.* 2009;49(9):1369-1377.
23. Bantick SJ, Wise RG, Ploghaus A, Clare S, Smith SM, Tracey I. Imaging how attention modulates pain in humans using functional MRI. *Brain.* 2002;125(Pt 2):310–319.
24. Kulkarni B, Bentley DE, Elliott R, et al. Attention to pain localization and unpleasantness discriminates the functions of the medial and lateral pain systems. *Eur J Neurosci.* 2005;21(11):3133–3142.
25. Miron D, Duncan GH, Bushnell MC. Effects of attention on the intensity and unpleasantness of thermal pain. *Pain.* 1989;39(3):345–352.
26. Tracey I, Ploghaus A, Gati JS, et al. Imaging attentional modulation of pain in the periaqueductal gray in humans. *J Neurosci.* 2002;22(7): 2748–2752.
27. Zampini M, Bird KS, Bentley DE, et al. 'Prior entry' for pain: attention speeds the perceptual processing of painful stimuli. *Neurosci Lett.* 2007;414(1): 75–79.
28. Goubert L, Crombez G, Van Damme S. The role of neuroticism, pain catastrophizing and pain-related fear in vigilance to pain: a structural equations approach. *Pain.* 2004;107(3):234–241.
29. Van Damme S, Crombez G, Bijttebier P, Goubert L, Van Houdenhove B. A confirmatory factor analysis of the Pain Catastrophizing Scale: invariant factor structure across clinical and non-clinical populations. *Pain.* 2002;96(3): 319–324.
30. Gracely RH, Geisser ME, Giesecke T, et al. Pain catastrophizing and neural responses to pain among persons with fibromyalgia. *Brain.* 2004;127(Pt 4): 835–843.
31. Drahovzal DN, Stewart SH, Sullivan MJ. Tendency to catastrophize somatic sensations: pain catastrophizing and anxiety sensitivity in predicting headache. *Cogn Behav Ther.* 2006;35(4):226–235.

32. Buenaver LF, Edwards RR, Smith MT, Gramling SE, Haythornthwaite JA. Catastrophizing and pain-coping in young adults: associations with depressive symptoms and headache pain. *J Pain.* 2008;9(4):311–319.
33. Radat F, Lanteri-Minet M, Nachit-Ouinekh F, et al. The GRIM2005 study of migraine consultation in France. III: Psychological features of subjects with migraine. *Cephalalgia.* 2009;29(3):338–350.
34. Holroyd KA, Drew JB, Cottrell CK, Romanek KM, Heh V. Impaired functioning and quality of life in severe migraine: the role of catastrophizing and associated symptoms. *Cephalalgia.* 2007;27(10):1156–1165.
35. Lucas C, Lanteri-Minet M, Massiou H, et al. The GRIM2005 study of migraine consultation in France II. Psychological factors associated with treatment response to acute headache therapy and satisfaction in migraine. *Cephalalgia.* 2007;27(12):1398–1407.
36. Thorn BE, Pence LB, Ward LC, et al. A randomized clinical trial of targeted cognitive behavioral treatment to reduce catastrophizing in chronic headache sufferers. *J Pain.* 2007;8(12):938–949.
37. Gu X, Han S. Attention and reality constraints on the neural processes of empathy for pain. *Neuroimage.* 2007;36(1):256–267.
38. Jackson PL, Brunet E, Meltzoff AN, Decety J. Empathy examined through the neural mechanisms involved in imagining how I feel versus how you feel pain. *Neuropsychologia.* 2006;44(5):752–761.
39. Loggia ML, Mogil JS, Bushnell MC. Empathy hurts: compassion for another increases both sensory and affective components of pain perception. *Pain.* 2008;136(1–2):168–176.
40. Singer T, Seymour B, O'Doherty J, Kaube H, Dolan RJ, Frith CD. Empathy for pain involves the affective but not sensory components of pain. *Science.* 2004;303(5661):1157–1162.
41. Goubert L, Vervoort T, Sullivan MJ, Verhoeven K, Crombez G. Parental emotional responses to their child's pain: the role of dispositional empathy and catastrophizing about their child's pain. *J Pain.* 2008;9(3):272–279.
42. Ahlberg J, Nikkila H, Kononen M, et al. Associations of perceived pain and painless TMD-related symptoms with alexithymia and depressive mood in media personnel with or without irregular shift work. *Acta Odontol Scand.* 2004;62(3):119–123.
43. Sipila K, Veijola J, Jokelainen J, et al. Association of symptoms of TMD and orofacial pain with alexithymia: an epidemiological study of the Northern Finland 1966 Birth Cohort. *Cranio.* 2001;19(4):246–251.
44. Burba B, Oswald R, Grigaliunien V, Neverauskiene S, Jankuviene O, Chue P. A controlled study of alexithymia in adolescent patients with persistent somatoform pain disorder. *Can J Psychiatry.* 2006;51(7):468–471.
45. Mehling WE, Krause N. Are difficulties perceiving and expressing emotions associated with low-back pain? The relationship between lack of emotional awareness (alexithymia) and 12-month prevalence of low-back pain in 1180 urban public transit operators. *J Psychosom Res.* 2005;58(1):73–81.
46. Lumley MA, Smith JA, Longo DJ. The relationship of alexithymia to pain severity and impairment among patients with chronic myofascial pain: comparisons with self-efficacy, catastrophizing, and depression. *J Psychosom Res.* 2002;53(3):823–830.

47. Lake AE, 3rd. Behavioral medicine for chronic headache: overview and practical tools for the practicing physician. *Continuum.* 2006;12(6):235–258
48. Afrell M, Biguet G, Rudebeck CE. Living with a body in pain—between acceptance and denial. *Scand J Caring Sci.* 2007;21(3):291–296.
49. Nicholson RA, Gramling SE, Ong JC, Buenaver L. Differences in anger expression between individuals with and without headache after controlling for depression and anxiety. *Headache.* 2003;43(6):651–663.
50. Arena JG, Bruno GM, Rozantine GS, Meador KJ. A comparison of tension headache sufferers and nonpain controls on the State-Trait Anger Expression Inventory: an exploratory study with implications for applied psychophysiologists. *Appl Psychophysiol Biofeedback.* 1997;22(3): 209–214.
51. Hatch JP, Schoenfeld LS, Boutros NN, Seleshi E, Moore PJ, Cyr-Provost M. Anger and hostility in tension-type headache. *Headache.* 1991;31(5): 302–304.
52. Materazzo F, Cathcart S, Pritchard D. Anger, depression, and coping interactions in headache activity and adjustment: a controlled study. *J Psychosom Res.* 2000;49(1):69–75.
53. Perozzo P, Savi L, Castelli L, et al. Anger and emotional distress in patients with migraine and tension-type headache. *J Headache Pain.* 2005;6(5):392–399.
54. Burns JW, Quartana P, Gilliam W, et al. Effects of anger suppression on pain severity and pain behaviors among chronic pain patients: evaluation of an ironic process model. *Health Psychol.* 2008;27(5):645–652.
55. Burns JW, Quartana PJ, Bruehl S. Anger management style moderates effects of emotion suppression during initial stress on pain and cardiovascular responses during subsequent pain-induction. *Ann Behav Med.* 2007;34(2):154–165.
56. Burns JW, Quartana PJ, Bruehl S. Anger inhibition and pain: conceptualizations, evidence and new directions. *J Behav Med.* 2008;31(3):259–279.
57. Fernandez E. The relationship between anger and pain. *Curr Pain Headache Rep.* 2005;9(2):101–105.
58. Graham JE, Lobel M, Glass P, Lokshina I. Effects of written anger expression in chronic pain patients: making meaning from pain. *J Behav Med.* 2008;31(3):201–212.
59. Bruehl S, Burns JW, Chung OY, Chont M. Pain-related effects of trait anger expression: neural substrates and the role of endogenous opioid mechanisms. *Neurosci Biobehav Rev.* 2009;33(3):475–491.
60. Bruehl S, Chung OY, Burns JW, Diedrich L. Trait anger expressiveness and pain-induced beta-endorphin release: support for the opioid dysfunction hypothesis. *Pain.* 2007;130(3):208–215.
61. Lake AE, 3rd. Medication overuse headache: biobehavioral issues and solutions. *Headache.* 2006;46(Suppl 3):S88–97.
62. Pull CB. Current empirical status of acceptance and commitment therapy. *Curr Opin Psychiatry.* 2009;22(1):55–60.
63. Vowles KE, McCracken LM, Eccleston C. Patient functioning and catastrophizing in chronic pain: the mediating effects of acceptance. *Health Psychol.* 2008;27(2 Suppl):S136–143.

64. McCracken LM, Vowles KE. Acceptance of chronic pain. *Curr Pain Headache Rep.* 2006;10(2):90–94.
65. Vowles KE, McCracken LM, Eccleston C. Processes of change in treatment for chronic pain: the contributions of pain, acceptance, and catastrophizing. *Eur J Pain.* 2007;11(7):779–787.
66. Viane I, Crombez G, Eccleston C, Devulder J, De Corte W. Acceptance of the unpleasant reality of chronic pain: effects upon attention to pain and engagement with daily activities. *Pain.* 2004;112(3):282–288.
67. Greenberg L. *The body broken: a memoir.* New York: Random House; 2009.
68. De Benedittis G, Lorenzetti A, Pieri A. The role of stressful life events in the onset of chronic primary headache. *Pain.* 1990;40(1):65–75.
69. Scher AI, Lipton RB, Stewart W. Risk factors for chronic daily headache. *Curr Pain Headache Rep.* 2002;6(6):486–491.
70. De Benedittis G, Lorenzetti A. The role of stressful life events in the persistence of primary headache: major events vs. daily hassles. *Pain.* 1992;51(1):35–42.
71. Tietjen GE, Brandes JL, Digre KB, et al. History of childhood maltreatment is associated with comorbid depression in women with migraine. *Neurology.* 2007;69(10):959–968.
72. Pereda N, Guilera G, Forns M, Gomez-Benito J. The prevalence of child sexual abuse in community and student samples: a meta-analysis. *Clin Psychol Rev.* 2009;29(4):328–338.
73. Briere J, Elliott DM. Prevalence and psychological sequelae of self-reported childhood physical and sexual abuse in a general population sample of men and women. *Child Abuse Negl.* 2003;27(10):1205–1222.
74. Lampe A. [The prevalence of childhood sexual abuse, physical abuse and emotional neglect in Europe]. *Z Psychosom Med Psychother.* 2002;48(4):370–380.
75. Sachs-Ericsson N, Blazer D, Plant EA, Arnow B. Childhood sexual and physical abuse and the 1–year prevalence of medical problems in the National Comorbidity Survey. *Health Psychol.* 2005;24(1):32–40.
76. Diaz-Olavarrieta C, Ellertson C, Paz F, de Leon SP, Alarcon-Segovia D. Prevalence of battering among 1780 outpatients at an internal medicine institution in Mexico. *Soc Sci Med.* 2002;55(9):1589–1602.
77. Felitti VJ. Long-term medical consequences of incest, rape, and molestation. *South Med J.* 1991;84(3):328–331.
78. Golding JM. Sexual assault history and headache: five general population studies. *J Nerv Ment Dis.* 1999;187(10):624–629.
79. Leserman J. Sexual abuse history: prevalence, health effects, mediators, and psychological treatment. *Psychosom Med.* 2005;67(6):906–915.
80. Romans S, Belaise C, Martin J, Morris E, Raffi A. Childhood abuse and later medical disorders in women. An epidemiological study. *Psychother Psychosom.* 2002;71(3):141–150.
81. Paras ML, Murad MH, Chen LP, et al. Sexual abuse and lifetime diagnosis of somatic disorders: a systematic review and meta-analysis. *Jama.* 2009;302(5):550–561.
82. Peterlin BL, Ward T, Lidicker J, Levin M. A retrospective, comparative study on the frequency of abuse in migraine and chronic daily headache. *Headache.* 2007;47(3):397–401.

83. Benish SG, Imel ZE, Wampold BE. The relative efficacy of bona fide psychotherapies for treating post-traumatic stress disorder: a meta-analysis of direct comparisons. *Clin Psychol Rev.* 2008;28(5):746–758.
84. Bisson JI, Ehlers A, Matthews R, Pilling S, Richards D, Turner S. Psychological treatments for chronic post-traumatic stress disorder. Systematic review and meta-analysis. *Br J Psychiatry.* 2007;190:97–104.
85. Domino JV, Haber JD. Prior physical and sexual abuse in women with chronic headache: clinical correlates. *Headache.* 1987;27(6):310–314.
86. Saper JR, Hamel RL, Lake AE, 3rd. Medication overuse headache (MOH) is a biobehavioural disorder. *Cephalalgia.* 2005;25(7):545–546.
87. Radat F, Creac'h C, Swendsen JD, et al. Psychiatric comorbidity in the evolution from migraine to medication overuse headache. *Cephalalgia.* 2005;25(7):519–522.
88. Radat F, Creac'h C, Guegan-Massardier E, et al. Behavioral dependence in patients with medication overuse headache: a cross-sectional study in consulting patients using the DSM-IV criteria. *Headache.* 2008;48(7):1026–1036.
89. American, Psychiatric, Association. *Diagnostic and Statistical Manual of Mental Disorders*, 4th *ed.*, *Text Revision (DSM-IV-TR).* Washington, DC: American Psychiatric Association; 2000.
90. Cupini LM, De Murtas M, Costa C, et al. Obsessive-compulsive disorder and migraine with medication-overuse headache. *Headache.* 2009;49(7):1005–1013.
91. Katsarava Z, Limmroth V, Finke M, Diener HC, Fritsche G. Rates and predictors for relapse in medication overuse headache: a 1–year prospective study. *Neurology.* 2003;60(10):1682–1683.
92. Katsarava Z, Muessig M, Dzagnidze A, Fritsche G, Diener HC, Limmroth V. Medication overuse headache: rates and predictors for relapse in a 4–year prospective study. *Cephalalgia.* 2005;25(1):12–15.
93. Andrasik F, Grazzi L, Usai S, Buse DC, Bussone G. Non-pharmacological approaches to treating chronic migraine with medication overuse. *Neurol Sci.* 2009;30(Suppl 1):S89–93.
94. Grazzi L, Andrasik F, D'Amico D, et al. Behavioral and pharmacologic treatment of transformed migraine with analgesic overuse: outcome at 3 years. *Headache.* 2002;42(6):483–490.
95. Grazzi L, Andrasik F, Usai S, Bussone G. Headache with medication overuse: treatment strategies and proposals of relapse prevention. *Neurol Sci.* 2008;29(2):93–98.
96. Lake AE, 3rd. Screening and behavioral management: medication overuse headache--the complex case. *Headache.* 2008;48(1):26–31.
97. Altieri M, Di Giambattista R, Di Clemente L, et al. Combined pharmacological and short-term psychodynamic psychotherapy for probable medication overuse headache: a pilot study. *Cephalalgia.* 2009;29(3):293–299.
98. Rothrock JF, Parada VA, Sims C, Key K, Walters NS, Zweifler RM. The impact of intensive patient education on clinical outcome in a clinic-based migraine population. *Headache.* 2006;46(5):726–731.
99. Dueland AN, Leira R, Burke TA, Hillyer EV, Bolge S. The impact of migraine on work, family, and leisure among young women—a multinational study. *Curr Med Res Opin.* 2004;20(10):1595–1604.

100. Lipton RB, Bigal ME, Kolodner K, Stewart WF, Liberman JN, Steiner TJ. The family impact of migraine: population-based studies in the USA and UK. *Cephalalgia.* 2003;23(6):429–440.
101. Smith R. Impact of migraine on the family. *Headache.* 1998;38(6):423–426.
102. Stang PE, Crown WH, Bizier R, Chatterton ML, White R. The family impact and costs of migraine. *Am J Manag Care.* 2004;10(5):313–320.

13

Nonpharmacological Treatments for Refractory Migraine

Acupuncture, Vitamins and Minerals, and Lifestyle Modifications

Christina Sun-Edelstein, MD, and Alexander Mauskop, MD

Introduction

Though a wide range of pharmacological therapies are now available for the treatment of migraine headaches, there remains a subset of patients with headaches that are refractory to traditional treatments. Offering nonpharmacological options may be particularly welcomed by this patient population, given the frustration associated with the failure of multiple medications, or their experiences with the intolerable side effects often associated with prescription medications. These patients may also express an interest in trying "natural" or nontraditional therapies as a new approach to treating their headaches. In this chapter, the evidence supporting the use of nonpharmacological therapies such as vitamins, supplements, and acupuncture in the treatment of refractory migraine headaches will be reviewed. Lifestyle modifications that can reduce headache frequency and severity are also discussed.

Acupuncture for RM

Acupuncture is a fundamental component of traditional Chinese medicine (TCM). Over the past few decades, interest in acupuncture in the Western world has grown, with 2.13 million people in the United States currently

Box 13-1 Key Points: Acupuncture in the Treatment of Migraine

1. Specific aspects of acupuncture methodology such as point selection, needling stimulation, and needling depth may not be as important as a regular needling schedule of approximately ten sessions done on a twice-weekly basis.
2. Psychological factors may play a significant role in the outcome of acupuncture treatment for migraine prevention.
3. The lack of differences found between verum and sham acupuncture suggests that unknown factors independent of acupuncture methodology must exist that provide a reduction in migraine symptoms.
4. Overall the evidence suggests that acupuncture is effective in reducing migraine pain and frequency, and is not inferior to a well-established pharmacological treatment (i.e., metoprolol) for migraine prevention.

undergoing treatment.[1] In 1997 the National Institutes of Health (NIH) convened a Consensus Development Conference on Acupuncture and concluded that acupuncture may be particularly effective in the treatment of postoperative and chemotherapy-induced nausea and vomiting, and postoperative dental pain. It may also have a role in the management of addiction, stroke rehabilitation, headache, menstrual cramps, tennis elbow, fibromyalgia, myofascial pain, osteoarthritis, low back pain, carpal tunnel syndrome, and asthma.[2] Headache treatment accounts for approximately 10% of visits to acupuncturists.[1]

The goal of treatment is to restore a state of equilibrium that has been disrupted by illness. The concept of *qi* refers to the life energy that normally flows through 12 organs and 12 meridians. Various illnesses and disorders are attributed to blockages in the flow of blood and *qi*. The activation of classic acupuncture points, which are distributed along the meridians, serves to clear the blockages, reestablishing the flow of *qi*. Recent studies have shown a more scientific explanation of the mechanism of action of acupuncture.

Mode of Action

While the mechanism by which acupuncture provides an analgesic effect in migraine treatment is not well understood, several theories have been postulated. Acupuncture has been shown to activate structures within the neuronal network involved in the control of pain perception, which includes the prefrontal cortex (PFC), the rostral anterior cingulate cortex (rACC), and the brain stem, as demonstrated by studies in which acupuncture-induced analgesia was inhibited by the experimental blockade of the pituitary gland,[3,4] the arcuate nucleus of the hypothalamus,[5,6] and the periaqueductal gray.[7] Other theories postulate that serotoninergic projections from the raphe nucleus to higher areas of the brain as well as descending projections to the spinal cord may contribute to the effectiveness of acupuncture,[8–10] and an anti-inflammatory effect of acupuncture may also be contributory.[11,12]

Nonetheless, when considering the potential mechanisms by which acupuncture reduces migraine headaches, one must also consider that studies (see later) have shown that both verum acupuncture and sham acupuncture are effective treatments. These findings imply that nonspecific physiological effects of sham acupuncture related to superficial skin penetration and the psychological effects of acupuncture play an important role in the efficacy of acupuncture.

Evidence Supporting the Use of Acupuncture in Migraine

In a 2001 Cochrane Review[13] of 16 randomized studies on acupuncture in the treatment of migraine, the authors concluded that a meta-analysis of the studies could not be conducted as a result of the heterogeneous nature of the available data, differences in the choice of acupuncture points used, small sample sizes, methodological problems, and insufficient reporting of study details. However, they were able to identify a trend in support of true acupuncture.

More recently, a 2007 review of RCTs on acupuncture and migraine published since the 2001 Cochrane report identified 10 studies.[14] These studies were also found to be heterogeneous in terms of the types of migraine studied, primary outcome measures, form of acupuncture studied, the nature of controls used, and types of placebo acupuncture. While nine of these studies investigated the use of acupuncture as a prophylactic therapy for migraine treatment, one study evaluated its use in the acute treatment of migraine attacks.[15] Subjects in that study received acupuncture, subcutaneous sumatriptan, or placebo (subcutaneous injection of NaCl solution), with approximately 60 patients per group. Though the acupuncture methodology was not well described, results showed that both acupuncture and sumatriptan prevented a full migraine attack in 35% to 36% of patients, as compared to only 18% in the placebo group. However, sumatriptan provided a faster response, and was also more effective when used as a second intervention in patients who developed a full attack. In practicality, patients are unlikely to seek acupuncture as acute treatment in the early stages of migraine, and acupuncture treatment on an emergency basis may not be readily available.[14]

Of the eight studies on the use of acupuncture in the preventative treatment of migraine, four[16–19] were underpowered or had methodological problems that limit the conclusions that can be made from their results.[14] A fifth study evaluated the use of acupuncture as part of a “treatment package” that also included herbal therapies and Qigong exercise and therefore study results cannot be attributed to acupuncture alone. Only the three remaining studies[20–22] utilized adequate methodology from which conclusions about the efficacy of acupuncture in migraine treatment could be drawn, as delineated in the review by Endres et al.[14] First, migraineurs showed a significant reduction in migraine symptoms as compared to their baseline at 6 months after the beginning of a 6-week course of acupuncture, or at 1 year after the start of a 3-month combination of acupuncture and standard medical care. Second, acupuncture is not inferior to a well-established pharmacological treatment (i.e., metoprolol) for migraine prevention. Lastly, no significant difference has been found between verum and sham acupuncture when considering the reduction in the number of migraine days.

Since 2007, several other randomized controlled trials (RCTs) investigating the use of acupuncture in migraine prevention have been published. One study[23] with 160 subjects compared the effectiveness of true acupuncture, standard mock acupuncture, ritualized mock acupuncture, and untreated controls in the treatment of migraine without aura. All groups also received rizatriptan at the onset of headaches. All groups experienced a decrease in the MIDAS (Migraine Disability Assessment Scale) Index (calculated based on the MIDAS score) at 3 and 6 months, but only the subjects in the true acupuncture groups demonstrated a significant improvement at both 3 and 6 months compared to the untreated controls. Ritualized mock acupuncture resulted in a transient improvement of the MIDAS Index at 3 months, but it was not sustained at 6 months.

In a smaller study,[24] with 37 participants, subjects received either 16 sessions of real acupuncture (RA) or sham acupuncture (SA) over 3 months. The primary end point was the percentage of subjects with at least a 50% reduction in migraine frequency in the second, third, fourth, fifth, and sixth months after treatment. Although the RA group showed significant improvement compared to the SA group at 2 months, these differences disappeared in the third month when subjects in the SA group began to demonstrate improvement as well. Both RA and SA groups also showed improvements in other migraine parameters, once again demonstrating the effects of sham acupuncture.

A third, large-scale study,[25] in which 15,056 patients were enrolled, sought to investigate the effectiveness of acupuncture in addition to routine care in primary headache patients as compared to treatment with routine care alone. The effect of acupuncture in randomized compared to nonrandomized patients was also studied. Of the 15,056 participants, 11,874 were openly treated with acupuncture in addition to standard care, while the remaining subjects were randomized to acupuncture or control groups. Patients in the control group did not receive any form of acupuncture. After 6 months, patients randomized to the acupuncture group showed a decrease in the number of headache days ($p < 0.001$) as well as improvements in pain intensity and quality of life ($p < 0.001$). Nonrandomized subjects showed outcome changes that were similar to those in the randomized group. This is the largest trial to date on the efficacy of acupuncture in primary headache. However, there were some methodological concerns with this study. First, the study groups included patients with migraine, tension-type headache, and a combination of both, and did not differentiate between the headache types when reporting the results. Second, the study was randomized but not blinded, and real acupuncture was not compared with a sham acupuncture procedure.[26]

Based on the aforementioned conclusions, it appears that specific aspects of acupuncture methodology such as point selection, needling stimulation, and needling depth may not be as important as a regular needling schedule of approximately 10 sessions done on a twice-weekly basis. Further, psychological factors may play a significant role in the outcome of acupuncture treatment for migraine prevention. Positive patient expectations about acupuncture, negative experiences with traditional pharmacologic therapy, the intensity of care provided by the acupuncturist as well as many other psychological variables may influence treatment outcome more so than the treatment itself. Given the lack of differences found between verum and sham acupuncture, unknown factors independent of acupuncture methodology must exist that provide a reduction in migraine symptoms.[14]

Acupuncture is a viable treatment alternative for migraine patients, especially those with contraindications to traditional pharmacological therapy or those with headaches that remain refractory to multiple trials of medications. Several studies have also demonstrated that is cost-effective in the treatment of headache.[27–29]

Vitamins and Other Supplements in the Treatment of RM (Table 13.1)

Magnesium

Magnesium is an essential cation that plays a vital role in multiple physiological processes, as a result of its central role in normal adenosine triphosphate (ATP) function and glucose metabolism. Deficits in magnesium are common[30] and can be seen in any chronic medical illness, including cardiovascular disease, diabetes, preeclampsia, eclampsia, sickle cell disease and alcoholism.[31] Chronic sleep deprivation has also been associated with autonomic imbalances and decreases in intracellular magnesium, which may precipitate cardiovascular events.[32] Even short-term exposure to stressors such as loud noise has been associated with increased urinary excretion of magnesium.[33] Symptoms of magnesium deficiency include premenstrual syndrome, leg muscle cramps, coldness of extremities, weakness, anorexia, nausea, digestive disorders, lack of coordination, and confusion. Given the multifaceted role played by magnesium deficiency in migraine pathophysiology as discussed later, supplementation with oral or intravenous magnesium may be an effective treatment option for migraine patients that are refractory to traditional medications.

Magnesium and Migraine Pathophysiology

Magnesium deficiency has been associated with many aspects of migraine pathophysiology, including cortical spreading depression (CSD) via its effects on the NMDA glutamate receptor,[34] neurotransmitter release,[35] platelet aggregation,[36] alterations in serotonergic activity, and vasoconstriction.[37,38]

Magnesium deficiency results in the generation and release of substance P,[39] which is believed to act on sensory fibers and produce headache pain.[40] Also, a decrease in the serum IMg^{2+} level and an elevation of the serum ratio of ionized calcium (ICa^{2+}) to IMg^{2+} may increase the affinity for cerebral vascular muscle serotonin receptor sites, potentiate cerebral vasoconstriction induced by serotonin,[41] and facilitate serotonin release for neuronal storage sites.[42] Further, magnesium may have an effect on circulating levels of CGRP.[43]

It has been speculated that during headaches, migraine sufferers excrete excessive amounts of magnesium as a result of stress, resulting in a transient worsening of serum hypomagnesemia.[44] Therefore, supplementation with magnesium may beneficially target various aspects of the neurogenic inflammation that occurs during migraine by counteracting vasospasm, inhibiting platelet aggregation, stabilization of cell membranes, and reducing the formation of inflammatory mediators. The use of magnesium in both acute and preventative headache treatment has been studied as a potentially simple, inexpensive, safe, and well-tolerated option.

Laboratory Assessment of Magnesium Deficiency

Though for many years magnesium deficiency has been suspected to play a role in the pathogenesis of migraine, research has been hindered by the lack of simple and reliable ways of measuring of magnesium content in various tissues. Low serum and tissue levels of total magnesium (TMg) have been reported in migraine patients,[45–47] although some of these findings were controversial in that both normal and low levels of Mg were found in the same tissues of migraine patients. The most likely reason for this inconsistency has been that although total magnesium levels have been measured, it is the ionized form of magnesium (IMg^{2+}) that truly reflects disturbed magnesium metabolism.[48–51]

Many studies have been undertaken to characterize the magnesium status of migraine sufferers. One study,[52] which utilized the magnesium load test, showed that magnesium retention occurred in patients with migraine after oral loading with 3000 mg of magnesium lactate during a 24-hour interictal period, suggesting a systemic magnesium deficiency. Other interictal studies on serum,[45,46,53–55] plasma,[47] and intracellular[46,47,55–57] Mg^{2+} levels in migraineurs and patients with tension-type headache have yielded inconsistent results. However, interictal levels of red blood cell (RBC) magnesium have been shown to be decreased in migraineurs with[56] and without aura,[46,47] as well as in juvenile migraine patients with and without aura.[58] These results were corroborated by a study[59] which showed low total magnesium in erythrocytes and low ionized magnesium in lymphocytes in migraine patients, both of which increased significantly after a 2-week trial of drinking mineral water containing 110 mg/L of magnesium. Therefore, given its commercial availability, the RBC magnesium assay may be a good way of assessing for deficiency.[58,60]

Treatment with Oral Magnesium

Three double-blind, placebo-controlled trials showed therapeutic efficacy of Mg^{2+} supplementation in headache patients. In the first, oral magnesium supplementation (360 mg magnesium pyrrolidone carboxylic acid) was given to 24 women with menstrual migraine on a daily basis from ovulation to the first day of flow.[47] In addition to a significant reduction of the number of days with headache ($p < 0.1$) and the total pain index ($p > 0.03$), patients receiving active treatment also showed improvement of the Menstrual Distress Questionnaire score. A second study, which involved 81 patients with migraine headaches, also showed significant improvement in patients on active therapy.[61] Attack frequency was reduced by 41.6% in the magnesium group and by 15.8% in the placebo group. The active treatment group received 600 mg of trimagnesium dicitrate in a water-soluble granular powder taken every morning. Most recently, a third randomized, double-blind, placebo-controlled study[62] showed that treatment with 600 mg of oral magnesium citrate resulted in a significant decrease in migraine attack frequency. An additional placebo-controlled, double blind trial showed no effect of oral magnesium on migraine.[63] This negative result has been attributed to the use of a poorly absorbed magnesium salt, since diarrhea occurred in almost half of patients in the treatment group.

Treatment with Intravenous Magnesium

Acute Migraine Treatment

Intravenous magnesium has been used in the treatment of acute migraine, though results from studies examining its use in this context have been conflicting. In a pilot study,[50] 40 patients received intravenous magnesium sulfate after a blood sample was drawn to measure ionized magnesium (IMg^{2+}) levels. An 85% correlation between the clinical response and the levels of serum IMg^{2+} was found ($p < 0.01$). Of the patients who had serum IMg^{2+} levels below 0.54 mmol/L, 86% had relief of pain and associated symptoms that was sustained over 24 hours. In contrast, of the patients who had serum IMg^{2+} levels greater than 0.54 mmol/L, only 16% experienced a similar degree of relief. Though the study was not double-blinded or placebo-controlled, both the researchers and subjects were blinded to the IMg^{2+} levels. Another study[51] subsequently showed that 1 gram of magnesium sulfate resulted in rapid headache relief in patients with low serum IMg^{2+} levels.

In a randomized, single-blind, placebo-controlled trial,[64] 30 patients with moderate to severe migraine attacks received either 1 gram of intravenous magnesium sulfate or 10 mL of saline intravenously. Treatment was superior to placebo in terms of both response rate (100% for magnesium sulfate vs. 7% for placebo) and pain-free rate (87% for magnesium sulfate and 0% for placebo). Although 87% had mild side effects including flushing and a burning sensation in the face and neck, none required discontinuation of treatment.

Further, none of the subjects reported headache recurrence during the 24 hours after treatment.

The efficacy of 1 gram of magnesium sulfate on the pain and associated symptoms in patients with migraine without aura and migraine with aura was assessed in a randomized, double-blind, placebo-controlled study.[65] There were no significant differences in pain relief or nausea between treatment and placebo in patients with migraine without aura, although a significantly lower intensity of photophobia and phonophobia was noted in patients receiving magnesium sulfate. However, patients with migraine with aura who received magnesium sulfate showed a statistically significant improvement in pain and all the associated symptoms when compared to those who received placebo.

Two randomized, double-blind, placebo-controlled studies[66,67] have been conducted in an emergency room setting, neither of which yielded positive results.

Treatment Recommendations

Magnesium plays a vital role in a multitude of cellular and physiological processes, and its involvement in the pathogenesis of migraine has also been well described. Although migraine attacks have been associated with magnesium deficiency, this is difficult to assess with routine blood testing. Treatment should therefore be considered in migraineurs based on clinical suspicion. Both oral and intravenous magnesium are simple, safe, inexpensive, and well tolerated, and may be especially effective in certain subsets of migraine patients. We recommend daily treatment with 400 mg of chelated magnesium, magnesium oxide, or slow-release magnesium in patients with symptoms suggestive of hypomagnesemia such as migraine headaches, premenstrual syndrome, cold extremities, and leg or foot muscle cramps. Some patients require and tolerate higher doses of oral magnesium, up to 1000 mg of magnesium oxide. Diarrhea and abdominal pain are the most commonly reported side effects.

We use intravenous magnesium for acute treatment of migraine, where it can be effective in up to 50% of patients, and in patients who do not tolerate, do not absorb, or are unable to comply with oral magnesium supplementation. Although concrete evidence has not yet been established by randomized, double-blind, placebo-controlled studies, we have observed that some patients with RM find great benefit from monthly (often premenstrual) prophylactic infusions of 1 gram of magnesium sulfate.

Riboflavin

Riboflavin, also known as vitamin B_2, is a precursor for flavin mononucleotides that are cofactors in the Krebs cycle. It is essential for membrane stability and the maintenance of energy-related cellular functions.[68] There has been one well-designed randomized controlled trial evaluating the use of riboflavin as a migraine prophylactic agent. Daily use of 400 mg riboflavin for 3 months

Table 13-1 Vitamins and Supplements in the Preventative Treatment of Migraine

Supplement	Recommended Daily Dosage	Side Effects
Chelated magnesium, slow-release magnesium, or magnesium oxide	400 mg	Diarrhea
Riboflavin (vitamin B2)	400 mg	Diarrhea, polyuria, urine discoloration
Coenzyme Q10	300 mg	GI disturbances, "cutaneous allergy"
α-Lipoic acid	600 mg	None reported
Feverfew *(Tanacetum parthenium)*	Unknown—preparations vary in strength and stability of active ingredient	GI disturbances Mouth ulcers Joint aches
Butterbur (*Petasites hybridus*)	150 mg	GI disturbances Eructation (burping)

resulted in a 50% reduction in attacks in 59% of patients, as compared to 15% for placebo. Two minor adverse reactions, diarrhea and polyuria, were reported in the treatment group.[69]

Coenzyme Q10

Coenzyme Q10 is an endogenous enzyme cofactor made by all cells in the body, functioning to promote mitochondrial proton-electron translocation. In an open-label study[70] in which 31 patients with migraine used 150 mg daily of CoQ10 for 3 months, 61% had at least a 50% reduction in migraine days without significant adverse events. Supplementation was effective within the first month of therapy. Later, a small randomized controlled trial[71] was conducted in which the treatment group received 100 mg of CoQ10 three times daily. Results showed that CoQ10 significantly decreased attack frequency, headache days, and days with nausea. Gastrointestinal disturbances and "cutaneous allergy" were reported, but at a low rate.

CoQ10 supplementation may be effective in the treatment of pediatric migraine. CoQ10 levels were measured in a study[72] of 1550 patients (mean age 13.3 ± 3.5 years) with frequent headaches, and found to be below the reference range in 32.9%. Supplementation with 1 to 3 mg/kg per day of CoQ10 in liquid gel capsule formulation resulted in an improvement in total CoQ10 levels, headache frequency, and degree of headache disability.

α-Lipoic Acid

Like riboflavin and CoQ10, α-lipoic acid (also known as thioctic acid) enhances mitochondrial oxygen metabolism and ATP production.[73] Its use in migraine prevention has been evaluated in one open pilot study (unpublished data, discussed in ref. 74) and one randomized placebo-controlled trial[74] to date.

Fifty-four patients were recruited into the randomized, placebo-controlled study, in which subjects received either 600 mg of α-lipoic acid or placebo daily for 3 months. Although there was a clear trend for reduction of migraine frequency after treatment with α-lipoic acid, the result was not significant. This result was attributed to the fact that the study was underpowered. However, within-group analyses did show a significant reduction in attack frequency, headache days, and headache severity in the treatment group.

Herbal Preparations

Feverfew *(Tanacetum parthenium)*

Feverfew is an herbal preparation that is available as the dried leaves of the weed plant *tanacetum parthenium.* It was used to treat headache, inflammation, and fever several centuries ago, and rediscovered in the late 20th century. The mechanism by which it works in migraine prophylaxis may be related to the parthenolides within the leaves. These may inhibit serotonin release from platelets and white blood cells, and inhibit platelet aggregation. Feverfew may also have anti-inflammatory action through the inhibition of prostaglandin synthesis and phospholipase A.[75–78]

Several randomized controlled studies have been conducted over the past decades with conflicting results,[79–84] including a meta-analysis[84] that did not recommend its use for headaches due to the paucity and low average quality of the existing randomized controlled trials on the subject. Inconsistencies in the results of those studies were probably related to wide variations in the strength of the active ingredient (parthenolide), and differences in the stability of feverfew preparations. Taking these differences into account, a new, more stable feverfew extract (MIG-99) was evaluated in a placebo-controlled trial involving 147 patients.[85] Although none of the doses were significant for the primary endpoint (number of migraine attacks in the last month of the 3-month study compared to baseline) relative to placebo, a subset of patients with high frequency of migraine attacks did seem to benefit. In a follow-up multicenter, double-blind, placebo-controlled study with 170 subjects,[86] those investigators evaluated 6.25 mg TID of MIG-99 versus placebo, and reported a statistically significant and clinically relevant reduction in migraine frequency in the MIG-99 group compared to placebo.

Side effects reported in clinical trials include gastrointestinal disturbances, mouth ulcers, and a "post-feverfew syndrome" of joint aches.

Butterbur *(Petasites hybridus)*

In recent years, *Petasites hybridus* root extract, also known as butterbur, has emerged as a potential new treatment in the prevention of migraine. The butterbur plant is a perennial shrub that was used in ancient times for its medicinal properties. *Petasites* is thought to act through calcium channel regulation and inhibition of peptide-leukotriene biosynthesis. Leukotrienes and other inflammatory mediators may have a role in the inflammatory cascade associated with migraine.[87,88] Though the butterbur plant itself contains pyrrolizidine alkaloids which are hepatotoxic and carcinogenic, these compounds are removed in the commercially available preparations.

A randomized, double-blind, placebo-controlled trial[89] using 50 mg of butterbur twice daily showed a significantly reduced number of migraine attacks and migraine days per month. Later, Lipton et al.[90] compared Petasites extract 75 mg twice daily, *Petasites* extract 50 mg twice daily, and placebo twice daily in a three-arm, parallel-group, randomized trial of 245 patients and found that the higher dose of *Petasites* extract was more effective than placebo in decreasing the number of monthly migraine attacks. A multicenter prospective open-label study[91] of butterbur in 109 children and adolescents with migraine resulted in 77% of all patients reporting a reduction in migraine frequency of at least 50%. In all three studies, butterbur was well tolerated and no serious adverse events occurred. The most frequently reported adverse reactions were mild gastrointestinal events, predominantly eructation (burping).

Lifestyle Modifications in the Management of RM

Sleep Hygiene

Sleep disturbances have been cited as a migraine trigger in up to 52% of migraine sufferers.[92–94] The mechanism by which this occurs is not fully understood but may be related to an interaction between sleep-related structures such as the suprachiasmatic nucleus and the medial preoptic nucleus with those structures involved in pain modulation, such as the noradrenergic neurons in the locus coeruleus and the serotoninergic neurons in the dorsal raphe. Sleep disturbances have been postulated to alter neuronal firing rate within these pathways, theoretically precipitating headaches.[95]

Box 13-2 Tips for Improved Sleep Hygiene

- Keep the bedroom cool, quiet, and dark.
- No reading or watching TV while in bed.
- Spend 30 minutes outside every morning within 90 minutes of awakening.
- Designate a bedtime that will allow 8 hours in bed each night.
- Wake up each morning at around the same time.
- Eliminate naps during the day.
- Eat dinner at least 4 hours prior to bedtime.
- No liquids within 2 hours of bedtime.
- No caffeine from mid-afternoon onwards.
- Don't look at the clock during the night.

Much of the literature on the relationship between sleep and migraine headaches has focused on the pediatric population. One study[96] showed that children and adolescents with migraine and tension-type headache were more likely to have short sleep duration, poorer sleep quality, more night awakenings, and more daytime somnolence when compared to controls. A follow-up randomized controlled study,[97] which evaluated the effect of poor sleep habits on several headache parameters, showed that mean duration and frequency of migraine attacks were significantly reduced in subjects who were instructed to follow directions to improve sleep hygiene, as compared to those who were not given directions for improving sleep. More recently, a study[98] with 69 adolescents complaining of headache showed that sleep complaints such as insufficient total sleep, daytime sleepiness, and difficulty falling and staying asleep were common in this population.

In adults, most studies have focused on the relationship between primary sleep disorders such as sleep apnea and chronic morning headaches. However, one study[99] showed that patients with chronic migraine had shorter sleep episodes and were more likely to complain of difficulty falling asleep and staying asleep when compared to those with episodic migraine. Also, nonrestorative sleep and poor sleep habits were found to be almost universally prevalent in a referral population of women with transformed migraine.[100] Later, in a small randomized, single-blind, placebo-controlled pilot study[101] of women with transformed migraine, targeted behavioral sleep intervention was associated with an improvement in headache frequency and headache index. In addition, a reversion to episodic migraine was noted. Behavioral sleep modifications (Box 13.2) included consistent bedtimes that allowed 8 hours of time in bed, elimination of TV, reading, and music in bed, visualization techniques to shorten the time to sleep onset, eating dinner at least 4 hours before bedtime, limiting fluids within 2 hours of bedtime, and the discontinuation of naps.

As yet, it is unclear whether headaches lead to sleep disturbances or vice versa. Nonetheless, some evidence suggests that improving sleep hygiene can improve migraine headaches and possibly revert transformed migraines to episodic patterns. Patients with frequent migraines should therefore be questioned about their sleep habits and educated about sleep hygiene where relevant.

Exercise

Exercise, particularly aerobic exercise, is frequently promoted as part of a multidisciplinary approach in the treatment of RM headaches. Several theories have been proposed to explain the relationship between migraine and exercise. One such theory relates to the large amounts of enkephalins and endorphins that are secreted during exercise. In one study,[102] cerebrospinal β-endorphin levels correlated with the severity of migraine, while another[103] showed that basal plasma β-endorphin levels were negatively correlated with headache duration. Others have proposed that the increase in nitric oxide production that occurs during exercise mediates the positive effect of exercise on migraine headaches,[104] and that regular exercise may protect endothelium by decreasing the levels of plasma norepinephrine,[105] vasoconstrictor prostanoids and free radicals.[106]

In contrast, exercise can precipitate headaches in some migraineurs, and was cited as a migraine trigger in 22% of subjects in a recent study.[107] Headache sufferers have also been shown to have less aerobic endurance and flexibility than healthy controls.[108] Further, even though exercise is frequently recommended as a preventative treatment for migraine, no clearcut guidelines exist for migraineurs regarding the optimal frequency, intensity, and duration of exercise programs. Toward this end, one group recently sought to develop and evaluate an exercise program for untrained patients with migraine, which could safely improve exercise capacity without exacerbating migraines. [109] Subjects underwent a moderate-intensity level aerobic training program consisting of three 40-minute sessions per week over 12 weeks. Sessions included warm-up, exercise, and cool-down periods. The program was well-tolerated with no reported increase in migraine, with some patients reporting an improvement in headaches and quality of life.

Despite the ubiquitous mandates to exercise regularly, the evidence supporting exercise in the treatment of migraine is based primarily on findings in anecdotal reports or observational studies. Some have shown that exercise can reduce headache frequency,[102,103,110] pain intensity,[102,103,111,112] and headache duration,[104] but others have shown no changes in those headache parameters.[111–113] Physical inactivity has also been strongly associated with headache disorders independent of economic and psychosocial factors.[114]

In a recent survey of the available studies and case reports on the therapeutic effect of exercise in the treatment of migraine,[115] the authors concluded that more studies are needed before exercise can recommended based on evidence-based medicine (EBM) criteria. In their review, which evaluated two randomized open-controlled studies, one "quasiexperimental and pseudorandomized" study, four observational studies with single cohorts and no control groups, and multiple case reports, they found that the majority of the studies did not show a significant reduction of headache attacks or headache duration, and only indicate a reduction of pain intensity. Further, most of the available studies were limited by methodological problems. Future trials should aim to quantify the analgesic effect of exercise in migraine and elucidate its role in migraine treatment, using randomized controlled designs.

Treatment Recommendations

- Acupuncture is a viable nonpharmacological treatment for RM. The acupuncture experience itself appears to be more important than the specifics of the acupuncture procedure such as needling depth, needling stimulation, and point selection.

- We recommend daily treatment with 400 mg of chelated magnesium, magnesium oxide or slow-release magnesium in patients with symptoms suggestive of hypomagnesemia such as migraine headaches, premenstrual syndrome, cold extremities, and leg or foot muscle cramps.
- We use intravenous magnesium for acute treatment of migraine. Although evidence has not yet been established by randomized, double-blind, placebo-controlled studies, we have observed that some patients with RM find great benefit from monthly (often premenstrual) prophylactic infusions of one gram of magnesium sulfate.
- Other vitamins and supplements with some evidence of efficacy in the preventative treatment of migraine include butterbur (*Petasites hybridus*), riboflavin, coenzyme Q10, feverfew (*Tanacetum parthenium*), and α-lipoic acid.
- Sleep hygiene is an important aspect of migraine management and may even be helpful in reverting transformed migraine back to episodic patterns.
- Although the data pertaining to the efficacy of aerobic exercise in the treatment or prevention of migraine does not meet EBM-based criteria, observational studies suggest that it may be helpful in reducing headache frequency, intensity, and duration. We usually recommend five 30-minute sessions of aerobic exercise per week in RM patients.

Conclusions

The treatment of RM remains a challenge for even the most seasoned headache specialist. Though there is a growing arsenal of acute and preventative medications for migraine treatment, a multidisciplinary approach that includes non-pharmacological therapies and lifestyle modifications may be most effective in minimizing the pain and disability associated with chronic, RM. With time, patience, and close follow-up, successful outcomes can be achieved.

References

1. Burke A, Upchurch DM, Dye C, Chyu L. Acupuncture use in the United States: findings from the National Health Interview Survey. *J Altern Complement Med.* 2006;12:639–648.
2. NIH Consensus Devlopement Conference on Acupuncture. http://consensus.nih.gov/1997/1997Acupuncture107html.htm
3. Pomeranz B, Cheng R, Law P. Acupuncture reduces electrophysiological and behavioral responses to noxious stimuli: pituitary is implicated. *Exp Neurol.* 1977;54:172–178.
4. Takeshige C, Kobori M, Hishida F, Luo CP, Usami S. Analgesia inhibitory system involvement in nonacupuncture point-stimulation-produced analgesia. *Brain Res Bull.* 1992;28:379–391.

5. Sato T, Usami S, Takeshige C. Role of the arcuate nucleus of the hypothalamus as the descending pain-inhibitory system in acupuncture point and non-point produced analgesia. In: Takeshige C, ed. *Studies on the Mechanism of Acupuncture Analgesia Based on Animal Experiments.* Tokyo: Showa University Press; 1986:542
6. Takeshige C, Zhao WH, Guo SY. Convergence from the preoptic area and arcuate nucleus to the median eminence in acupuncture and nonacupuncture point stimulation analgesia. *Brain Res Bull.* 1991;26:771–778.
7. Wang QA, Mao LM, Han JS. The role of periaqueductal gray in mediation of analgesia produced by different frequencies electroacupuncture stimulation in rats. *Int J Neurosci.* 1990;53:167–172.
8. McLennan H, Gilfillan K, Heap Y. Some pharmacological observations on the analgesia induced by acupuncture in rabbits. *Pain.* 1977;3:229–238.
9. Cheng RS, Pomeranz B. Monoaminergic mechanism of electroacupuncture analgesia. *Brain Res.* 1981;215:77–92.
10. Han CS, Chou PH, Lu CC, Lu LH, Yang TH, Jen MF. The role of central 5-hydroxytryptamine in acupuncture analgesia. *Sci Sin.* 1979;22:91–104.
11. Lao L, Zhang RX, Zhang G, Wang X. Berman BM, Ren K. A parametric study of electroacupuncture on persistent hyperalgesia and Fos protein expression in rats. *Brain Res.* 2004;1020:18–29.
12. Ceccherelli F, Gagliardi G, Ruzzante L, Giron G. Acupuncture modulation of capsaicin-induced inflammation: effect of intraperitoneal and local administration of naloxone in rats. A blinded controlled study. *J Altern Complement Med.* 2002;8:341–349.
13. Melchart D, Linde K, Fischer P, et al. Acupuncture for idiopathic headache. Cochrane Database Syst Rev 2001; 1; CD001218.
14. Endres HG, Diener H-C, Molsberger A. Role of acupuncture in the treatment of migraine. *Expert Rev Neurother.* 2007;7:1121–1134.
15. Melchart D, Thormaehlen J, Hager S, Liao J, Linde K, Weidenhammer W. Acupuncture versus placebo versus sumatriptan for early treatment of migraine attacks: a randomized controlled trial. *J Intern Med.* 2003;253:181–188.
16. Linde M, Fjell A, Carlsson J, Dahlof C. Role of the needling per se in acupuncture as prophylaxis for menstrually-related migraine: a randomized placebo-controlled study. *Cephalalgia.* 2005;25:41–47.
17. Alecrim-Andrade J, Maciel-Junior JA, Cladellas XC, Correa-Filho HR, Machado HC. Acupuncture in migraine prophylaxis: a randomized sham-controlled trial. *Cephalalgia.* 2006;26:520–529.
18. Streng A, Linde K, Hoppe A, et al. Effectiveness and tolerability of acupuncture compared with metoprolol in migraine prophylaxis. *Headache.* 2006;46:1492–1502.
19. Allais G, De Lorenzo C, Quirico PE, et al. Acupuncture in the prophylactic treatment of migraine without aura: a comparison with flunarizine. *Headache.* 2002;42:855–861.
20. Diener HC, Kronfeld K, Boewing G, et al. Efficacy of acupuncture for the prophylaxis of migraine: a multicentre randomized controlled clinical trial. *Lancet Neurol.* 2006;5:310–316.
21. Linde K, Streng A, Jurgens S, et al. Acupuncture for patients with migraine: a randomized controlled trial. *JAMA.* 2005;23:2118–2125.

22. Vickers AJ, Rees RW, Zollman CE, et al. Acupuncture for chronic headache in primary care: large, pragmatic, randomized trial. *Br Med J.* 2004;328:744–749.
23. Facco E, Liguori A, Petti F, Zanette G, Coluzzi F, De Nardin M, Mattia C. Traditional acupuncture in migraine: a controlled, randomized study. *Headache.* 2008;48:398–407.
24. Alecrim-Andrade J, Maciel-Junior JA, Carne X, Severino Vasconcelos GM, Correa-Filho HR. Acupuncture in migraine prevention: a randomized sham controlled study with 6-months posttreatment follow-up. *Clin J Pain.* 2008;24:98–105.
25. Jena S, Witt CM, Brinkhaus B, Wegscheider K, Willich SN. Acupuncture in patients with headache. *Cephalalgia.* 2008;28:969–979.
26. Diener H-C. Editorial: Acupuncture for the treatment of headaches: more than sticking needles into humans? *Cephalalgia.* 2008;28:911–913.
27. Vickers AJ, Rees RW, Zollman CE, et al. Acupuncture of chronic headache disorders in primary care: randomized controlled trial and economic analysis. *Health Technol Assess.* 2004;8:1–35.
28. Wonderling D, Vickers AJ, Grieve R, McCarney R. Cost effectiveness analysis of a randomized trial of acupuncture from chronic headache in primary care. *BMJ.* 2004;328:747.
29. Witt CM, Reinhold T, Jena S, Brinkhaus B, Willich SN. Cost-effectiveness of acupuncture treatment in patients with headache. *Cephalalgia.* 2008;28:334–345.
30. Schimatschek HF, Rempis R. Prevalence of hypomagnesemia in an unselected German population of 16,000 individuals. *Magnes Res.* 2001;14:283–290.
31. Laires MJ, Monteiro CP, Bicho M. Role of cellular magnesium in health and human disease. *Front Biosci.* 2004;1:262–276.
32. Takase B, Akima T, Satomura K, et al. Effects of chronic sleep deprivation on autonomic activity by examining heart rate variability, plasma catecholamine, and intracellular magnesium levels. *Biomed Pharmacother.* 2004;58(Suppl 1):S35–39.
33. Mocci F, Canalis P. The effect of noise on serum and urinary magnesium and catecholamines in humans. *Occup Med.* 2001;51:56–61.
34. Mody I, Lambert JD, Heinemann U. Low extracellular magnesium induces epileptiform activity and spreading depression in rat hippocampal slices. *J Neurophysiol.* 1987;57:869–888.
35. Coan EJ, Collingridge GL. Magnesium ions block an *N*-methyl D-aspartate receptor-mediated component of synaptic transmission in rat hippocampus. *Neurosci Lett.* 1985;53:21–26.
36. Baudouin-Legros M, Dard B, Guichency P. Hyperreactivity of platelets from spontaneously hypertensive rats. Role of external magnesium. *Hypertension.* 1986;8:694–699.
37. Altura BT, Altura BM. Withdrawal of magnesium causes vasospasm while elevated magnesium produced relaxation of tone in cerebral arteries. *Neurosci Lett.* 1989;20:323–327.
38. Altura BT, Altura BM. The role of magnesium in etiology of strokes and cerebrovasospasm. *Magnesium.* 1982;1:277–291.
39. Weglicki WB, Phillips TM. Pathobiology of magnesium deficiency: a cytokine/neurogenic inflammation hypothesis. *Am J Physiol.* 1992; 263(pt 2): R734–737.

40. Moskowitz MA. The neurobiology of vascular head pain. *Ann Neurol.* 1984;16:157–168.
41. Altura BM, Turlapaty PDMV. Withdrawal of magnesium enhances coronary arterial spasm produced by vasoactive agents. *Br J Pharmacol.* 1982;77:649–659.
42. Peters JA, Hales TG, Lambert JJ. Divalent cations modulate 5-HT3 receptor-induced currents in N1E-115 neuroblastoma cells. *Eur J Pharmacol.* 1988;151:491–495.
43. Myrdal U, Leppert J, Edvinsson L, et al. Magnesium sulphate infusion decreases circulating calcitonin gene-related peptide (CGRP) in women with primary Raynaud's phenomenon. *Clin Physiol.* 1994;14:539–546.
44. Durlach J. Neurological manifestations of magnesium imbalance. In: Vinken PJ, Bruyn GW, eds. *Handbook of Clinical Neurology*, Vol. 28. Amsterdam: North-Holland;1976:545–579.
45. Sarchielli P, Coata G, Firenze C, Morucci P, Abbritti G, Gallai V. Serum and salivary magnesium levels in migraine and tension-type headache. Results in a group of adult patients. *Cephalalgia.* 1992;12:21–27, 42.
46. Schoenen J, Sianard-Gainko J, Lenaerts M. Blood magnesium levels in migraine. *Cephalalgia.* 1991;11:97–99.
47. Facchinetti F., Sances G., Borella P., Genazzani A.R., Nappi G. Magnesium prophylaxis of menstrual migraine: effects on intracellular magnesium. *Headache.* 1991;31:298–301.
48. Altura BT, Shirley T, Young CC, Dell'Ofrano K, Handwerker SM, Altura BM. A new method for the rapid determination of ionized Mg^2+ in whole blood, serum and plasma. *Methods Find Exp Clin Pharmacol.* 1992;14(4):297–304.
49. Altura BT, Shirley TL, Young CC, et al. Characterization of a new ion selective electrode for ionized magnesium in whole blood, plasma, serum and aqueous samples. *Scand J Clin Lab Invest.* 1994;54(Suppl 217):21–36.
50. Mauskop A, Altura BT, Cracco RQ, et al. Intravenous magnesium sulfate relieves migraine attacks in patients with low serum ionized magnesium levels: a pilot study. *Clin Sci.* 1995;89:633–636.
51. Mauskop A, Altura BT, Cracco RQ, Altura BM. Intravenous magnesium sulfate rapidly alleviates headaches of various types. *Headache.* 1996;36:154–160.
52. Trauninger A, Pfund Z, Koszegi T, Czopf J. Oral magnesium load test in patients with migraine. *Headache.* 2002;42:114–119.
53. Gallai V, Sarchielli P, Costa G, et al. Serum and salivary magnesium levels in migraine. Results in a group of juvenile patients. *Headache.* 1992;32: 132–135.
54. Mauskop A, Altura BT, Cracco RQ, Altura BM. Deficiency in serum ionized magnesium but not total magnesium in patients with migraines. Possible role of ICa2+/IMg2+ ratio. *Headache.* 1993;33:135–138.
55. Thomas J, Thomas E, Tomb E. Serum and erythrocyte magnesium concentrations and migraine. *Magnes Res.* 1992;5:127–130.
56. Gallai V, Sarchielli P, Morucci P, Abbritti G. Red blood cell magnesium levels in migraine patients. *Cephalalgia.* 1993;13:94–98.
57. Gallai V, Sarchielli P, Morucci P, Abbritti G. Magnesium content of monomuclear blood cells in migraine patients. *Headache.* 1994;34:160–165.
58. Soriani S, Arnaldi C, De Carlo L, et al. Serum and red blood cell magnesium levels in juvenile migraine patients. *Headache.* 1995;35:14–16.

59. Thomas J, Millot JM, Sebille S, Delabroise AM, et al. Free and total magnesium in lymphocytes of migraine patients- effect of magnesium-rich mineral water intake. *Clin Chim Acta.* 2000;295:64–75.
60. Touitou Y, Godaud JP, Ferment O, et al. Prevalence of magnesium and potassium deficiencies in the elderly. *Clin Chem.* 1987;33:518–523.
61. Peikert A, Wilimzig C, Kohne-Volland R. Prophylaxis of migraine with oral magnesium: results from a prospective, multi-center, placebo-controlled and double-blind randomized study. *Cephalalgia.* 1996;16:257–263.
62. Koseoglu E, Talashoglu A, Gonul AS, Kula M. The effects of magnesium prophylaxis in migraine without aura. *Magnes Res.* 2008;21:101–108.
63. Pfaffenrath V, Wessely P, Meyer C, et al. Magnesium in the prophylaxis of migraine-A double-blind, placebo-controlled study. *Cephalalgia.* 1996;16:436–440.
64. Demirkaya S, Vural O, Dora B, Topcuoglu MA. Efficacy of intravenous magnesium sulfate in the treatment of acute migraine attacks. *Headache.* 2001;41:171–177.
65. Bigal ME, Bordini Ca, Tepper SJ, Speciali JG. Intravenous magnesium sulphate in the acute treatment of migraine without aura and migraine with aura. A randomized, double-blind, placebo-controlled study. *Cephalalgia.* 2002;22:345–353.
66. Corbo J, Esses D, Bijur PE, Iannaccone R, Gallagher EJ. Randomized clinical trial of intravenous magnesium sulfate as an adjunctive medication for emergency department treatment of migraine headache. *Ann Emerg Med.* 2001;38:621–627.
67. Cete Y, Dora B, Ertan C, Ozdemir C, Oktay C. A randomized prospective placebo-controlled study of intravenous magnesium sulphate vs. metoclopramide in the management of acute migraine attacks in the emergency department. *Cephalalgia.* 2005;25:199–204.
68. Evans RW, Taylor FR. Expert opinion: "Natural" or alternative medications for migraine prevention. *Headache.* 2006;46:1012–1018.
69. Schoenen J, Jacquy J, Lanaerts M. Effectiveness of high-dose riboflavin in migraine prophylaxis. *Neurology.* 1998;50:466–470.
70. Rozen TD, Oshinsky ML, Gebeline CA, Bradley KC, Young WB, Schechter AL, Silberstein SD. Open label trial of Coenzyme Q10 as a migraine preventive. *Cephalalgia.* 2002;22:137–141.
71. Sandor PS, DiClemente L, Coppola G, et al. Efficacy of coenzyme Q10 in migraine prophylaxis: a randomized controlled trial. *Neurology.* 2005;64:713–715.
72. Hershey AD, Powers, SW, Vockell AB, et al. Coenzyme Q10 deficiency and response to supplementation in pediatric and adolescent migraine. *Headache.* 2007;47:73–80.
73. Matalon R, Tumpf DA, Kimberlee M, et al. Lipoamide dehydrogenase deficiency with primary lactic acidosis: favorable response to treatment with oral lipoic acid. *J Pediatr.* 1984;104:65–69.
74. Magis D, Ambrosini A, Sandor P, et al. A randomized double-blind placebo-controlled trial of thioctic acid in migraine prophylaxis. *Headache.* 2007;47:52–57.
75. Heptinstall S, White A, Williamson L, Mitchell JRA. Extracts of feverfew inhibit granule secretion in blood platelets and polymorphonuclear leukocytes. *Lancet.* 1985;1:1071–1074.

76. Heptinstall S, Goenewegen WA, Spangenberg P, Loesche W. Extracts of feverfew may inhibit platelet behaviour via neutralisation of suphydryl groups. *J Pharm Pharmacol.* 1987;39:459–465.
77. Pugh WH, Sambo K. Prostaglandin synthetase inhibitors in feverfew. *J Pharm Pharmacol.* 1988;40:743–745.
78. Makheja AM, Bailey JM. A platelet phospholipase inhibitor from the medicinal herb feverfew (*Tanacetum parthenium*). *Prostaglandins Leukotrienes Med.* 1982;8:653–660.
79. Johnson ES, Kadam, NP, Hylands DM, Hylands PJ. Efficacy of feverfew as prophylactic treatment of migraine. *BMJ.* 1985;291:569–573.
80. Murphy JJ, Heptinstall S, Mitchell JR. Randomised double-blind placebo-controlled trial of feverfew in migraine prevention. *Lancet.* 1988;2:189–192.
81. Kuritzky A, Elhacham Y, Yerushalmi Z, Hering R. Feverfew in the treatment of migraine: its effect on serotonin uptake and platelet activity. *Neurology.* 1994;44(Suppl): 293P.
82. De Weerdt CJ, Bootsma HPR, Hendricks H. Herbal medicines in migraine prevention: randomized double-blind placebo-controlled crossover trial of feverfew preparation. *Phytomoedicine.* 1996;3:225–230.
83. Palevitch D, Earon G, Carasso R. Feverfew (*Tanacetum parthenium*) as a prophylactic treatment for migraine: a placebo-controlled double-blind study. *Phytother Res.* 1997;11:508–511.
84. Vogler BK, Pittler BK, Ernst E. Feverfew as a preventive treatment for migraine: a systematic review. *Cephalalgia.* 1998;18:704–708.
85. Pfaffentreath V, Diener HC, Fisher M, Friede M, Henneicke-von Zepelin HH. The efficacy and safety of *Tanacetum parthenium* (feverfew) in migraine prophylaxis—a double-blind, multicentre, randomized placebo-controlled dose-response study. *Cephalalgia.* 2002;22:523–532.
86. Diener HC, Pfaffenrath V, Schnitker J, et al. Efficacy and safety of 6.25 mg tid feverfew CO2 extract (MIG-99) in migraine prevention—a randomized, double-blind, multicenter, placebo-controlled study. *Cephalalgia.* 2005;25:1031–1041.
87. Sheftell F, Rapoport A, Weeks R, Walker B, Gammerman I, Baskin S. Montelukast in the prophylaxis of migraine: a potential role for leukotriene modifiers. *Headache.* 2000;40:158–163.
88. Pearlman EM, Fisher S. Preventive treatment for childhood and adolescent headache: role of once-daily montelukast sodium. *Cephalalgia.* 2001;21:461.
89. Grossman M, Schmidrams H. An extract of *Petasites hybridus* is effective in the prophylaxis of migraine. *Int J Clin Pharmacol Ther.* 2000;38: 430–435.
90. Lipton RB, Gobel H, Einhaupl KM, Wilks K, Mauskop A. *Petsites hybridus* root (butterbur) is an effective preventive treatment for migraine. *Neurology.* 2004;63:2240–2244.
91. Pothmann R, Danesch U. Migraine prevention in children and adolescents: results of an open study with a special butterbur root extract. *Headache.* 2005;45:196–203.
92. Robbins L. Precipitating factors in migraine: a retrospective review of 494 patients. *Headache.* 1994;34:214–216.
93. Scharff L Turk DC, Marcus DA. Triggers of headache episodes and coping responses of headache diagnostic groups. *Headache.* 1995;35:397–403.

94. Turner LC, Molgaard CA, Gardner CH, et al. Migraine triggers in non-clinical Mexican-American population in San Diego county: implications for etiology. *Cephalalgia.* 1995;15:523–530.
95. Martin VT, Behbehani MM. Toward a rational understanding of migraine trigger factors. *Med Clin North Am.* 2001;85:911–941.
96. Bruni O, Fabrizi P, Ottaviano S, et al. Prevalence of sleep disorders in childhood and adolecents with headache. A case-control study. *Cephalalgia.* 1997;17:492–498.
97. Bruni O, Galli F, Guidetti V. Sleep hygiene and migraine in children and adolescents. *Cephalalgia.* 1999;19(Suppl 25):57–59.
98. Gilman DK, Palermo TM, Kabbouche MA, Hershey AD, Powers SW. Primary headache and sleep disturbances in adolescents. *Headache.* 2007;47:1189–1194.
99. Kelman L, Rains JC. Headache and sleep: examination of sleep patterns and complaints in a large clinical sample of migraineurs. *Headache.* 2005;45:904–910.
100. Calhoun AH, Ford S, Finkel AG, Kahn KA, Mann JD. The prevalence and spectrum of sleep problems in women with transformed migraine. *Headache.* 2006;46:604–610.
101. Calhoun AH, Ford S. Behavioral sleep modification may revert transformed migraine to episodic migraine. *Headache.* 2007;47:1178–1183.
102. Genazzani AR, Nappi G, Facchinetti F, et al. Progressive impairment of CSF -EP levels in migraine sufferers. *Pain.* 1984;18:127–133.
103. Koseoglu E, Akboyrz A, Soyeur A, Ersoy AO. Aerobic exercise and plasma beta endorphin levels in patients with migrainous headache without aura. *Cephalalgia.* 2003;23:972–976.
104. Narin SO, Pinar L. The effects of exercise and exercise-related changes in blood nitric oxide level on migraine headache. *Clin Rehab.* 2003;17: 624–630.
105. Higashi Y, Sasaki S, Kurisu S, et al. Clinical abstracts: vascular disease. *Modern Med.* 1999;67:30.
106. Varin R, Mulder P, Richard V, Tamion F. Exercise improves flow-mediated vasodilatation of skeletal muscle arteries in rats with chronic heart failure: role of nitric oxide, prostanoids, and oxidant stress. *Circulation.* 1999;99:2951–2957.
107. Kelman L. The triggers or precipitants of the acute migraine attack. *Cephalalgia.* 2007;27:394–402.
108. Neususs K, Neumann B, Steinhoff BJ, Thegeder H, Bauer A, Reimers D. Physical activity and fitness in patients with headache disorders. *Int J Sports Med.* 1997;18:607–611.
109. Varkey E, Cider A, Carlsson J, Linde M. A study to evaluate the feasibility of an aerobic exercise program in patients with migraine. *Headache.* 2008 (Epub ahead of print].
110. Grimm L, Douglas D, Hanson P. Aerobic training in the prophylaxis of migraine. *Med Sci Sports Exerc.* 1981;13:98.
111. Fitterling JM, Martin JE, Gramling S, Cole P, Milan MA. Behavioral management of exercise training in vascular headache patients: an investigation of exercise adherence and headache activity. *J Appl Behav Anal.* 1988;21:9–19.

112. Norlander E, Cider A, Carlsson J, Linde M. Improvement of exercise capacity in patients with migraine—methodological considerations. *Cephalalgia.* 2007;27:575–579.
113. Lockett DM, Campbell JF. The effects of aerobic exercise on migraine. *Headache.* 1992;32:50–54.
114. Molarius A, Tegelberg A, Ohrvik J. Socio-economic factors, lifestyle, and headache disorders- a population-based study in Sweden. *Headache.* 2008;48:1426–1437.
115. Busch V, Gaul C. Exercise in migraine therapy—is there any evidence for efficacy? A critical review. *Headache.* 2008;48:890–899.

14

Women with Refractory Migraine

Elizabeth Loder, MD, MPH, Luzma Cardona, MD, and Paul Rizzoli, MD

Introduction

Though mostly indirect, the evidence is convincing that sex hormones, particularly estrogen, might initiate, aggravate, or maintain migraine (Table 14.1). It is thus understandable that hormonal factors receive great scrutiny in women with refractory migraine (RM). Being female increases the risk of developing migraine and increases the likelihood that it will become chronic. Women with migraine also have headache attacks that are, on average, more severe and disabling than migraine attacks in men.[1,2] As one expert has noted, "The femaleness of migraine and its modulation by ovarian steroid hormones is inescapable."[3]

This chapter reviews how to determine whether hormonal factors are involved in a particular woman's RM problem, and details the hormonal strategies that can be considered if that is the case. It also discusses important sex-specific considerations in the care of women with RM. These include advice on contraception and hormone replacement therapy and the management of RM in pregnancy and the puerperium.

Menstrual Exacerbations of Migraine

Attacks of migraine that occur in predictable relation to the menstrual period are termed "menstrual migraine." The *International Classification of*

Table 14-1 Evidence that Hormonal Factors Influence the Expression of Migraine in Women

- The prevalence of migraine is higher in females than in males at all ages after puberty, and the discrepancy is most marked in the reproductive years
- The incidence (new cases) of migraine in women peaks during the early reproductive years.
- The late luteal phase decline in estrogen levels is a well-characterized trigger of migraine; migraine often improves with the stable estrogen levels characteristic of mid and late pregnancy.
- The incidence of migraine is elevated during the pill-free week of traditional combination estrogen-progesterone oral contraceptive use.
- The erratic hormonal swings of perimenopause may worsen migraine, while established menopause may improve it.

Headache Disorders (ICHD) distinguishes between pure menstrual migraine and menstrually related migraine. In pure menstrual migraine, headache attacks occur during a menstrual window of 2 days before through 3 days after the onset of bleeding, and at no other time of the month. In menstrually related migraine, attacks occur predictably during the –2 to +3 window and also at other times of the month.[4] In women who have very frequent headaches it can be difficult to define the contribution of the menstrual cycle to the headache problem. In some cases a link between headaches and the menstrual cycle will become more apparent as headaches decrease in frequency with successful prophylactic treatment.

Are Hormones Part of the Problem?

Evidence of a link between headache worsening and the menstrual cycle or other hormonal events, in the form of a headache diary or calendar, is probably the best means of establishing whether hormonal factors play a significant role in a woman's headaches. Common sense suggests that several months' worth of diary information is needed to establish a clear link between headaches and hormonal factors. The diary should track occurrence of menstrual bleeding or the use of hormonal contraception, and the frequency and severity of headache.

Other corroborating evidence might include a close temporal relationship between headache and hormonal events such as menarche, pregnancy or its termination, or the initiation of exogenous hormones for contraception, infertility treatment, or menopause. If headaches are frequent and severe, it can be hard to identify headache changes attributable to hormones because of the high level of background headache activity.[5] In these cases it might be useful to track medication intake or emergency department visits in relation to hormonal changes.

Table 14-2 Evidence that Hormonal Contributions to Headache Are Important and May Warrant Specific Attention in Individual Women with Refractory Migraine[a]

- The headaches occur in predictable, repeated temporal relationship to hormonal events, as indicated by carefully kept headache diaries.
- There is a plausible biologic explanation for a change in migraine in relation to that event.
- Removal or avoidance of the suspected hormonal event (when possible) results in improvement in headache (e.g., menstrually connected headaches improve during pregnancy and resume once cycles resume postpartum).
- Subjective measurements of headache severity change in concert with objective measures such as medication intake, work-related disability, medication intake, or emergency department visits.

[a]Tests of ovarian or pituitary function generally are not useful.

Tests of ovarian or pituitary hormone levels generally are not useful in identifying hormonal causes or contributors to refractory headache problems. Despite the commonly expressed belief that "there must be something wrong with my hormones," there is no evidence of treatable hormonal abnormalities in most women with hormonally influenced migraine, although menorrhagia and endometriosis seem to be more common in women attending specialty headache centers.[6] For example, there is no evidence of an increased risk of migraine in women with polycystic ovarian syndrome or other infertility disorders (although infertility *treatment* can provoke migraine).[7] Rather, all of the available evidence points to exaggerated sensitivity of the "migraine-prone brain" to normally fluctuating levels of hormones.

In addition to the fact that hormonal abnormalities are unlikely to be the cause of hormonally connected migraine, measurement of such hormones also is impractical. Blood or urine levels of ovarian hormones are difficult to measure and are not easily correlated with headache activity or useful in selecting or monitoring treatment. Instead, in most cases we look for circumstantial evidence that hormones are involved, which includes worsening or predictable occurrence in connection with hormonal fluctuations. Typically, stable levels of estrogen, regardless of level, protect against headache activity, while a decline in estrogen level seems to provoke headache.[8]

Table 14.2 lists some features that can stand as circumstantial evidence of an important hormonal contribution to headaches in an individual patient. Sometimes headache severity will increase in a predictable pattern in relation to the natural menstrual cycle or during the hormone-free period of estrogen-containing contraceptives.[9] The more individual items that are present in a particular case, the stronger the case that hormonal treatment might be warranted.

A Note of Caution

Despite strong evidence that hormonal factors influence migraine expression in women in general, individual susceptibility to migraine triggers varies considerably. It is unlikely that hormonal factors play a significant role in all women with RM. Overemphasis on the hormonal aspects of migraine may divert attention from more likely causes of headache or from nonhormonal treatments with a more favorable harm to benefit balance. In some cases, an unfounded belief in hormonal causes of headache may lead to unnecessary surgery or to the use of treatments that are dangerous or unproven, with unknown long-term health risks.

Some well-intentioned hormonal treatment strategies may even make migraine worse; evidence suggests, for example, that oophorectomy worsens, rather than improves, migraine.[10] All hormonal treatments can cause potentially serious side effects and complications, so their empirical use generally should be avoided.

A cultural predisposition to blame hormones for a wide variety of physical and emotional ailments may increase the tendency of both patients and doctors to accept spurious or weak evidence that hormonal factors play an important role in an individual woman's headache problem.[11,12] For all of these reasons there should be convincing evidence that hormonal triggers contribute substantially to an individual woman's migraine problem before the potential risks of hormonal treatment are incurred. Table 14.3 lists some useful questions to ask before embarking on hormonal treatment of headaches.

What Strategies Might Be Tried if Hormonal Aspects of Headache Warrant Specific Attention?

Treatment Options for Menstrual Migraine

Even if hormonal factors are determined to play an important role in a woman with RM, it does not follow that treatment must be hormonal in nature. Likewise, treatment of hormonal headache does not always have to be targeted at the hormonally influenced exacerbations of migraine. As hormones are likely to be only one of many triggers in a case of RM, general treatment strategies aimed at the overall migraine problem may well be more appropriate.[13] Those treatments are covered in other chapters. There is a perception, however, that hormonal headaches may not respond as well as nonhormonal headaches to general treatment measures. A common clinical experience is that general prophylaxis for migraine eliminates many headaches but that menstrually related headaches may remain troublesome nonetheless.

Still, there is good evidence that some nonhormonal treatment strategies are effective when used to target hormonally connected headaches. In fact, the quality of evidence supporting the scheduled use of triptans or nonsteroidal anti-inflammatory agents for menstrual migraine is higher than the quality of evidence supporting the use of hormonal treatment strategies.[14]

Nonhormonal treatment strategies aimed at hormonally influenced headaches usually seek to interfere with the headache in its early stages of

Table 14-3 Should Hormonal Treatment Be Tried? Five Questions to Ask

Question	Comment
On review of the patient's headache history, is there clear evidence that headaches are sensitive to hormonal fluctuations?	This could take the form of clear worsening around menstrual periods, ideally based on diary information; improvement during pregnancy; worsening on oral contraceptives or peri-menopausally or a strong history in female relatives of hormonal sensitivity
Is the patient significantly disabled by headache despite aggressive use of appropriate nonhormonal therapy?	Given the potential harms and tolerability problems of some hormonal treatment regimens, as well as their off-label status, it is harder to defend hormonal treatment attempts when other more traditional methods of treatment have not been exhausted.
Is the patient free of medical contraindications to the use of hormonal regimens?	Estrogen and perhaps progesterone is associated with an increased risk of breast cancer. If the woman has aura or is over 35 the increased risk of ischemic stroke attributable to estrogen is generally considered unacceptable. This risk is amplified by other CV risk factors such as hypertension or tobacco use.
Does the patient understand the experimental nature of the treatment and the uncertain and probably modest nature of any benefits? In particular, the potential for unknown harms and risks?	The legal standard for consent to treatment is that a patient has been told of risks that a "reasonable person" would want disclosed. Women should understand that there are no large randomized, controlled trials that demonstrate and quantify the benefits of these treatment strategies. In contrast to this uncertainty about treatment benefit, harms of treatment, including elevated risks of stroke and breast cancer from estrogen, are better understood.
Is the patient able to keep track of headaches, compliant with treatment, and able to manage complex treatment regimens?	Many hormonal treatment regimens are complex, and some depend upon accurate timing of menstrual cycles or adherence to daily medication.

development, or even to preempt a predictable headache by taking medication on a scheduled basis during the period of headache susceptibility.

Available evidence suggests that stable levels of estrogen have a beneficial effect on headache. Hormonal treatment strategies for RM thus aim to achieve and maintain stable levels of estrogen. While this may seem a simple and straightforward goal, in practice it is not always easy to achieve. There are also important safety and tolerability concerns that make hormonal treatment an approach of last resort. Finally, we lack information from well-designed trials about which strategies and doses are most helpful, the magnitude of any benefits, and whether those benefits outweigh harms.

Table 14.4 lists some commonly used strategies for the treatment of menstrual migraine along with comments relevant to the use of each in women with RM. A detailed discussion of each regimen is beyond the scope of this chapter; readers interested in the details of each strategy are referred to the original publications.

Why Don't They Work Well?

Despite the strong evidence that hormonal factors play an important role in migraine in many women, most studies of hormonal treatment show only modest, if any, treatment benefits. One possible explanation for this paradox is that hormonal factors provoke migraine activity that is self-perpetuating. In other words, the central nervous system mechanisms through which hormones aggravate migraine may not be fully reversible.

Another possible explanation is that the interventions we have are crude or poorly timed, either with respect to small month-to-month variations in the cycle of an individual woman, or with relation to the timing of such treatments in the course of a woman's reproductive life. It is possible, for example, that hormonal interventions might be more effective if used early in the course of migraine. As with many other sorts of treatment, there may be a limited window of time during which treatment can influence disease activity. This could explain why, as with many other treatments, hormonal therapies are minimally effective in women with RM.

A final reason that hormonal treatments of migraine may be ineffective is that the degree or type of hormonal manipulation necessary to help with headaches is not feasible or tolerated. It is possible, for example, that higher doses of estrogen in combination oral contraceptives might more effectively suppress endogenous ovarian function.[28] Such high dose regimens, though, incur a risk of thromboembolic events that is usually judged unacceptable in comparison to the risks of lower dose regimens.

Contraceptive Advice for Women with RM

Most patients with RM are women of childbearing potential who will need to make decisions about contraception. Combination estrogen-progesterone contraceptives are the most reliable method of birth control, but guidelines suggest that exogenous estrogen should be avoided in women of any age who have migraine with aura, and avoided in women who have migraine without aura after the age of 35.[29–31] This recommendation is based on worries about the safety of estrogen in women who already have one risk factor (migraine) for ischemic stroke. Evidence suggests that stroke risk in

Table 14-4 Short-term Preventive Strategies for Menstrual Migraine

Strategy	Example	Comments
Scheduled use of NSAIDs, triptans, or their combination to pre-empt expected menstrual attacks of migraine	Naproxen sodium 550 mg orally twice daily for 5–7 days[15]; Naratriptan 2.5 mg twice orally for 5 days[16]; Frovatriptan loading dose of 5 mg orally twice daily then 2.5 mg orally twice daily for 5 days [17]	Treatment benefits are modest, but evidence of benefit is consistent and based on high-quality randomized controlled trials; tripans are not approved by the U.S. FDA for this indication.
Modified contraceptive regimens	Extended duration or continuous estrogen/ progesterone combination contraception.[18] This approach minimizes or eliminates the pill-free portion of traditional combined contraceptive regimens, in the hope that estrogen withdrawal symptoms, including headache, will be minimized.	Extended duration or continuous contraceptive regimens are not approved by the FDA for the treatment of migraine. Evidence of specific benefit in migraine is weak and based on trials of limited quality which examined general measures of "headache" activity, not migraine. Benefits on general headache activity appear modest. Exogenous estrogens are contraindicated in women who have aura or women with migraine older than 35.
Estrogen Supplementation With or Without Ovarian Suppression	Estradiol gel, patches or injections are commonly used. Regimens vary but typically are timed to prevent or minimize he expected estrogen nadir in naturally occurring menstrual cycles or in contraceptive cycles. Gonadotropin releasing hormone agonists may be administered with or without add-back estrogen.	Hypoestrogenic side effects are an important long-term concern if add-back estrogen is not used. If add-back estrogen regimens are used, it can be difficult to prevent variations in estrogen level even with transdermal formulations. In one study, many women with migraine proved sensitive to even small drops in estrogen levels while using a patch formulation of estrogen in combination with a GNRH agonist.[19]

(*Continued*)

Table 14-4 Continued

Strategy	Example	Comments
Oophorectomy		Oophorectomy as a treatment for refractory migraine is not recommended because available evidence, although of low quality, suggests headache may worsen rather than improve.[20]
Magnesium	1–2 grams of magnesium sulfate intravenously one week prior to menstruation; magnesium 360 mg orally daily during the luteal phase of the menstrual cycle[21]	Evidence of benefit in small trials and case series
Phytoestrogens		The evidence supporting the use of phytoestrogens to treat hormonally related headaches is of extremely low quality.[22, 23]
Danazol	200 mg danazol twice daily, administered for 25 days/month[24]	Not approved by the FDA for this indication. Evidence of benefit comes from small, open-label trials.
Tamoxifen	20 mg/day[25–27]	Not approved by the FDA for this indication. Evidence of benefit comes from uncontrolled case series and case reports. A case report suggests tamoxifen may worsen migraine. Tamoxifen increases the risk of blood clots, uterine cancer, and produces hypoestrogenic side effects such as hot flashes.

women with migraine and aura is increased compared with women who have no migraine or migraine without aura; the addition of estrogen-containing contraceptives or smoking elevated the risk further.[32]

Aside from the safety risks of estrogen-containing contraceptives, tolerability problems must also be considered. High-quality evidence of the impact of various contraceptives on headache activity in women with preexisting migraine is lacking.[33] Circumstantial evidence suggests, though, that estrogen-containing combination contraceptives may worsen migraine. The large Norwegian Head-HUNT study found a higher prevalence of migraine in women using estrogen containing contraceptives but not in women using progestin-only contraceptives.[34] Progestin-only contraceptives also do not increase the risk of stroke and thus are not contraindicated in women with migraine. Other options for contraception that do not aggravate migraine or increase stroke risk include physical or chemical methods such as foam and condoms, or intrauterine devices.

Because the influence of estrogen-containing contraceptives on the clinical course of migraine is uncertain, it may be prudent to avoid their use in women with RM. The fact that female sex is a risk factor for increased frequency of migraine suggests that estrogen itself may predispose to chronification of headaches; in someone where headaches are already difficult to control even this theoretical risk may warrant use of other forms of contraception. If estrogen-containing contraceptives cannot be avoided or if a woman decides that in her case the benefits outweigh potential risks, monophasic contraceptives with 35 micrograms of estrogen or less should be used. Extended duration contraceptive regimens (in which the traditional monthly pill-free week is shortened or eliminated) may minimize estrogen withdrawal headaches but the impact seems modest, and breakthrough bleeding is a common side effect that limits compliance. Likewise, "add-back" estrogen, for example, 0.1 mg of transdermal estradiol can be used during the pill-free week of traditional oral contraceptives. If women develop new-onset aura or worsening headache in close association with the use of estrogen-containing contraceptives, the treatment should probably be stopped.

Pregnancy, the Puerperium, and Lactation in Women with RM

Preconception Planning

Women with RM may hesitate to undertake pregnancy because of uncertainty about whether migraine or medications need to treat it will have a negative effect on pregnancy outcome. They may also worry that refractory headaches will make it difficult to meet the responsibilities of parenthood. Because pregnancy in a woman with RM has so many implications, clinicians should emphasize the desirability of planning pregnancy and provide advice on appropriate contraceptive methods. To reduce the risk of neural tube defects, all women of childbearing potential should be encouraged to use a daily multivitamin supplement containing at least 400 μg of folate.

There is no evidence that migraine affects fertility, but with delayed childbearing the need for infertility treatments is becoming more common, and there is evidence that the exaggerated hormonal fluctuations of infertility treatment have a negative effect on migraine.[35] This is especially undesirable in women with RM, so that severe migraine might be an argument for immediately attempting oocyte retrieval and extrauterine fertilization, in preference to repeated episodes of ovulation induction and intrauterine insemination.

The Impact of Pregnancy on RM

Evidence suggests that, in general, about three quarters of women with migraine will experience headache improvement or cessation in pregnancy. It is not clear, though, whether these findings apply to women with RM. Even in the general population of women with migraine, not all improve during pregnancy; in fact, some experience worsening of headache. It is also the case that "improvement" in someone with refractory headache at baseline may not be substantial enough to allow discontinuation or avoidance of medications during pregnancy. There is some evidence that increased parity may be associated with a higher prevalence of migraine, but a causal link is uncertain. It is possible that the stresses and lifestyle changes associated with having more children are responsible for this association.[36]

Thus it is useful for women who are contemplating pregnancy to consider how they might deal with the "worst case scenario" of continued severe headaches during pregnancy. Some are prepared to accept the risks associated with a continued need for medications, while others hope to forgo or minimize medication despite bad headaches. Other approaches to coping with bad headaches during pregnancy include curtailed work and home responsibilities and more aggressive use of nonpharmacological or complementary methods of headache treatment.

The Impact of RM and Its Treatment on Pregnancy Complications and Adverse Outcomes

Some complications of pregnancy are more common in women with migraine (Table 14.5). Preeclampsia is one serious complication that is more common in women who have migraine, especially those who have migraine with aura.[37] Risk may be even higher in women with poorly controlled or frequent headaches.[38] Preeclampsia is the most common cause of maternal morbidity and mortality in developed countries. Its initial presentation can be subtle, and headache is a common symptom that, in women with RM, might easily be missed. Thus a high index of suspicion for preeclampsia is appropriate in women with migraine.

Table 14-5 Pregnancy Complications that May Be More Common or Severe in Women with Migraine

- Preeclampsia/eclampsia
- Reversible vasoconstrictive syndromes[39]
- Postpartum stroke[40]
- Low-pressure headache following unintended dural puncture with epidural anesthesia. Refractory migraine does not increase the chance that headache from unintended dural puncture will occur, but the addition of this headache to migraine may increase the overall burden of RM.[41]

There is no good quality evidence that migraine itself increases the risk of birth defects or congenital anomalies, but some medications used to treat it have been associated with birth defects or other problems. The U.S. Food and Drug Administration (FDA) rating system is a commonly used method of determining the pregnancy risks of drugs. In this system, drugs are assigned a rating of A, B, C, D, or X, depending upon evidence of harms. Drugs with ratings of D or X should generally be avoided; for others decisions must be individualized. The FDA rating system is much criticized; some experts prefer the use of other methods of risk assessment such as that of the Teratogen Information Service (TERIS). Table 14.6 lists some commonly used headache medications and their FDA and TERIS ratings, along with other considerations relevant to their use in women with RM.

Whichever method of risk assessment is used to evaluate the potential harms of a drug, it has to be recognized that, with few exceptions, definitive evidence of harm or safety is lacking for any drug. As a general rule, when medication is used in pregnancy it is prudent to choose those with a longer track record of use in pregnancy and those for which there is no good theoretical reason to suspect potential harm.

There is little good evidence regarding the pregnancy safety of nontraditional headache treatments such as vitamins, herbs and nutritional supplements, and these should be avoided in pregnancy. An exception to this is magnesium, which may be appropriate for use. The pregnancy effects of botulinum toxin for headache are also unknown and it should also be avoided.

In most cases, though, difficult decisions will have to be made about balancing uncertain risks and benefits of drug therapy. Shared decision-making that involves the patient and her partner is desirable, and discussions should be carefully documented in the patient's record. It may be useful to refer the patient to teratogen information or other counseling services for expert advice about drug risks.

The Puerperium and Lactation

Even if it has improved during pregnancy, migraine commonly recurs shortly after delivery. Headaches are common after delivery.[44] In this setting, it can be

Table 14-6 Considerations Relevant to The Use of Some Common Headache Drugs in Pregnant Women with Refractory Migraine

Drug	FDA rating[a]/TERIS rating[b]	Comment
Acetaminophen	B/None	Also compatible with lactation; not usually very helpful on its own for headache, but may augment effects of other analgesics when used in combination.
Amitriptyline		
Aspirin	C/None–Minimal	NSAIDs should be avoided near term because of the risk of premature closure of the ductus arteriosus.
Divalproex	D/Small–Moderate	Best avoided because of the risk of neural tube defects
Ergotamine/DHE	X/Undetermined	
Indomethacin	B (D in 3d trimester)/Undetermined	Indomethacin is a potent prostaglandin inhibitor and use near term should be avoided.
Opioids	Morphine, Methadone, butorphanol are B/ Minimal but D if prolonged or near term	Withdrawal syndromes can occur in the newborn with frequent maternal use.
Propranolol	C/Undetermined	May affect fetal size and weight; no evidence of teratogenicity.
Topiramate	C/Undetermined	Preliminary reports from pregnancy registries suggest a possible increase in congenital defects in women who have used topiramate, but evidence is insufficient to draw firm conclusions at present.[39]
Triptans	C/Undetermined	Some triptans are considered compatible with lactation; the best evidence of pregnancy effects is for sumatriptan. To date, the large sumatriptan pregnancy registry shows no signal of teratogenicity but evidence is insufficient to make definitive recommendations.[40]

[a]US FDA pregnancy ratings:

A = Controlled human studies show no risk.

B = No evidence of risk in humans, but no controlled studies.

C = Risk to humans has not been ruled out (risk vs. benefit in prescribing).

D = Positive evidence of risk to humans from human or animal studies.

X = Contraindicated in pregnancy.

[b]TERIS ratings: Risk is categorized as none, minimal, small, moderate, high or undetermined.

difficult to distinguish a return or worsening or preexisting migraine from some other postpartum complications that may present with headache. These include post-partum preeclampsia, cerebral vasoconstrictive syndromes, postdural puncture headaches and cerebral venous thrombosis. A high index of suspicion for these problems is appropriate in women with RM, since some of these disorders are also more common in migraineurs. Because vasoconstrictive medications such as the triptans or ergots may increase the risk of vasoconstrictive syndromes they should generally be avoided in the immediate postpartum period; the authors' practice is to avoid their use until 6 weeks following delivery.[45,46]

Lactation in Women with RM

The benefits of breastfeeding are substantial for mother and baby, so lactation should be encouraged. Lactation does not seem to aggravate migraine; if breastfeeding is consistent and exclusive it may delay the return of ovulatory menstrual cycles. In most cases, it is possible to find medications that are compatible with lactation, so that women rarely have to choose between breastfeeding and treatment of their headaches. It is unwise to assume that different members of the same drug class are equally safe in pregnancy or lactation. For example, sumatriptan is considered compatible with lactation, but the safety of other triptans in lactation is less certain. The preventive drug propranolol can typically be used during pregnancy and lactation, but atenolol has an FDA black box warning against use in pregnancy or lactation because of the risks of fetal bradycardia and hypoglycemia.[47] In general, the amount of drug that passes into breast milk is heavily dependent upon its lipophilicity. The American Academy of Pediatrics rates the compatibility of various drugs with lactation and their current information on a particular drug should be consulted before prescribing it.[48]

General Principles of RM Treatment in Pregnancy

The general principles of migraine treatment during pregnancy (Table 14.7) are the same whether a woman has treatment-responsive or RM, but the harm to benefit balance of some interventions is probably different. For example, women with infrequent, treatment-responsive migraine may also be more responsive to alternative, nonpharmacological methods of treatment than are women with RM. They are generally able to forgo prophylactic treatment in pregnancy, and may also be successful in avoiding or minimizing the use of drugs for individual migraine attacks. Instead, they might rest at home or use nonspecific therapies to cope with an attack.

In contrast, a woman with RM may have more need to continue prophylactic treatments during pregnancy. Even if prophylaxis does not fully control the problem, headaches may be even worse in its absence. Women with RM

Table 14-7 General Principles of Pregnancy Management in Women with RM

- Encourage planned pregnancies. Think through and discuss possible scenarios with the patient and her partner.
- Minimize work and home responsibilities.
- Minimize medication use, especially during the first trimester, but remember that complete avoidance may not be feasible or humane.
- When medication is needed, choose those with the best evidence of safety in pregnancy.
- Be alert for complications of pregnancy that are more common in migraineurs and that might correlate with disease activity.
- Expect a postpartum flare of headache.
- Avoid the use of vasoconstrictive medications in the puerperium.
- Encourage breast-feeding if appropriate; many medications are compatible with lactation

commonly have little success with nonpharmacological treatment methods as well as drug treatments. These women may not be able to function at all without headache treatment of some kind. It is probably unrealistic to expect that a woman with RM will be able to avoid use of all abortive or prophylactic medication for headache for the duration of pregnancy.

Menopause in Women with RM

Many women with RM have been told by friends or physicians that their headaches will improve after menopause, but in fact it is not uncommon for RM to persist well beyond menopause. Headaches may be especially troublesome during the perimenopause, perhaps because of erratic swings in estrogen levels.[7,49] Perimenopause may be associated with irregular periods or symptoms such as hot flashes, night sweats and sleep disturbance.

The effect of hormone replacement therapy on preexisting migraine is uncertain. Evidence from the large Norwegian Head-HUNT study and from the U.S. Women's Health study shows that women using hormone replacement therapy are more likely to report migraine, but it is not possible to be certain whether hormone replacement therapy is causing headache or might be used in an effort to treat it.[50,51] Some women report headache improvement with continuous replacement regimens, but it does not have FDA approval for this indication.

Hormonal therapy is sometimes needed to control severe vasomotor symptoms. Because of emerging evidence of stroke and cardiovascular risks associated with hormone replacement therapy, it should generally be used at the lowest possible dose for the shortest amount of time needed to control symptoms. As with estrogen-containing contraceptives, estrogen use after menopause is generally felt to be contraindicated in women with migraine because of the risk of stroke.[31] If used, nonoral routes of administration, particularly transdermal routes, seem less likely to provoke or aggravate headaches. Transdermal estrogen patches delivering 0.05 to 0.1 mg of estrogen are often used continuously. Progesterone is used concomitantly in women with a uterus; it is omitted in women without a uterus. Postmenopausal estrogen use may provoke visual aura, so this and its effect on headache should be monitored.[49]

References

1. Lipton RB, Bigal ME. Migraine: epidemiology, impact, and risk factors for progression. *Headache.* 2005;45(Suppl 1):S3–S13.
2. Hu XH, Markson LE, Lipton RB, Stewart WF, Berger ML. Burden of migraine in the United States: disability and economic costs. *Arch Intern Med.* 1999; 159(8):813–818.
3. Welch KM, Brandes JL, Berman NE. Mismatch in how oestrogen modulates molecular and neuronal function may explain menstrual migraine. *Neurol Sci.* 2006;27 Suppl 2:S190–192.
4. Headache Classification Subcommittee of the International Headache Society. The *International Classification of Headache Disorders,* 2nd ed. *Cephalalgia.* 2004;24 (Suppl 1):9–160.
5. Johannes CB, Linet MS, Stewart WF, Celentano DD, Lipton RB, Szklo M. Relationship of headache to phase of the menstrual cycle among young women: a daily diary study. *Neurology.* 1995;45(6):1076–1082.
6. Tietjen GE, Conway A, Utley C, Gunning WT, Herial NA. Migraine is associated with menorrhagia and endometriosis. *Headache.* 2006;46(3): 422–428.
7. Pourabolghasem S, Najmi S, Arami MA. Polycystic ovary syndrome and migraine headache, is there any correlation?. *Eur Neurol.* 2009;61(1):42–45.
8. Somerville BW. The role of estradiol withdrawal in the etiology of menstrual migraine. *Neurology.* 1972;22(4):355–365.
9. Sulak PJ, Scow RD, Preece C, Riggs MW, Kuehl TJ. Hormone withdrawal symptoms in oral contraceptive users. *Obstet Gynecol.* 2000;95(2):261–266.
10. Neri I, Granella F, Nappi R, Manzoni GC, Facchinetti F, Genazzani AR. Characteristics of headache at menopause: a clinico-epidemiologic study. *Maturitas.* 1993;17(1):31–37.
11. Sheldrake P, Cormack M. Variations in menstrual cycle symptom reporting. *J Psychosom Res.* 1976;20(3):169–177.
12. McFarland C, Ross M, DeCourville N. Women's theories of menstruation and biases in recall of menstrual symptoms. *J Pers Soc Psychol.* 1989;57(3): 522–531.
13. Loder E, Rizzoli P, Golub J. Hormonal management of migraine associated with menses and the menopause: a clinical review. *Headache.* 2007;47(2): 329–340.
14. Martin VT. Menstrual migraine: a review of prophylactic therapies. *Curr Pain Headache Rep.* 2004;8(3):229–237.
15. Sances G, Martignoni E, Fioroni L, Blandini F, Facchinetti F, Nappi G. Naproxen sodium in menstrual migraine prophylaxis: a double-blind placebo controlled study. *Headache.* 1990;30(11):705–709.

16. Newman L, Mannix LK, Landy S, et al. Naratriptan as short-term prophylaxis of menstrually associated migraine: a randomized, double-blind, placebo-controlled study. *Headache.* 2001;41(3):248–256.
17. Silberstein SD, Elkind AH, Schreiber C, Keywood C. A randomized trial of frovatriptan for the intermittent prevention of menstrual migraine. *Neurology.* 2004; 27;63(2):261–269.
18. Sulak PJ, Cressman BE, Waldrop E, Holleman S, Kuehl TJ. Extending the duration of active oral contraceptive pills to manage hormone withdrawal symptoms. *Obstet Gynecol.* 1997;89(2):179–183.
19. Martin V, Wernke S, Mandell K, et al. Medical oophorectomy with and without estrogen add-back therapy in the prevention of migraine headache. *Headache.* 2003;43(4):309–321.
20. Neri I, Granella F, Nappi R, Manzoni GC, Facchinetti F, Genazzani AR. Characteristics of headache at menopause: a clinico-epidemiologic study. *Maturitas.* 1993;17(1):31–37.
21. Mauskop A, Altura BT, Altura BM. Serum ionized magnesium levels and serum ionized calcium/ionized magnesium ratios in women with menstrual migraine. *Headache.* 2002;42(4):242–248.
22. Ferrante F, Fusco E, Calabresi P, Cupini LM. Phyto-oestrogens in the prophylaxis of menstrual migraine. *Clin Neuropharmacol.* 2004;27(3): 137–140.
23. Burke BE, Olson RD, Cusack BJ. Randomized, controlled trial of phytoestrogen in the prophylactic treatment of menstrual migraine. *Biomed Pharmacother.* 2002; 56(6):283–288.
24. Lichten EM, Bennett RS, Whitty AJ, Daoud Y. Efficacy of danazol in the control of hormonal migraine. *J Reprod Med.* 1991;36(6):419–424.
25. O'Dea JP, Davis EH. Tamoxifen in the treatment of menstrual migraine. *Neurology.* 1990;40(9):1470–1471.
26. Powles T. Prevention of migrainous headaches by tamoxifen. *Lancet.* 1986;ii: 1334.
27. Mathew P, Fung F. Recapitulation of menstrual migraine with tamoxifen. *Lancet.* 1999;353(9151):467–468.
28. Sulak PJ. Ovulation suppression of premenstrual symptoms using oral contraceptives. *Am J Manag Care.* 2005;11(16 Suppl):S492–497.
29. ACOG Committee on Practice Bulletins-Gynecology. ACOG practice bulletin. No. 73: Use of hormonal contraception in women with coexisting medical conditions. *Obstet Gynecol.* 2006;107(6):1453–1472.
30. Gaffield ME, Curtis KM, Mohllajee AP, Peterson HB. Medical eligibility criteria for new contraceptive methods: combined hormonal patch, combined hormonal vaginal ring and the etonogestrel implant. *Contraception.* 2006; 73(2):134–144.
31. Bousser MG, Conard J, Kittner S, et al. Recommendations on the risk of ischaemic stroke associated with use of combined oral contraceptives and hormone replacement therapy in women with migraine. The International Headache Society Task Force on Combined Oral Contraceptives & Hormone Replacement Therapy. *Cephalalgia.* 2000;20(3):155–156.
32. Tzourio C, Kittner SJ, Bousser MG, Alperovitch A. Migraine and stroke in young women. *Cephalalgia.* 2000;20(3):190–199.

33. Loder EW, Buse DC, Golub JR. Headache as a side effect of combination estrogen-progestin oral contraceptives: a systematic review. *Am J Obstet Gynecol.* 2005;193(3 Pt 1):636–649.
34. Aegidius K, Zwart JA, Hagen K, Schei B, Stovner LJ. Oral contraceptives and increased headache prevalence: the Head-HUNT Study. *Neurology.* 2006; 66(3):349–353.
35. Amir BY, Yaacov B, Guy B, Gad P, Itzhak W, Gal I. Headaches in women undergoing in vitro fertilization and embryo-transfer treatment. *Headache.* 2005;45(3):215–219.
36. Aegidius K, Zwart JA, Hagen K, Stovner L. The effect of pregnancy and parity on headache prevalence: the Head-HUNT study. *Headache.* 2009;49(6): 851–859.
37. Adeney KL, Williams MA. Migraine headaches and preeclampsia: an epidemiologic review. *Headache.* 2006;46(5):794–803.
38. Adeney KL, Williams MA, Miller RS, Frederick IO, Sorensen TK, Luthy DA. Risk of preeclampsia in relation to maternal history of migraine headaches. *J Matern Fetal Neonatal Med.* 2005;18(3):167–172.
39. Modi M, Modi G. Case reports: postpartum angiopathy in a patient with chronic migraine with aura. *Headache* 2000; 40(8):677-681.
40. James AH, Bushnell CD, Jamison MD, Myers ER. Risk factors for stroke in pregnancy and the puerperium. *Obstet Gynecol* 2005;106(3):509-516.
41. Corbey MP, Bach AB, Lech K, Frorup AM. Grading of severity of postdural puncture headache after 27-gauge Quincke and Whitacre needles. *Acta Anaesthesiol Scand* 1997; 41(6):779-784.
42. Hunt S, Russell A, Smithson WH, et al. Topiramate in pregnancy: preliminary experience from the UK Epilepsy and Pregnancy Register. *Neurology.* 2008; 71(4):272–276.
43. Loder E. Safety of sumatriptan in pregnancy: a review of the data so far. *CNS Drugs.* 2003;17(1):1–7.
44. Goldszmidt E, Kern R, Chaput A, Macarthur A. The incidence and etiology of postpartum headaches: a prospective cohort study. *Can J Anaesth.* 2005;52(9):971–977.
45. Sato S, Shimizu M, Endo K, Homma M, Yamamoto T. Postpartum cerebral angiopathy--a case report the vasculopathy associated with co-administration of two vasoconstrictives, methylergometrine maleate and sumatriptan. *Rinsho Shinkeigaku.* 2004;44(2):96–101.
46. Granier I, Garcia E, Geissler A, Boespflug MD, Durand-Gasselin J. Postpartum cerebral angiopathy associated with the administration of sumatriptan and dihydroergotamine—a case report. *Intens Care Med.* 1999; 25(5):532–534.
47. Schimmel MS, Eidelman AI, Wilschanski MA, Shaw D, Jr, Ogilvie RJ, Koren G. Toxic effects of atenolol consumed during breast feeding. *J Pediatr.* 1989; 114(3):476–478.
48. Ressel G. AAP updates statement for transfer of drugs and other chemicals into breast milk. American Academy of Pediatrics. *Am Fam Physician.* 2002; 65(5):979–980.
49. Prior JC. Ovarian aging and the perimenopausal transition: the paradox of endogenous ovarian hyperstimulation. *Endocrine.* 2005;26(3):297–300.

50. Aegidius KL, Zwart JA, Hagen K, Schei B, Stovner LJ. Hormone replacement therapy and headache prevalence in postmenopausal women. The Head-HUNT study. *Eur J Neurol.* 2007;14(1):73–78.
51. Misakian AL, Langer RD, Bensenor IM, et al. Postmenopausal hormone therapy and migraine headache. *J Womens Health (Larchmt).* 2003;12(10):1027–1036.
52. MacGregor EA, Barnes D. Migraine in a specialist menopause clinic. *Climacteric.* 1999;2(3):218–223.

15

Refractory Headaches in Children and Adolescents

Andrew D. Hershey, MD, PhD, FAHS

Introduction

Refractory migraine (RM) has recently received increased attention by physicians interested in headache treatment. Many gaps remain in our understanding of this entity, especially for children and adolescents. As discussed in the chapter defining RM, these headaches must meet the *International Classification of Headache Disorders*, 2nd ed. (ICHD-II) criteria for migraine or chronic migraine (CM), and be unresponsive to standard treatment—both acute and preventative. The definition requires the failure of three out of four preventative classes, as well as a lack of response to acute treatments including both migraine specific (i.e., triptans and dihydroergotamine [DHE]) as well as nonspecific agents (i.e., nonsteroidal anti-inflammatory drugs [NSAIDs] and combination analgesics). In addition, the definition included modifiers for medication overuse headaches (MOH) and for associated disability. Other primary headaches and secondary headaches may refractory, but are not defined.

Application of this RM definition in the pediatric and adolescent population poses additional challenges. CM in children is less well studied than in adults, including its epidemiology and prognosis. Many of the treatments in children and adolescents, although presumed effective, lack rigorous study in CM and RM patients and none are U.S. Food and Drug Administration (FDA) approved for those younger than the age of 18. As for the modifiers, MOH is clearly present in children and adolescents. An instrument Pediatric Migraine Disability Assessment [PedMIDAS]) has been used to define the impact of pediatric and adolescent migraine, and reflect disability.

Given these limitations, a logical starting point in the study of RM in children is the study of unresponsiveness to acute medication and to the presence of CM. In children and adolescents, there are additional unique contributors that may influence the responsiveness to treatment and need to be addressed when these young patients do not respond to treatment.

Epidemiology

The prevalence of RM and other refractory headaches in children and adolescents is unknown. The best estimate is that these children make up a small fraction of children with chronic daily headache (CDH), including CM. Limited studies have addressed this question, but CDH appears to occur less frequently in children and adolescents than adults, occurring with a prevalence rate of 1% to 2%.[1–3] In tertiary specialty headache centers, however, CDH may represent a significant proportion of the children seen.

In a survey of the Cincinnati Children's Headache Center database of more than 5000 children and adolescents, 41.3% had CDH defined as 15 or more headaches per month at their initial evaluation. Of this group of patients 39.7% continued to have CDH at 1 year, while 39.2% continue to have CDH at 2 years. These patients had all been treated with multiple preventative agents and continued to have CDH. Some of these patients may have met the criteria for RM. Further analysis of RM patients is needed to help define the contributors to their refractory nature.

The frequency of MOH in the general population of children and adolescents is also largely unknown, but may occur in up to 50% of the patients with CDH seen in tertiary headache centers. In the initial ICHD-II definition of MOH, criteria required 2 months of cessation of the overused analgesics. Under this definition, only those patients that had a significant reduction in their headache frequency could be defined as MOH, while those that did not respond were classified as not having MOH. This has been modified to exclude this 2-month observation period, and the view that most MOH patients respond to cessation of analgesics, but not all. In one estimate of children that were overusing analgesic, it appears that approximately 50% of these patients responded to cessation of analgesic overuse. The group that does not improve may provide a glimpse of the patient that may evolve into the RM.

Characteristics of CDH and CM

Some of the risk factors for development of CDH/CM in adults have been identified. These contributing factors in adults may allow extrapolation to children. Several studies have investigated the characteristics of CDH/CM in children.[4–9] The majority of these are derived from specialty headache centers. A common observation is that the majority of these patients have migraine features with their CDH. In one study, it was observed that these groups of patients could be subdivided into daily continuous (i.e., the patient always has a headache), daily intermittent (i.e., a headache every day, but not continuously), and frequent but not daily.[4] This led to two observations: (1) as the patients improved, the features of their headaches were more clearly migraine and (2) the CDHs were the most resistant to treatment. The majority, however, did eventually respond to a multidisciplinary treatment approach, leaving a small number of patients that may have had RM, providing the other criteria of the definition were met.

Medication Unresponsiveness

Although several well controlled studies evaluated the efficacy of the acute and preventative medications have been performed in adolescents with migraine, none are approved by the FDA for the treatment of pediatric or adolescent migraine. A recent practice parameter acknowledged that only flunarizine had the rigorous studies to substantiate Grade I evidence as being effective. A detailed review of the studies on acute and preventative treatment of pediatric and adolescent migraine is beyond the scope of this chapter, but can be reviewed elsewhere.[10] The studies of CDH and CM are even more limited, largely to anecdotal, retrospective reports.

The underlying etiology to this unresponsiveness is not known, but barriers to treatment that are unique to children are evident (Table 15.1). Recognizing these barriers and overcoming them is essential to overcome the refractoriness of acute treatments.

When patients do not respond to their home treatment plan, parenteral treatment may be necessary. This typically requires intravenous medications and can include dopamine antagonist (prochlorperazine) in combination with NSAIDs (ketorolac). If this is unsuccessful, just as in adults, DHE can be employed.

Disability

Disability is a common result of migraine headaches in children and adolescents. Several instruments have been developed to address this question in adults. For children and adolescents PedMIDAS was developed to address this question.[11,12] This instrument is similar to MIDAS for adults,[13–15] but addresses the more pervasive impact of headaches on school and social activities.

Table 15-1 Barriers to Acute Treatment in Children

- School barriers
  - Zero tolerance restrictions (cannot have the medications with them)
  - Absent or limited access to school nurse
  - Teachers doubting headache
  - Requirement for doctor's note
- Patient barriers
  - Not recognizing the onset of headache
  - Ability to attenuate or "play through the pain"
  - Reliance on adult caregivers to administer the medications
- Family barriers
  - Parents doubting that children can have headaches
  - Unwillingness to "medicate" their child
- Medical barriers
  - No FDA-approved headache treatments for children and adolescents
  - Limited education in medical school/residencies in headaches

The corresponding grading scale, although similar to MIDAS with four grades of disability, has a larger range of scores within each grade to reflect the greater spectrum of activities that children and adolescents may fail to attend. From the studies that have been done in children using PedMIDAS, a significant proportion of children may have high PedMIDAS scores. Preliminary analysis had demonstrated that those children with a PedMIDAS score above 150 may have an increased risk of psychological factors contributing to their headache intractability. When such a score is observed additional involvement of psychiatry and psychology including behavioral therapy may be necessary.

Contributing Factors to RM in Children and Adolescents

The factors that may contribute to the development of RM are only speculative. In adults these factors are only beginning to be addressed and are discussed elsewhere in this text. It is unclear whether any of these factors are translatable to the pediatric and adolescent population.

Some of the potential contributors (Table 15.2) may include a biological predilection to RM that may be either genetic based or induced by ineffective management. Other factors include psychological and personality factors that may be either a sign of an underlying biological condition or behaviorally related, including relationships to parents, friends, and school. All of these may work in a synergistic manner to contribute to RM and therefore must be addressed.

Biological Basis

It is clear that migraine in children and adolescents have a genetic basis.[16] What specific genes contribute to this headache type is unknown. This genetic

Table 15-2 Factors Contributing to RM in Children

- Biological factors
  - Genetic predisposition
  - Biobehavioral factors
    - Skipping meals
    - Poor eating habits
    - Lack of sleep or changes in sleep patterns
  - Nutritional deficiencies
    - Riboflavin
    - Coenzyme Q10
- Medication factors
  - Inappropriate dosing
  - Adherence to treatment plan
- Psychological factors
  - Lack of coping skills for a chronic illness
  - Anxiety
    - School avoidance due to frequent absences
    - Disease related due to fear of headache interrupting activities
    - Social anxiety due to withdrawal from peer groups

predisposition may serve as a biological risk factor for the development of CDH. A preliminary genomic analysis of gene expression patterns in children and adolescents with CDH has revealed a unique gene expression pattern.[17] This suggests that the phenotypic expression of CDH has a unique gene expression pattern that may help understand the biological contribution. When the identification of RM patients is improved in children and adolescents, a unique gene expression pattern may be found in this group of patient to explain the underlying biological contribution.

What biological process contributes to the development of MOH is unclear. In animal studies, it has been noted that there is an alteration in serotonin transporters.[18] The more relevant question in RM is whether there is a different biological marker that differentiates those MOH patients respond to cessation of analgesics from those who do not. The identification of these factors in children and adolescents may help us understand why some patients are refractory after they have initiated their treatment for migraine with MOH.

Psychological Factors

Although some studies have suggested that there may be a psychological or personality factors that lead to the development of CDH in children and adolescents, these studies are inconsistent, small and limited in their controls. Some of these features may include anxiety related disorders, oppositional-defiant personalities, and depressive symptoms. These observations may suggest that there are some psychological mechanisms that underlie RM, although CDH is defined differently. Sorting out whether the underlying chronic pain condition generates this mood disorder or whether this is from an independent comorbid condition, is difficult. Although migraine and mood affect each other in a bidirectional fashion, the best way to sort this issue is through long-term treatment and outcome analysis. If the psychological features resolve purely through the successful treatment of the CDH, it is likely that in those patients the features are more a reflection of their chronic pain condition. In any case, mood must be addressed and managed appropriately.

A psychological and behavioral assessment and management plan needs to be an essential component in the evaluation and long-term treatment of patients with RM. This can not only address the underlying contributors to the RM, but also establish treatment strategies for these conditions. It has recently been noted that adolescents with migraine have an increased risk of suicidal ideation.[19] This assessment and management must include a discussion of this issue. Asking if the patient has thoughts of hurting themselves should be done in a direct fashion, if possible, in private. In adolescents with RM, this relationship needs to be studied further.

Anxiety can have a significant impact on disability in school-aged children, often resulting in school absences. This compounds the levels of complexity that contribute to these absences and impacts the child's learning and life successes. Severe headaches in school are disruptive to learning. They impair concentration, may require leaving class for treatment, or even absence from school. Prevention of headaches and elimination of road blocks to treatment in school are paramount. The practitioner and parents serving as advocates for the student is the first step in minimizing the impact of headache and the associated anxiety. In children prone to anxiety, however, the anticipation of having a headache in school can itself be disruptive. Overcoming this anxiety through the inclusion of coping skills and desensitization may minimize this effect.

When the child is missing school, a greater degree of anxiety may evolve into school avoidance. This is complicated further by social isolation that develops as the child loses contact with friends and fellow students. This has potential dire consequences, as social isolation has been noted as one of the major contributors to teen suicide.

In children with RM, all of these factors may come together: lack of consistent effective acute treatment, ineffective preventative medication, and an underlying anxiety or depression. It is therefore essential to minimize this with the development of a coping strategy for the child to utilize when they have an acute headache as well when school anxiety is experienced. Part of this strategy requires a return to school plan and rejecting any plan that leads to social withdrawal. This is often made difficult by a well intentioned response from school systems which mandates home schooling or tutoring.

Management of these psychological and behavioral factors may require intensive psychological and biobehavioral intervention in close coordination of pharmacological management. This requires the involvement of the child, but should also include the parents, teachers, and possibly even friends.

Management of RM in Children and Adolescents

Once it appears that a child or adolescent may have RM, a multidisciplinary treatment approach is necessary that incorporates the child as the focus, along with the inclusion of practitioners (headache medicine specialist, psychologist, nursing, and social work), teachers, and family. It is essential that the plan revolves around the child. They must have a full understanding of the plan, goals and outcomes. Realistic expectations need to be incorporated from the beginning along with continued encouragement Close contact with frequent visits and discussions are essential.

This treatment plan needs to include an acute treatment strategy that ensures that MOH does not develop. This can be done by providing a NSAID at an appropriate dose, but in a limited frequency, with the inclusion of a triptan for severe headaches. At the Cincinnati Children's Headache Center, we often have the child determine which NSAID is most effective for them (ibuprofen, naproxen sodium, or for those older than 15, aspirin) to be used at the onset of a headache or in the case of continuous headaches at the onset of headache worsening, but only on Monday, Wednesday, and Friday. In this way we limit the use to no more than 3 days per week, focused on school days, to minimize the impact on school headache and absences. Once the headaches begin to respond, and the child does not have a headache requiring treatment on one of these 3 days, he or she then has the flexibility of using the NSAID on another day of the week, as long as he or she keeps the use at 3 or fewer times per week. For those children with occasional severe headaches the addition of a triptan or DHE may be required, but with limits employed to avoid the overuse of these agents.

Behavioral treatment can also be employed to treat these acute exacerbations. This can include biofeedback, assisted relaxation therapy,[20] and hydration with sports drinks.

Preventative therapy is also important in the treatment plan. Given the limited evidence of effectiveness of a wide variety of agents in children and adolescents for the prevention of CM, this may require a trial of a variety of different medications. These medications may lead to a stepwise improvement in the child's headache and disability. This can be assessed through headache diaries as well as routine disability assessment using tools such as PedMIDAS. For all of these agents, a strategy of slow initiation to minimize side effects, to a presumed effective dose, and sustaining this dose for an adequate duration (typically at least 3 months) is important to ensure success as well as avoid the phenomenon of "already used everything." As studies have not been done for RM in children, the effective dose is unknown, but can be guided by experience in episodic prevention studies. Polypharmacy may be required.

Biobehavioral strategies also need to be employed. This includes a discussion of the maintenance of healthy habits (adequate fluid hydration without caffeine, an exercise program, nutritional plan including both regular meals and healthy food choices, and a sleep plan that includes regular and adequate sleep). All of these issues need to be regularly addressed to develop a mechanism to resolve particular barriers. The biobehavioral treatment also requires a discussion of the importance of adherence to the treatment plan. This requires that not only does the child understand the treatment plan but agrees with the plan and actively participates. Frustration develops, especially in children with RM, when they are excluded from the treatment plan development. Further interventions that incorporate the child in the decision-making component of the treatment plan may assist with resolving this barrier to outcome.

When there are identifiable mood disorders, each must be addressed in its own way. These factors may be reflected as an elevated PedMIDAS score that reflects school and social absences. When the child becomes socially withdrawn due to either the headaches or the comorbid anxiety, it is essential to include a pain psychologist, a psychiatrist, and a counselor. The incorporation of all of these services needs to be individualized, and may become time consuming for both the patient and the care providers.

Conclusions

From the experience of tertiary headache centers, it is clear a subset of children and adolescents with migraine will develop RM. The understanding and recognition of these patients is incomplete. It is important that these RM patients be identified early, so that treatment strategies can be employed to minimize the impact of this condition and prevent long-term negative outcomes. Further research in pediatric and adolescent patients is essential. Only when there is optimal recognition of RM can the risk factors, and the underlying the biological etiologies, be effectively be identified and managed.

References

1. Sillanpää M, Piekkala P, Kero P. Prevalence of headache at preschool age in an unselected child population. *Cephalalgia.*1991;11:239–242.
2. Abu-Arafeh I, Russell G. Prevalence of headache and migraine in schoolchildren. *BMJ.*1994;309:765–769.
3. Wang SJ, Fuh JL, Lu SR, Juang KD. Chronic daily headache in adolescents: prevalence, impact, and medication overuse. *Neurology.* 2006;66(2):193–197.
4. Hershey AD, Powers SW, Bentti AL, LeCates S, deGrauw TJ. Characterization of chronic daily headaches in children in a multidisciplinary headache center. *Neurology.* 2001;56(8):1032–1037.
5. Koenig MA, Gladstein J, McCarter RJ, Hershey AD, Wasiewski W. Chronic daily headache in children and adolescents presenting to tertiary headache clinics. *Headache.* 2002;42(6):491–500.
6. Bigal ME, Lipton RB, Winner P, Reed ML, Diamond S, Stewart WF. Migraine in adolescents: association with socioeconomic status and family history. *Neurology.* 2007 69(1):16–25.

7. Wiendels NJ, van der Geest MC, Neven AK, Ferrari MD, Laan LA. Chronic daily headache in children and adolescents. *Headache.* 2005;45(6):678–683.
8. Scalas C, Calistri L. Chronic daily headache in a paediatric headache centre. *J Headache Pain.* 2005;6(4):274–276.
9. Bigal ME, Rapoport AM, Tepper SJ, Sheftell FD, Lipton RB. The classification of chronic daily headache in adolescents—a comparison between the second edition of the international classification of headache disorders and alternative diagnostic criteria. *Headache.* 2005;45(5):582–589.
10. Hershey A, Powers S, Winner P, Kabbouche M. *Pediatric Headaches in Clinical Practice.* West Sussex, UK: John Wiley & Sons; 2009.
11. Hershey AD, Powers SW, Vockell AL, LeCates S, Kabbouche MA, Maynard MK. PedMIDAS: development of a questionnaire to assess disability of migraines in children. *Neurology.* 2001;57(11):2034–2039.
12. Hershey AD, Powers SW, Vockell AL, LeCates SL, Segers A, Kabbouche MA. Development of a patient-based grading scale for PedMIDAS. *Cephalalgia.* 2004;24(10):844–849.
13. Stewart WF, Lipton RB, Dowson AJ, Sawyer J. Development and testing of the migraine disability assessment (MIDAS) questionnaire to assess headache-related disability. *Neurology.* 2001;56(6 Suppl 1):S20–28.
14. Bigal ME, Rapoport AM, Lipton RB, Tepper SJ, Sheftell FD. Assessment of migraine disability using the migraine disability assessment (MIDAS) questionnaire: a comparison of chronic migraine with episodic migraine. *Headache.* 2003;43:336–342.
15. Stewart WF, Lipton RB, Kolodner K. Migraine disability assessment (MIDAS) Score: Relation to headache frequency, pain intensity, and headache symptoms. *Headache.* 2003;43:258–265.
16. Hershey AD. Genetics of headache in children: where are we headed? *Curr Pain Headache Rep.* 2008;12(5):367–372.
17. Tang Y, Hershey AD, Powers SW, et al. Genomic abnormalities in patients with migraine and chronic migraine: preliminary blood gene expression suggests platelet abnormalities. *Headache.* 2004;44(10):994–1004.
18. Srikiatkhachorn A, Tarasub N, Govitrapong P. Effect of chronic analgesic exposure on the central serotonin system: a possible mechanism of analgesic abuse headache. *Headache.* 2000;40(5):343–350.
19. Wang SJ, Fuh JL, Juang KD, Lu SR. Migraine and suicidal ideation in adolescents aged 13 to 15 years. *Neurology.* 2009;72(13):1146–1152.
20. Powers SW, Hershey AD. Biofeedback for childhood migraine. In: Maria BL, ed. *Current Management in Child Neurology*, 2nd ed. Hamilton, Ontario: BC Decker; 2002:83–85.

16

Nerve Blocks, Neurostimulation, and *Botulinum* Toxin Injection Treatment for Refractory Migraine

Avi Ashkenazi, MD, and Morris Levin, MD

Introduction

Patients with refractory migraine either do not respond to, or are unable to use traditional prophylactic and acute agents.[1] Many patients have had unacceptable adverse effects related to these approaches. In some, many pharmaceutical approaches may be hazardous due to concomitant cardiovascular, cerebrovascular, or peripheral vascular disease; hepatic or renal disease; pregnancy; or psychiatric conditions. In addition, in many of these patients, medication interactions may prove insurmountable. For many of them, peripheral nerve procedures, such as nerve blocks, nerve stimulation, or other local injection techniques can be dramatically effective and should be included in the management repertoire.

Nerve Blocks

Background

Local anesthetic procedures have unfortunately not been well studied in controlled sham placebo trials. One study[2] did compare pericranial nerve blocks with cognitive therapy in treatment for headache. The results were not striking and the numbers of subjects in each group who completed the study were very low. In addition, classification of headache type was not clear. Adding to the difficulty of assessing these procedures, it is well known that injections for pain carry a significant placebo effect.[3]

Local anesthetic procedures for pain suppression are useful because of the ability of these agents to selectively block sensory fibers (sparing motor function) in mixed nerves at relatively low concentrations. The duration of the block depends on the dose and the pharmacokinetic properties of the particular local anesthetic(s), but a longer than expected duration of all or some benefits has been a common observation. Moreover, blockade of a number of nerves in the head and neck can produce beneficial effects in pain affecting regions outside of the territory served by the anesthetized nerve. This is often explained by the concept of convergence in the nociceptive system of the head and neck (i.e., higher order levels in the nociceptive pathway receive input from multiple areas), but not all observations can be accounted for by this mechanism.

Local Anesthetic Blockade: Pharmacology and General Techniques

Local anesthetics (LAs) are divided into the ester and amide categories. All LAs have hydrophilic components, which make them easily absorbable, as well as lipophilic components, which allow passage across nerve membranes. The ester LAs were discovered and utilized first but are more allergenic. This is because a metabolite of all ester LAs is the allergen *para*-aminobenzoic acid (PABA). Ester LAs include procaine and cocaine and tend to be shorter acting than the amide LAs. Amide LAs include lidocaine, mepivacaine, bupivacaine, and prilocaine. Amide LAs tend to be hypoallergenic and well tolerated. LAs inhibit neural activity by interfering with sodium and potassium currents (probably by binding to voltage-gated sodium channels), thus preventing depolarization. The diffusion of LA agents across nerve membranes is related to myelin thickness. This is why motor function (subserved by the most thickly myelinated Aα fibers) is spared compared with sensation (in typical nerve block doses). All LAs are eventually absorbed systemically. The most severe effects, which include dizziness, nausea, cardiac arrhythmias, seizures, and alterations in consciousness, occur only when systemic levels of anesthetic agents are high. Generally, these consequences can be avoided by taking measures aimed at avoiding intravascular injection. Technically, this is usually not a challenge if one consistently makes sure to pull back the plunger of the syringe and injects only if there is no blood return (implying that the needle tip is not intravascular). However, this is not entirely reliable when using small-gauge needles (30 and smaller) or if back pressure is applied too forcefully.

Amide LAs are metabolized by the hepatic cytochrome P-450 3A enzyme systems. A number of pharmacological agents, including antiarrhythmics, antibiotics, antiepileptics, calcium channel blockers, beta-blockers, and antidepressants) can inhibit this system, leading to increased anesthetic levels due to delayed disposal. In some situations, this could lead to adverse central nervous system (CNS) effects with only minimal intravascular absorption. Ester LAs are metabolized by hydrolysis, which is a function of the plasma enzyme pseudocholinesterase. Rarely, a patient will have a genetic defect in this enzyme that leads to elevated levels of anesthetic and possible toxicity. Other adverse effects resulting from LA injection include local infection, nerve damage with later neuroma formation, hematoma (particularly in patients with a bleeding diathesis), and local injury to adjacent structures, depending on the site of injection.

Potential Adverse Effects of Nerve Blockade

- Local: infection, hematoma, damage to adjacent structures
- Dizziness
- Nausea
- Cardiac arrhythmias (rare)
- Seizures (rare)
- Allergic reactions (rare with amide local anesthetics)

Individual anatomical features, such as skull defects, local infection, and/or previous surgery, must be identified, and avoided. Direct trauma to peripheral nerves is rare but can occur. Patients will usually report lancinating pain if nerves are directly impinged upon, at which point the needle should be redirected. In the case of nerve irritation, local measures to reduce inflammation, such as local cold application, are usually sufficient. Skin injection tends to distort anatomy, so it is important to ascertain geographical markers carefully and even mark the skin appropriately. Because LAs tend to diffuse well throughout the dermis, multiple injection sites are often unnecessary. Sensation testing after an appropriate time interval should reveal an area of anesthesia corresponding to the usual distribution of the nerve(s) injected. If further anesthesia is thought to be indicated, inserting the needle through already anesthetized skin is usually possible and relatively comfortable for the patient.

LA agents available for local injection include bupivacaine, lidocaine, mepivacaine, and prilocaine, all of which have been used to treat head pain. The latter three have similar potency (about one-fourth that of bupivacaine) and a mid-range duration of action. Lidocaine in the 1% solution, with an onset of action at around 4 to 8 minutes after injection and duration of about 1 to 3 hours, is the most common choice. Bupivacaine in a 0.25% or 0.50% solution offers more prolonged action, with onset in about 8 to 12 minutes and duration between 4 and 8 hours, but tends to be slightly more painful, perhaps because of its generally lower pH (Table 16.1). Combining lidocaine with bupivacaine is another option. Anesthetic formulations with epinephrine (used in surgical procedures to reduce local bleeding) are neither necessary nor recommended for nerve blocks. Some practitioners add a corticosteroid

Table 16-1 Pharmacological Profile of the Two Most Commonly Used Local Anesthetics

	Lidocaine	Bupivacaine
Commonly used concentration	1%–2%	0.25%–0.5%
Duration of anesthetic effect after SC injection	1–3 hours	4–8 hours
Max. dose for SC injection	300 mg	175 mg
Toxic plasma concentration	>5 μg/mL	>1.5 μg/mL

SC = subcutaneous.

Adapted from: Barrett J, Harmon D, Loughnane F, Finucane B, Shorten G. Local anesthetics. In: Barrett J, Harmon D, Loughnane F, Finucane B, Shorten G (edis), *Peripheral Nerve Blocks and Perioperative Pain Relief.* Edinburgh: Saunders, 2004, pp. 11–18

medication such as triamcinolone (Kenalog) or methylprednisolone (Depo-Medrol), but Ashkenazi et al. in 2008 found that there was no difference in outcome between patients given greater occipital nerve blocks for headache with either (1) lidocaine and bupivacaine alone or (2) the same agents with the addition of a steroid medication.[4]

Specific Nerve Block Techniques and Efficacy

Although many scalp nerves and ganglia are accessible to blockade with local anesthetic, several have been targeted for the treatment of migraine and other primary headache disorders. These include the greater and lesser occipital nerves, the auriculotemporal nerve, the supraorbital and supratrochlear nerves, and the sphenopalatine ganglion.

Peripheral Nerves/Ganglions that Have Been Targeted for Blockade in Headache Treatment

- Greater occipital nerve
- Lesser occipital nerve
- Auriculotemporal nerve
- Supratrochlear nerve
- Supraorbital nerve
- Sphenopalatine ganglion

Greater Occipital Nerve Block

The greater occipital nerve (GON) is the primary branch of the second cervical (C2) root and innervates the scalp from the level of the external occipital protuberance to the vertex . For the purposes of injection, its trunk is located approximately two-thirds of the distance on a line drawn from the center of the mastoid to the external occipital protuberance (see Fig. 16.1). It is adjacent to the occipital artery and can also be located by palpating for this artery.

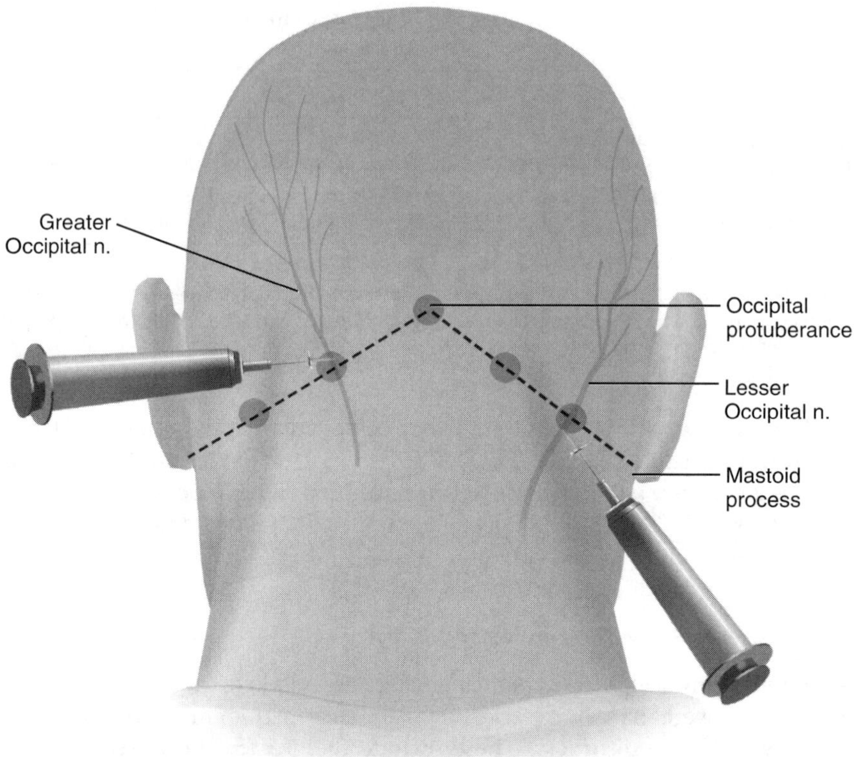

Figure 16-1 Greater and lesser occipital nerve blocks.[21] (Used with permission of Oxford University Press.)

Injecting approximately 2 cm lateral to the external occipital protuberance is another useful approach. Approximately 2 to 3 mL of bupivacaine or lidocaine, or a mixture of the two, injected in the area of the GON should be sufficient to anesthetize this nerve. If a mixture is selected, a common ratio is 1:1. Several unusual adverse effects of GON block have been reported, including local alopecia[5] and Cushing's syndrome.[6]

The two conditions commonly treated with GON blocks are occipital neuralgia (or "neuritis") and so-called cervicogenic headache. GON block seems to be effective in many patients with migraine, although controlled studies have not been done. In a study of 19 patients with acute migraine and allodynia, headache was relieved in 17, and allodynia decreased in all patients.[7] Another study of 25 migraine patients found that 60% of subjects had significant improvement of migraine pain within 5 minutes of injection.[8] Long-lasting relief was seen in 26 of 54 migraine patients who received a unilateral GON block with lidocaine and methylprednisolone.[9] GON blockade also appears to be effective in the acute, and possibly prophylactic, treatment of cluster headache.[9–11] In one study of GON block in migraine and cluster headaches patients, tenderness around the GON seemed to be predictive of a good response to GON block in both groups.[9]

Although studies of GON block in refractory migraine per se have not been attempted yet, a comparative controlled study of the benefits of GON block in chronic daily headache was positive.[4] Interestingly, GON block has also been successful in other headache types. In 2008, Matute reported successful GON block in post-lumbar puncture headache.[12] Weatherall reported response to GON block in refractory trigeminal neuralgia.[13] Refractory hemiplegic migraine may also respond to GON.[14] Interestingly, chronic tension type headache seems not to respond to GON block.[15]

Lesser Occipital Nerve Block

The lesser occipital nerve (LON) is primarily derived from the cervical plexus (C3, C2) and supplies the posterior–inferior scalp and skin of the upper neck. This nerve can be blockaded by injecting approximately 2 to 3 mL of bupivacaine or lidocaine, or a mixture of the two, one-third of the way from the center of the mastoid to the greater occipital protuberance, on the same line used for GON block (Fig. 16.1). There are no data supporting the use of LON blockade in headache disorders, but there are reports of successful trigger point injection therapy in the region of the LON, including migraine patients refractory to other forms of treatment.

Auriculotemporal Nerve Block

The auriculotemporal nerve (ATN) is a branch of the mandibular division of the trigeminal nerve, and supplies sensation over the ear and temporalis muscle. Blockade can be done by injecting approximately 2 to 3 mL of bupivacaine and/or lidocaine, superior to the posterior portion of the zygoma just anterior to the ear (Fig. 16.2). If this block is successful, anesthesia is obtained over the temporal fossa. Although evidence for the effectiveness of ATN blockade in any headache disorder is lacking, selected patients have benefitted.

Supraorbital and Supratrochlear Nerve Block

The supraorbital and supratrochlear nerves are branches of the ophthalmic division of the trigeminal nerve, and innervate the frontalis region. They both pass through the orbit above the orbital ridge and are easily accessible to neural blockade. The supratrochlear nerve (STN) is blocked by inserting the needle just above the eyebrow over its medial border and injecting approximately 1 to 2 mL of bupivacaine or lidocaine or a mixture (Fig. 16.3). To anesthetize the supraorbital nerve (SON), which runs approximately 2 cm lateral to the supratrochlear nerve, the injection can be done here, or the needle can be advanced laterally through the same puncture that was used for the supratrochlear nerve, with injection of 1 to 2 mL of anesthetic (Fig. 16.3)

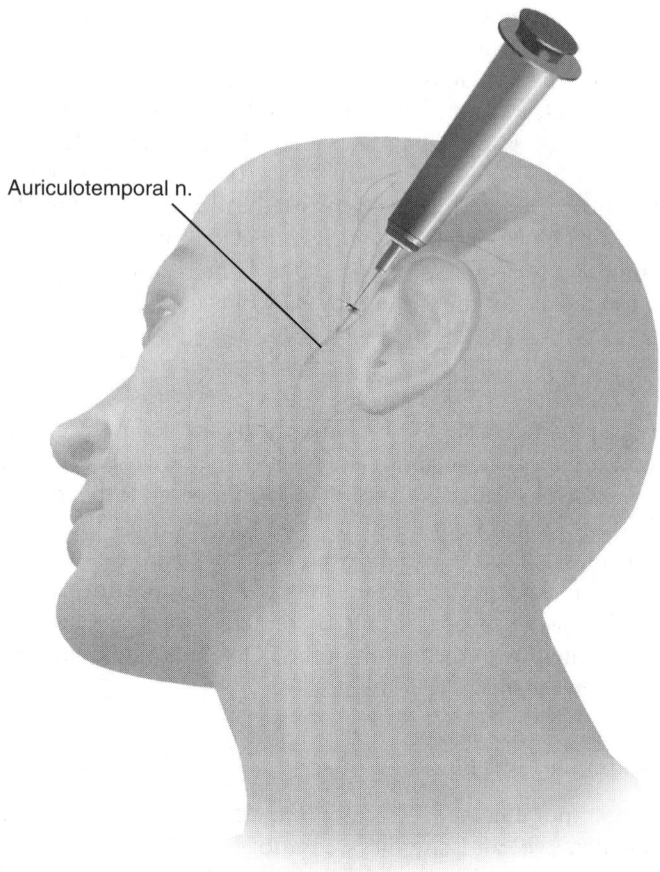

Figure 16-2 Auriculotemporal nerve block.[21] (Used with permission from Oxford University Press.)

The SON and STN are prone to traumatic injury due to their superficial locations, and headaches after frontal trauma with pain and/or tenderness localized to this area should raise a high level of suspicion for the diagnosis of neuralgia involving these nerves. This can then be confirmed (and treated) with SON/STN blockade. In a study of SON and/or GON blockade in 29 patients with migraine, 25 patients (85%) had a favorable response. However, this report did not include the data for those who received only SON blocks.[16]

Other Nerve Blocks

Sphenopalatine ganglion block, cervical facet/medial branch blocks, and cervical dorsal root blockade have all been proposed for intractable headache

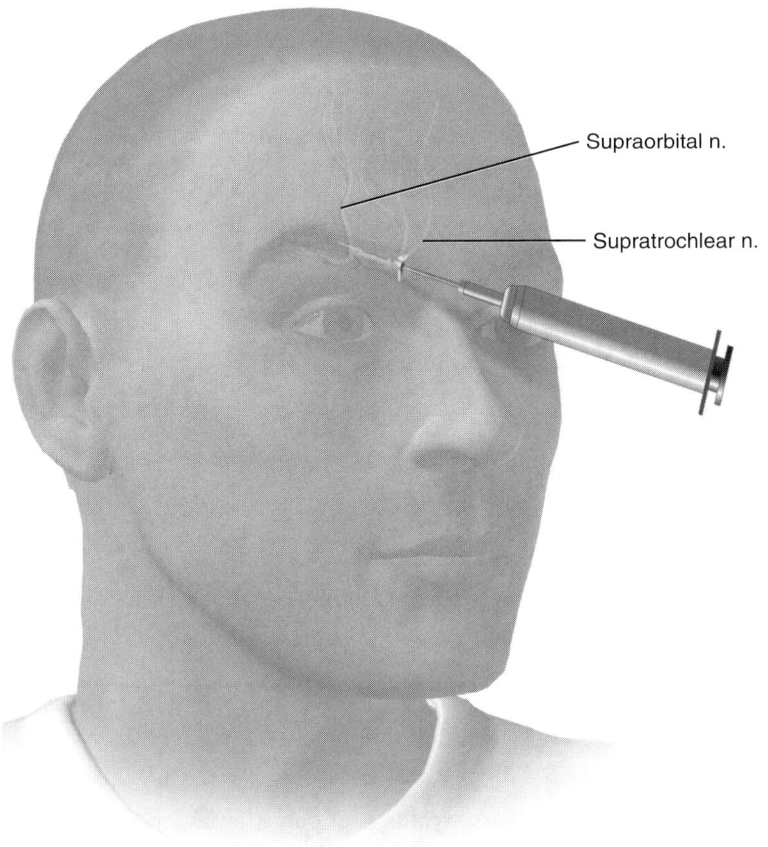

Figure 16-3 Supratrochlear and supraorbital nerve blocks.[21] (Used with permission from Oxford University Press.)

disorders. Sphenopalatine ganglion blockade has been used in cases of refractory cluster headache, and only rarely of migraine. However, when performed via topical application of lidocaine to the lateral posterior recess of the nasal cavity (Fig. 16.4) it is quite benign and may be worth experimenting with in selected refractory migraine patients. Upper cervical facet injections have been proposed for the treatment of refractory headaches, where pain generation in the upper cervical spine is postulated. The second cervical root has been proposed as a target in some headaches, particularly those in which GON block was of some benefit. The third cervical root has also been proposed as a target in some headaches, generally those thought to be caused by cervical injury or other pathology. These techniques require fluoroscopy and experienced injectors. Adverse effects that may occur after facet or root blocks include local hemorrhage, infection, nerve trauma with persistent

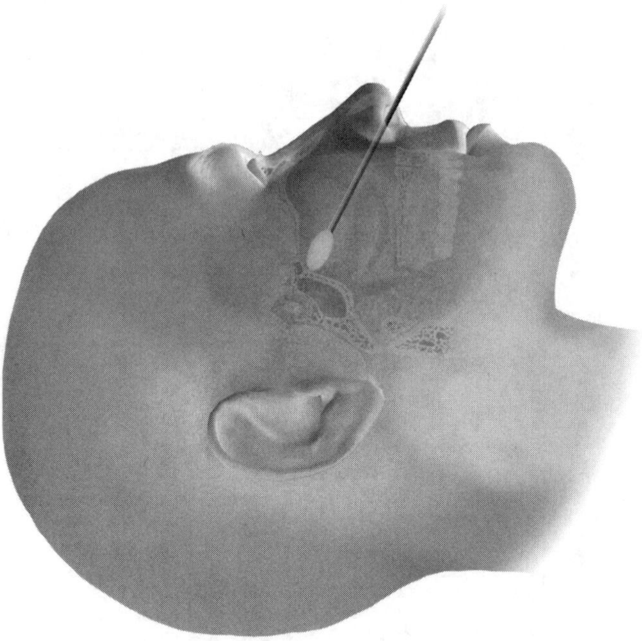

Figure 16-4 Sphenopalatine ganglion block.[21] (Used with permission from Oxford University Press.)

neuropathic pain, sensory loss, weakness or paresthesias, and injury to vascular structures such as carotid or vertebral arteries.

Mechanisms of Nerve Block Effects in Primary Headache

The mechanisms by which these procedures work are not clear. Migraine is believed to be a centrally mediated primary neuropathic phenomenon, and it is unclear how blocking trigeminal and upper cervical nerve branches might affect it. Clearly, nociceptive physiology must be affected at higher levels, if these peripheral procedures truly improve migraine pain.

For acute pain relief, the mechanism may stem from a reduction in afferent "tone," leading to a lessening of activity at the level of the trigeminal nucleus caudalis and cervical dorsal horn. This reduction in transmission at the first synapse of the nociceptive pathways governing head pain might conceivably reduce pain perception in a much broader area than that served by the blocked nerve because of the organization of primary and secondary neurons serving head regions. For example, there is good evidence that convergence between the cervical and trigeminal systems happens at this level and that changes in one component can modulate the other.[17–20] More puzzling, however, is the question of how long-term improvement could result from anesthesia that only lasts some 4 to 6 hours. Many clinicians have observed that in cases of refractory pain, it is crucially important to "break the pain cycle." Perhaps this interruption of ongoing refractory pain helps to reverse central sensitization and allow a "winding-down" of nociceptive activity.

Peripheral Neurostimulation

Background

Peripheral neurostimulation has long been used in pain management.[21,22] The scientific rational for the use of this technique for pain is based, in part, on the fact that diverse peripheral inputs to the spinal dorsal horn can exert an inhibitory effect on pain transmission.[23] Based on this concept, transcutaneous electrical nerve stimulation (TENS) has been used for headache treatment for decades. More recently, there has been increased interest in the use of implanted electrodes to stimulate various peripheral nerves in an attempt to relieve head pain. The most commonly targeted nerve for this purpose has been the greater occipital nerve (GON). Attempts have also been made to stimulate the vagus and the supraorbital nerves for pain relief. Because nerve stimulation using implantable electrodes is an invasive procedure, it has been offered to patients with chronic headache who were refractory to other treatment modalities. This treatment option requires cooperation between the headache clinician and the neurosurgeon who performs the procedure. Although clinical experience is still limited, it appears that some patients with refractory chronic daily headache (CDH) may benefit from this treatment. Technical problems, such as lead migration and early battery depletion, need to be addressed to make this treatment modality more satisfactory to patients.

Transcutaneous Electrical Nerve Stimulation

Transcutaneous electrical nerve stimulation (TENS) is the stimulation of primary afferents by low-voltage electrical pulses through electrodes applied to the skin. This technique has long been used in the management of various pain syndromes. However, there are few controlled studies on its efficacy in headache treatment. TENS constitutes a potential treatment modality for the

Advantages of TENS in Headache Treatment

- Noninvasive
- Technically easy to perform
- High tolerability
- Few contraindications
- High safety profile
- Does not interfere with other treatments for headache

refractory migraine patient that is safe, noninvasive, and usually tolerable. Although a complete theory to explain the mechanisms of the antinociceptive effect of TENS is lacking, it is thought that the afferent activity induced by TENS inhibits nociceptive transmission in the spinal cord.[24] It has also been suggested that TENS exerts an analgesic effect through activation of the endogenous opioid system.[25]

Technical Aspects

Various pulse patterns have been used for TENS (high-frequency [50–120 Hz], low-frequency [1–4 Hz], or a combination of the two). No stimulus pattern has been shown to be superior to others. It is also unknown what stimulus pattern is optimal for any specific pain syndrome. A typical TENS session lasts 30 to 45 minutes. The patient may experience pain relief during the session only, or for several hours after the treatment as well. Patients who experience allodynia at the painful area may not be able to tolerate high-frequency stimulation.

Data from Clinical Studies

Data on the efficacy of TENS for migraine and other headache are scarce. Solomon and Guglielmo examined the efficacy of high-frequency TENS on head pain in 62 patients with migraine or "muscle contraction headache".[26] Patients were randomly assigned to three treatment arms: TENS at a level just above tactile perception (perceived stimuli); TENS at a level just below tactile perception (subliminal stimuli); and placement of electrodes without stimulation (sham procedure). After perceived stimuli, 55% of patients reported on headache improvement, compared with 28% and 18% of patients in the subliminal stimuli and the sham procedure groups, respectively. The decrease in headache intensity was, however, only slight to moderate in the majority of patients. In an open-label study, Allais et al. examined the effect of TENS, laser therapy, and acupuncture on headache in 60 women with transformed migraine (TM), a chronic daily headache pattern thought to represent evolution from intermittent migraine.[27] TENS electrodes were applied to the frontal, temporal, and occipital areas, and to the dorsal aspect of the hand. The treatment resulted in a significant decrease in headache frequency, an effect that lasted for 3 months. Farina et al. examined in an uncontrolled study the efficacy of TENS in 60 patients with cervicogenic headache, occipital neuralgia, and "muscle contraction" or mixed headache.[28] TENS electrodes were applied to cervical tender points. TENS treatment decreased headache severity and frequency in the three headache groups.

Percutaneous electrical nerve stimulation (PENS) is performed by using acupuncture-like needles that are inserted to a depth of 1 to 3 cm subcutaneously at specific points. Ahmed et al. showed that PENS was more effective than a sham procedure in decreasing pain scores of 30 patients with tension-type headache (TTH), migraine, or post-traumatic headache (PTH).[29] Ghoname et al. used a similar technique to study the effect of PENS on five patients with post-electroconvulsive therapy (ECT) headache.[30] PENS was delivered at the temporal, occipital, cervical, and upper thoracic areas bilaterally. All patients responded favorably to treatment, with either elimination of or marked improvement in ECT-associated headache.

In summary, the efficacy of TENS and PENS in headache treatment is still debated. Larger controlled trials are needed to clarify the role of this treatment in headache management, including refractory forms. However, the procedure is noninvasive, safe, and easy to perform, and some patients may benefit from it.

Neurostimulation Using Implantable Electrodes

The use of implantable electrodes to stimulate nerves in the head and neck for pain relief is relatively new.[21] The most common targets for this purpose have been the GON and the suboccipital area. Currently, data on the efficacy of these procedures for headache relief come from retrospective uncontrolled studies. Therefore, although some encouraging results have been reported, they should be taken with caution.

Nerves that Have Been Targeted for Neurostimulation in Headache Treatment

- Greater occipital nerve and suboccipital area (by far the most common target)
- Vagus nerve
- Supraorbital nerve

Neurostimulation of the Greater Occipital and Other Upper Cervical Nerves

As mentioned earlier, clinical and scientific data suggest that the upper cervical roots and the trigeminal nerve are connected.[31] Migraine patients often experience pain not only in trigeminally innervated areas, but also in upper cervical dermatomes (i.e., the occiput and the posterior neck). Further, blocking the GON, a nerve that arises mostly from the C2 root, often results in pain relief in trigeminal dermatomes.[7] Supporting these observations, animal studies have shown evidence for convergence of sensory input from upper cervical and trigeminal afferents into second order trigeminal nucleus caudalis (TNC) neurons.[17] Stimulation of the GON has been shown to increase metabolic activity in the TNC and in the upper cervical dorsal horn in cats.[32] Moreover, stimulation of the GON has a facilitating effect on C2 neuronal response to dural stimulation, supporting not only an anatomic connection, but also functional interactions between the trigeminal and the upper cervical systems.

Based on these data, several studied have been performed to examine the efficacy of GON or upper cervical root stimulation on head pain in migraine and other headaches[21] (Table 16.2). In an uncontrolled study, Popeney and Aló evaluated the effect of neurostimulation at the upper cervical (C1–C3) distribution on head pain and disability in 25 patients with refractory TM.[33] Electrodes were placed under fluoroscopic guidance subcutaneously at the posterior cervical area, and were connected to an implantable pulse generator. After neurostimulation, the average number of days with headache decreased from 25 to 13 per month, and the average headache severity (on an 11-point verbal scale) decreased from 9 to 6. Disability, as measured by the Migraine Disability Assessment (MIDAS) score, decreased by 89%. Complications included electrode migration (nine patients [36%]) and infection (one patient [4%]). Matharu et al. studied the effect of suboccipital stimulation on head pain in eight patients with chronic migraine (CM).[34] The stimulating electrodes were implanted in the vicinity of the GON, at the level of C1. Four patients had an excellent response, with complete headache suppression; two had a "very good" response, with suppression of headache most of the time; and two had a "good" response, with headache severity decreased 50% to 75%. All patients maintained the response to treatment throughout a follow-up period averaging 18 months. Three patients had electrode lead migration necessitating revision, and one had an abdominal hematoma at the site of generator implantation. Positron emission tomography (PET) studies in these patients showed significant changes in regional cerebral blood flow in the dorsal rostral pons, anterior cingulate gyrus, and cuneus, which correlated with pain scores. Schwedt et al. reported on a retrospective study of 15 patients with intractable CM ($n = 8$), cluster headache (CH) ($n = 3$), hemicrania continua ($n = 2$), and PTH ($n = 2$) who underwent implantation of stimulating electrodes over the GON.[35] Eight patients underwent bilateral- and seven had unilateral lead placement. Patients were evaluated before and 5 to 42 months after implantation. After treatment, there was a significant decrease in headache frequency and severity, and significant improvement from baseline in MIDAS, Headache Impact Test-6 (HIT-6) and Beck Depression Inventory II scores. The majority of patients (60%) required lead revision within 1 year, and all patients required it by 3 years post-implantation. One patient required generator revision.

Several recent studies examined the effect of occipital nerve stimulation (ONS) in patients with refractory CH. Magis et al. reported on eight patients with drug-resistant CH who underwent implantation of a suboccipital neurostimulator ipsilateral to the attacks.[36] Two patients were pain-free after a follow-up of 16 and 22 months, three had a 90% reduction in attack frequency, and two had improvement of 40%. Mean follow-up was 15 months. Interruption of stimulation was followed within days by recurrence or increase of attacks. There were no serious adverse events. Burns et al. recently reported on 14 patients with intractable chronic CH (CCH) who were treated with bilateral suboccipital neurostimulation.[37] At a median follow-up of 18 months,

Table 16-2 Studies of Occipital Nerve Stimulation for Migraine

Study Design	Diagnosis (*n*)	Intervention	Results	Adverse Effects (n)	Reference
Case series	TM (25)	Implanted stimulating electrodes at the C1 level bilaterally.	Decrease in headache frequency, headache severity and headache-related disability.	Lead migration (9) Infection (1)	Popeney and Aló 2004[35]
Case series	CM (8)	Bilateral suboccipital stimulation using implanted electrodes.	"Excellent" response - 4 "Very good" response - 2 "Good" response - 2	Lead migration (3) Abdominal hematoma (1)	Matharu et al. 2004[36]
Case series	CM (8), CH (3) HC (2), PTH (2)	Implanted subcutaneous electrodes at the C1 level (uni- or bilaterally).	A significant decrease in headache frequency, headache severity and headache-related disability.	Lead migration[a] (8/8) Battery depletion[a] (5/8)	Schwedt et al. 2007[37]

[a]At 3 years postimplantation.

CH = cluster headache; HC = hemicrania continua; CM = chronic migraine; PTH = post traumatic headache TM = transformed migraine. *n* = number of patients

10 (71%) patients reported on headache improvement (three of whom had marked improvement, three had moderate improvement, and four had mild improvement). Similar to the study by Magis et al., patients reported that attacks recurred when the device was off. Adverse effects included lead migration and battery depletion. These studies suggest that GON stimulation may be an effective treatment for drug resistant CCH. The delay of 2 months or more between implantation and significant clinical improvement suggests that the procedure acts via slow neuromodulatory processes, possibly at upper brain stem or diencephalic centers.

In summary, current data suggest that ONS may be effective in the treatment of intractable headaches, including CM, CCH, and possibly other headache types. This treatment modality offers potential benefit to patients who are refractory to other treatment modalities. However, current data should be taken with reservation because they are derived from uncontrolled studies. Data from ongoing large controlled trials are expected to help us better understand the role of ONS in headache treatment.

Vagal Nerve Stimulation

Vagal nerve stimulation (VNS) has been used as a treatment for some patients with epilepsy. There are little data on the effect of this treatment on headaches.[38–40] Hord et al. examined retrospectively the effect of VNS on head pain in four epileptic patients who had concomitant migraine.[38] All four patients reported on reduction in headache frequency and severity after VNS implantation, one of them experiencing complete headache relief. Improvement in headache started 1 to 3 months after VNS implantation. Sadler et al. reported on a 42-year-old man with intractable seizures and migraine.[40] After VNS implantation, there was a significant decrease in migraine attack frequency, with prolonged periods of time when he was headache free. Mauskop reported on the effect of VNS on head pain and related symptoms in six patients with chronic refractory headaches (four with migraine and two with CH).[39] Two of the four migraine patients and the two CH patients experienced significant improvement in headaches after VNS. One migraine patient could not tolerate VNS due to nausea, and another experienced only temporary headache relief.

Data from these studies suggest a possible beneficial effect of VNS on migraine and CH. However, these studies were not controlled and the number of patients was small. Until the results of controlled prospective studies are available, no conclusions can be made regarding the efficacy of VNS in headache treatment.

Supraorbital Nerve Stimulation

Amin et al. examined the efficacy of supraorbital nerve (SON) stimulation in the treatment of refractory supraorbital neuralgia (SN).[41] Of 16 patients with refractory SN who underwent a trial of SON stimulation, 10 elected to undergo a permanent electrode implantation. Mean headache severity and opioid consumption decreased significantly after electrode implantation (from 7.5 ± 0.4 before implantation to 3.5 ± 1.2 after it), and this effect was maintained for the entire follow-up period of 30 weeks. Three patients required lead revision, including two who had local infection. The authors concluded that SON stimulation may be an effective treatment for selected patients with refractory SN. No studies have been done on chronic or refractory migraine.

Botulinum Neurotoxin Injections

Background

Botulinum neurotoxin (BoNT) has long been used to treat dystonia and other disorders associated with increased muscle tone. The toxin inhibits the release of acetylcholine from nerve terminals at the neuromuscular junction, thereby causing muscle relaxation. Anecdotal observations of an analgesic effect of BoNT when given for other indications led to attempts of using the drug for various pain disorders, including headaches. Scientific data support these observations: the toxin was shown to inhibit the release of pain neurotransmitters, such as substance P, glutamate, and calcitonin gene related peptide, from presynaptic nerve terminals.[42–44] BoNT may also affect the activity of muscle spindles, thereby modulating afferent pathways. It has also been suggested that by decreasing muscle contraction, BoNT decreases the levels of metabolites that have pro-nociceptive properties, contributing to its analgesic effect.

Proposed Mechanisms of the Analgesic Effect of Botulinum Neurotoxin

- Inhibition of the presynaptic release of substance P
- Inhibition of CGRP release from trigeminal nerve terminals
- Inhibition of glutamate release
- Modulation of afferent pathways through an effect on muscle spindles
- Decreased levels of pro-nociceptive metabolites in muscle through its muscle relaxation effect

CGRP = calcitonin gene related peptide.

Over the past decade, BoNT (and particularly BoNT serotype A [BoNT-A]), has been studied extensively as a potential treatment for various types of headache, including chronic migraine.[21,45] Despite positive clinical experience with the toxin as a treatment for some headache patients, the results of the majority of large clinical studies were negative or equivocal. However, in some studies, specific subgroups of patients (e.g., those who were not taking other headache preventive mediations, and those who were not overusing acute pain medications) showed a positive response.[46,47] The most widely used serotype of BoNT in migraine treatment is BoNT-A. BoNT type B (BoNT-B) is also used occasionally for this purpose.

The pharmacological profile of BoNT makes it an attractive candidate as a migraine preventive drug for refractory patients. Its long duration of action (of 3 months on average) is particularly appealing to patients who are unable or unwilling to adhere to the commitment to take daily oral preventives. BoNT also has a more favorable adverse effect profile compared with many oral migraine preventive drugs, with little or no effect on weight, cognition or alertness.

Favorable Pharmacological Properties of Botulinum Neurotoxin for Headache Prevention

- Long duration of action (typically 2–4 months)
- Few adverse effects
- Little or no effect on weight
- Few interactions with oral headache preventive drugs
- High safety profile

Technical Aspects

BoNT-A is available in the United States as Botox® (Allergan, Irvine, CA). It is marketed in a purified sterile vacuum-dried form in vials containing 100 units (U). Before injections, the toxin needs to be reconstituted and diluted, typically with 4 mL of saline, creating a solution of 25 U/mL. The solution is then transferred to four 1-mL syringes. A 30-gauge needle is used for the intramuscular injections. There is no standardized dosage and injection-site regimen for the use of BoNT in headache treatment. The toxin may be injected in either a "fixed-site" or a "follow the pain" approach, or a combination of the two. A commonly used fixed-site regimen for migraine treatment is shown in Figure 16.5, and the doses for the various injection sites are shown in Table 16.3.

Data from clinical studies of BoNT for the treatment of chronic daily headache

The effect of BoNT in patients with CDH, most of whom had CM, was evaluated in several well-designed studies[47,48–50] (Table 16.4). Ondo et al. examined the effect of BoNT-A injections on 60 patients with CDH.[49] The patients were randomized to receive either BoNT-A (200 U), injected in a "follow-the-pain" approach, or placebo. The primary end-point (number of headache-free days at week 12 compared to baseline) was not met. However, the number of headache-free days in the BoNT-A group improved significantly from week 8 to 12, and patients' global impression improved in the BoNT-A group.

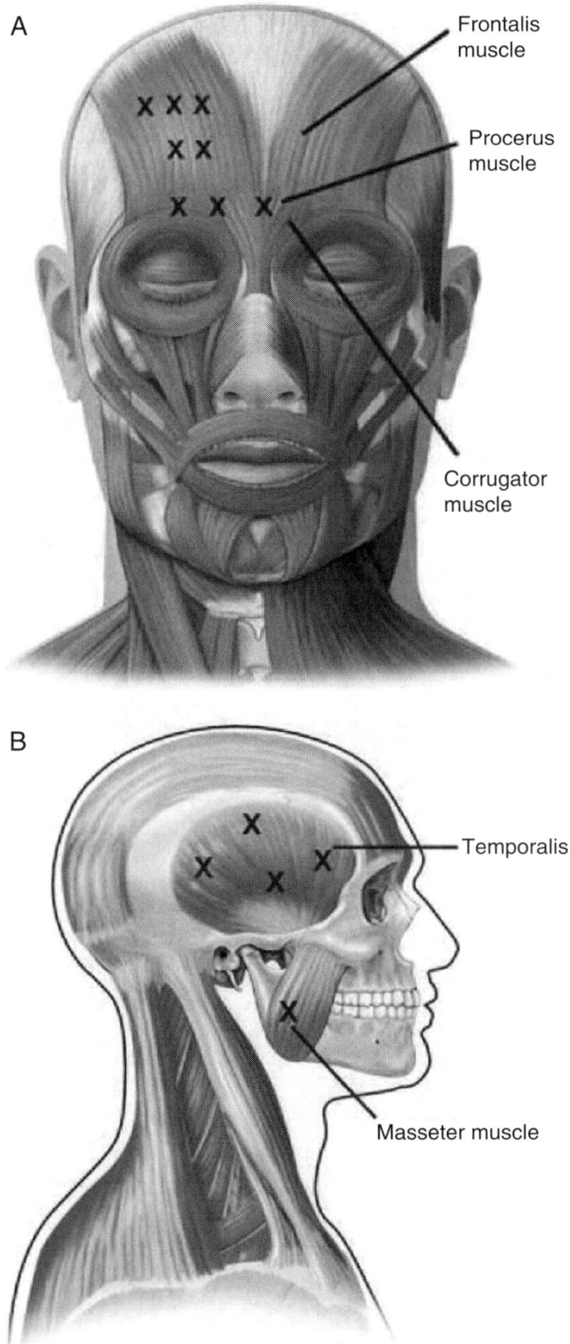

Figure 16-5 Injection sites for botulinum neurotoxin for headache treatment. (**A**) Frontal area. (**B**) Lateral area. (**C**) Posterior area. (Reprinted with permission from Blumenfeld AM, et al. *Headache.* 2003;43:884–891.)

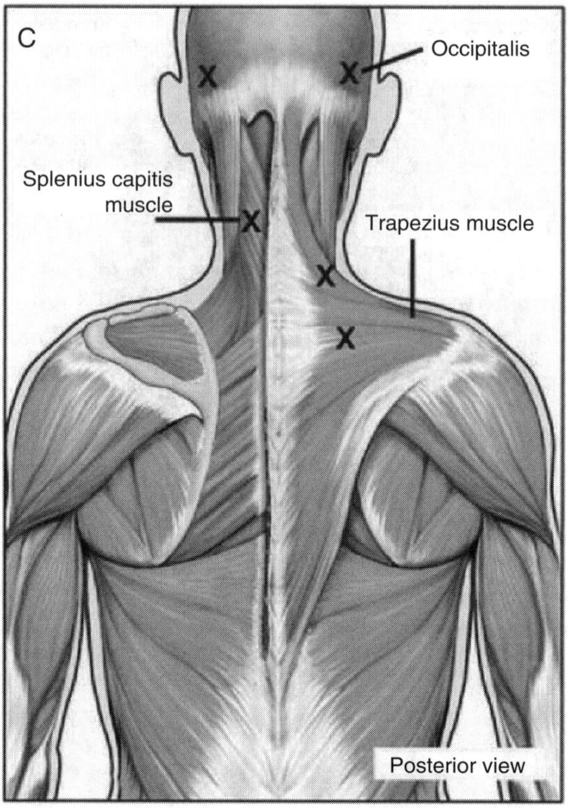

Figure 16-5 (Continued)

Table 16-3 A Proposed Fixed-Site Injection Paradigm of Botulinum Neurotoxin Type A (BoNT-A) for Migraine

Muscle (no.)	Injections per Muscle	BoNT-A Units per Injection	Dose per Muscle	Total Dose
Procerus (1)	1	5	5	5
Corrugator (2)	2	2.5	5	10
Frontalis (2)	5	2.5	12.5	25
Temporalis (2)	4	2.5	10	20
Masseter (2) (optional)	1	2.5	2.5	5
Occipitalis (2)	1	2.5	2.5	5
Splenius capitis (2)	1	5	5	10
Trapezius (2)	2	5	10	20

Adapted from Blumenfeld AM et al. *Headache.* 2003;43:884–891.

Mathew et al. examined the efficacy of BoNT-A in the prophylactic treatment of 355 patients with CDH and a history of migraine or probable migraine.[48] Patients were randomized to receive either BoNT-A, using a follow-the-pain approach at a dose range of 105 to 260 U every 3 months for a total of three treatment cycles, or placebo. At 6 months post-treatment, the primary end point of the study (the differences between the BoNT-A and the placebo groups in the increase in mean number of headache-free days per 30 days) was not met. However, significantly more patients in the BoNT-A group experienced a greater than 50% decrease in headache days 6 months after enrollment. Also, the mean decrease from baseline in headache frequency was significantly greater in the BoNT-A group compared with the placebo group. BoNT-A treatment was well tolerated. A subgroup analysis of data from this study for patients who did not use concurrent headache preventive drug was done by Dodick et al.[46] They found that in this subgroup, BoNT-A was significantly superior to placebo in reducing the mean frequency of headaches per month after two treatment cycles. BoNT-A treatment was also associated with a significantly greater increase in the number of headache-free days per month compared with placebo. Silberstein et al. examined the prophylactic effect of BoNT-A in a large study of patients with CDH (the majority of whom had TM).[50] Patients were treated with BoNT-A (at doses of 225, 150, or 75U, given at fixed predetermined sites), or placebo. Three treatment sessions were given at 3-month intervals. The mean change from baseline in the number of headache-free days per month (the study primary end-point) did not differ significantly among the patient groups. BoNT-A, at doses of 150 and 225 U, was slightly superior to placebo in decreasing migraine headache frequency. The sample of this study consisted of particularly difficult to treat patients, with long standing CDH (average disease duration of 13.7 years), 42% of whom were overusing pain medications.

In summary, the results of these studies are mostly negative, although they suggest that specific subgroups of patients with CDH may benefit from the use of BoNT. The American Academy of Neurology (AAN) has recently published recommendations for the use of BoNT in headache treatment.[51] Based on a review of the literature, the AAN expert panel stated that there was no consistent or strong evidence to permit drawing conclusions on the efficacy of BoNT in CDH, and that BoNT-A is probably ineffective in the treatment of episodic migraine (and of TTH, see later).

Data from clinical studies of BoNT for the treatment of tension type headache

TTH has been associated with increased pericranial muscle tone, although the significance of this finding in the pathogenesis of the disease has been debated. Since BoNT has muscle relaxation effect, it has been speculated that the toxin may be effective in the treatment of TTH. Based on this rational, BoNT-A has been examined as a potential treatment for chronic TTH (CTTH) in a number of studies.[21] Early results from small open-label studies and a small

Table 16-4 Studies of Botulinum Neurotoxin for the Prevention of Chronic Daily Headache

Study Design	Diagnosis (*n*)	Patients with Medication Overuse	Injection Paradigm	BoNT Serotype and Dose (Units)	Results	Reference
Prospective double-blind randomized placebo-controlled	CM (14) CTTH (46)	Included	Follow the pain	Type A (Botox®), 200 U	Primary end-point (change in number of headache-free days) not met. Patients' global impression improved with BoNT-A	Ondo et al. 2004[49]
Prospective double-blind randomized placebo-controlled	CDH (355) (most patients had TM)	Included	Follow the pain	Type A (Botox®), 105–260 U	Primary end-point (change in number of headache-free days) not met. More patients with BoNT-A had >50% decrease in headache frequency at 6 months, compared with placebo.	Mathew et al. 2005[48]
Prospective double-blind randomized placebo-controlled	CDH (228) (a subgroup of patients from study by Mathew et al. who were not using other preventive drugs)	Included	Follow the pain	Type A (Botox®), 105–260 U	BoNT-A superior to placebo in reducing the mean frequency of headaches per month. BoNT-A also associated with a greater increase in number of headache-free days per month compared with placebo.	Dodick et al.2005[46]
Prospective double- blind randomized placebo-controlled	TM (375) CTTH (89) NDPH (16) Other or not classified CDH (222)	Included	Fixed site	Type A (Botox®), 225 U, 150 U, or 75 U	Primary end-point (change in number of headache-free days) not met. BoNT-A slightly superior to placebo in decreasing total headache frequency and migraine headache frequency.	Silberstein et al. 2005[50]

(*n* = number of patients). CDH = chronic daily headache; CM = chronic migraine; CTTH = chronic tension type headache; NDPH = new daily persistent headache; TM = transformed migraine.

Adapted with permission from: Ashkenazi A, Levin M, Dodick DW. Peripheral procedures: nerve blocks, peripheral neurostimulation and botulinum toxin injections. In: Silberstein SD, Lipton RB, Dodick DW, eds. *Wolff's Headache and Other Head Pain.* New York: Oxford University Press; 2007:767–792.

controlled study suggested that BoNT may alleviate TTH pain. However, larger controlled studies conducted subsequently failed to confirm this. The AAN recommendations state that BoNT is probably ineffective in the treatment of chronic CTTH.[51]

Safety

With clinical experience of more than two decades, BoNT-A has proved to be a safe drug. Based on animal studies, the lethal dose in humans is estimated at approximately 3000 U.[52] The doses used for headache treatment are therefore unlikely to be toxic. An antitoxin is available in the event of accidental overdose.[53] BoNT should be used with caution in patients with neuromuscular junction diseases (e.g., myasthenia gravis). It is contraindicated in patients who take aminoglycosides or other drugs that impair neuromuscular transmission. Rarely, a therapeutic injection of the toxin may cause generalized muscle weakness and even full-blown botulism.[54] Allergic reactions after BoNT injection may rarely occur. There is little data on the safety of BoNT in pregnant and lactating women. Therefore, it is not recommended for use in these circumstances.

Assessment of the Data

A key question in the debate over the use of BoNT for migraine is patient selection. Many headache clinicians have seen patients who responded well to BoNT injections. The mostly negative results of large clinical trials of this drug for migraine may be explained, in part, by failure to select the patients who would best respond to it.[21] Factors to be considered in this regard include the following: (1) The use of concurrent preventive medications: there are data suggesting that patients who do not use concurrent headache preventive drugs may respond better to BoNT treatment.[46] (2) Pain medication overuse: data from one retrospective study suggest that patients who do not overuse pain medications may benefit more from BoNT treatment than those who do.[55] Prospective studies however, did not confirm this. (3) Disease duration: Eross et al. found that disease duration greater than 30 years adversely affected outcome after BoNT-A treatment in their migraine patients.[56] (4) Headache characteristics: Jakubowski et al. found that most of their migraine patients who improved after BoNT-A treatment described their headache as a pressure from outside (imploding headache) or as a feeling of eye-popping (ocular headache). Conversely, the majority of those who did not improve after BoNT treatment described their headache as a pressure building up from inside (exploding headache).[57] Based on current data, BoNT cannot be recommended as a standard treatment for headache prevention. Further studies are needed to examine the effect of BoNT on headache in selected patients with refractory migraine. In addition, the optimal approach for the administration of BoNT to headache patients remains to be determined.

Factors that May Improve the Therapeutic Response of Migraine Patients to Botulinum Neurotoxin

- No use of concurrent migraine preventive drugs
- No overuse of pain medications
- Shorter disease duration
- "Imploding" or ocular headache

Conclusions

Although there is limited evidence from controlled studies, peripheral nerve blocks are a viable treatment option for selected groups of headache patients, particularly those with intractable headache or neuralgic type pain. Local tenderness overlying superficial nerves of the scalp and face might be predictive of good results with local nerve blockade but this too is not yet clear.

Greater occipital nerve block, the most widely used local anesthetic procedure in headache conditions, is safe and relatively easy to perform in the office. Adverse effects are few and infrequent. The procedure can result in rapid relief of pain and allodynia, and effects may last for several weeks. There is less clear evidence to support the usefulness of neurostimulation of the GON or other nerves but compelling anecdotal reports are abundant in cases of intractable occipital neuralgia, chronic migraine, and chronic cluster headache.

Botulinum toxin therapy has many advantages over traditional pharmaceutical treatment of refractory migraine and other intractable headache conditions, in particular its safety and duration of action. However, despite many compelling clinical successes, clear evidence for its efficacy has proven elusive.

However, the refractory migraine group is desperate for alternatives, so blinded, sham-controlled studies are needed to establish the efficacy of nerve blocks, neurostimulation, and botulinum toxin therapy in refractory migraine.

References

1. Schulman EA, Lake AE, Goadsby PJ, et al. Defining refractory migraine and refractory chronic migraine: proposed criteria from the Refractory Headache Special Interest Section of the American Headache Society. *Headache.* 2008;48:778–782.
2. Gale G, Nussbaum D, Rothbart P, Hann B, Leung V, Kanetz G. A randomized treatment study to compare the efficacy of repeated nerve blocks with cognitive therapy for control of chronic head and neck pain. *Pain Res Manag.* 2002;7:185–189.
3. de Craen AJ, Tijssen JG, de GJ, Kleijnen J. Placebo effect in the acute treatment of migraine: subcutaneous placebos are better than oral placebos. *J Neurol.* 2000;247:183–188.

4. Ashkenazi A, Matro R, Shaw JW, Abbas MA, Silberstein SD. Greater occipital nerve block using local anesthetics alone or with triamcinolone for transformed migraine: a randomized comparative study. *J Neurol Neurosurg Psychiatry.* 2008;79:415–417.
5. Shields KG, Levy MJ, Goadsby PJ . Alopecia and cutaneous atrophy after greater occipital nerve infiltration with corticosteroid. *Neurology.* 2004;63:2193–2194.
6. Lavin PJ, Workman R. Cushing syndrome induced by serial occipital nerve blocks containing corticosteroids. *Headache.* 2001;41:902–904.
7. Ashkenazi A, Young WB. The effects of greater occipital nerve block and trigger point injection on brush allodynia and pain in migraine. *Headache.* 2005;45:350–354.
8. Cook BL, Malik SN, Shaw JW, Oshinsky ML, Young WB. Greater occipital nerve (GON) block successfully treats migraine within five minutes. *Neurology.* 2006;66:A42 (Abstr).
9. Afridi SK, Shields KG, Bhola R, Goadsby PJ. Greater occipital nerve injection in primary headache syndromes—prolonged effects from a single injection. *Pain.* 2006;122:126–129.
10. Peres MF, Stiles MA, Siow HC, Rozen TD, Young WB, Silberstein SD. Greater occipital nerve blockade for cluster headache. *Cephalalgia.* 2002;22:520–522.
11. Ambrosini A, Vandenheede M, Rossi P, Aloj F, Sauli E, Pierelli F, Schoenen J. Suboccipital injection with a mixture of rapid- and long-acting steroids in cluster headache: a double-blind placebo-controlled study. *Pain.* 2005;118:92–96.
12. Matute E. Bilateral greater occipital nerve block for post-dural puncture headache. *Anaesthesia.* 2008;63(5):557–558.
13. Weatherall MW. Idiopathic trigeminal neuropathy may respond to greater occipital nerve injection. *Cephalalgia.* 2008;28(6):664–666.
14. Rozen T. Cessation of hemiplegic migraine auras with greater occipital nerve blockade. *Headache.* 2007;47(6):917–919.
15. Leinisch-Dahlke E, Jurgens T, Bogdahn U, Jakob W, May A. Greater occipital nerve block is ineffective in chronic tension type headache. *Cephalalgia.* 2005; 25:704–708.
16. Caputi CA, Firetto V. Therapeutic blockade of greater occipital and supraorbital nerves in migraine patients. *Headache.* 1997;37:174–179.
17. Bartsch T, Goadsby PJ. Stimulation of the greater occipital nerve induces increased central excitability of dural afferent input. *Brain.* 2002;125: 1496–1509.
18. Bartsch T, Goadsby PJ. Increased responses in trigeminocervical nociceptive neurons to cervical input after stimulation of the dura mater. *Brain.* 2003;126: 1801–1813.
19. Busch V, Jakob W, Juergens T, Schulte-Mattler W, Kaube H, May A. Functional connectivity between trigeminal and occipital nerves revealed by occipital nerve blockade and nociceptive blink reflexes. *Cephalalgia.* 2006;26: 50–55.
20. Piovesan EJ, Kowacs PA, Tatsui CE, Lange MC, Ribas LC, Werneck LC. Referred pain after painful stimulation of the greater occipital nerve in humans: evidence of convergence of cervical afferences on trigeminal nuclei. *Cephalalgia.* 2001;21:107–109.

21. Ashkenazi A, Levin M, Dodick DW. Peripheral procedures: nerve blocks, peripheral neurostimulation and *Botulinum* neurotoxin injections. In: Silberstein SD, Lipton RB, Dodick DW, eds. *Wolff's Headache and Other Head Pain.* New York: Oxford University Press; 2007:767–792.
22. Weiner RL. Peripheral nerve neurostimulation. *Neurosurg Clin North Am.* 2003;14:401–408.
23. Woolf CJ, Salter MW. Plasticity and pain: role of the dorsal horn. In: McMahon SB, Koltzenburg M, eds. *Wall and Melzac's Textbook of Pain.* Philadelphia: Elsevier;2006: 91–105.
24. Sluka KA, Walsh D. Transcutaneous electrical nerve stimulation: basic science mechanisms and clinical effectiveness. *J Pain.* 2003;4:109–121.
25. Barlas P, Lundeberg T. Transcutaneous electrical stimulation and acupuncture. In: McMahon SB, Koltzenburg M, eds. *Wall and Melzack's Textbook of Pain.* Philadelphia: Elsevier; 2006:583–590.
26. Solomon S, Guglielmo KM. Treatment of headache by transcutaneous electrical stimulation. *Headache.* 1985;25:12–15.
27. Allais G, De Lorenzo C, Quirico PE, Lupi G, Airola G, Mana O, Benedetto C. Non-pharmacological approaches to chronic headaches: transcutaneous electrical nerve stimulation, laser therapy and acupuncture in transformed migraine treatment. *Neurol Sci.* 2003;24 (Suppl 2):S138–S142.
28. Farina S, Granella F, Malferrari G, Manzoni GC. Headache and cervical spine disorders: classification and treatment with transcutaneous electrical nerve stimulation. *Headache.* 1986;26:431–433.
29. Ahmed HE, White PF, Craig WF, Hamza MA, Ghoname ES, Gajraj NM. Use of percutaneous electrical nerve stimulation (PENS) in the short-term management of headache. *Headache.* 2000;40:311–315.
30. Ghoname EA, Craig WF, White PF. Use of percutaneous electrical nerve stimulation (PENS) for treating ECT-induced headaches. *Headache.* 1999;39:502–505.
31. Goadsby PJ, Bartsch T, Dodick DW. Occipital nerve stimulation for headache: mechanisms and efficacy. *Headache.* 2008;48:313–318.
32. Goadsby PJ, Hoskin KL, Knight YE. Stimulation of the greater occipital nerve increases metabolic activity in the trigeminal nucleus caudalis and cervical dorsal horn of the cat. *Pain.* 1997;73:23–28.
33. Popeney CA, Alo KM. Peripheral neurostimulation for the treatment of chronic, disabling transformed migraine. *Headache.* 2003;43:369–375.
34. Matharu MS, Bartsch T, Ward N, Frackowiak RS, Weiner R, Goadsby PJ. Central neuromodulation in chronic migraine patients with suboccipital stimulators: a PET study. *Brain.* 2004;127:220–230.
35. Schwedt TJ, Dodick DW, Hentz J, Trentman TL, Zimmerman RS. Occipital nerve stimulation for chronic headache--long-term safety and efficacy. *Cephalalgia.* 2007;27:153–157.
36. Magis D, Allena M, Bolla M, De Pasqua V, Remacle JM, Schoenen J. Occipital nerve stimulation for drug-resistant chronic cluster headache: a prospective pilot study. *Lancet Neurol.* 2007;6:314–321.
37. Burns B, Watkins L, Goadsby PJ. Treatment of intractable chronic cluster headache by occipital nerve stimulation in 14 patients. *Neurology.* 2009;72:341–345.

38. Hord ED, Evans MS, Mueed S, Adamolekun B, Naritoku DK. The effect of vagus nerve stimulation on migraines. *J Pain.* 2003;4:530–534.
39. Mauskop A. Vagus nerve stimulation relieves chronic refractory migraine and cluster headaches. *Cephalalgia.* 2005;25:82–86.
40. Sadler RM, Purdy RA, Rahey S. Vagal nerve stimulation aborts migraine in patient with intractable epilepsy. *Cephalalgia.* 2002;22:482–484.
41. Amin S, Buvanendran A, Park KS, Kroin JS, Moric M. Peripheral nerve stimulator for the treatment of supraorbital neuralgia: a retrospective case series. *Cephalalgia.* 2008;28:355–359.
42. Aoki KR. Evidence for antinociceptive activity of botulinum toxin type A in pain management. *Headache.* 2003;43(Suppl 1):S9–15.
43. Cui M, Khanijou S, Rubino J, Aoki KR. Subcutaneous administration of botulinum toxin A reduces formalin-induced pain. *Pain.* 2004;107:125–133.
44. Durham PL, Cady R. Regulation of calcitonin gene-related peptide secretion from trigeminal nerve cells by botulinum toxin type A: implications for migraine therapy. *Headache.* 2004;44:35–42.
45. Ashkenazi A, Silberstein SD. Botulinum toxin and other new approaches to migraine therapy. *Annu Rev Med.* 2004;55:505–518.
46. Dodick DW, Mauskop A, Elkind AH, DeGryse R, Brin MF, Silberstein SD. Botulinum toxin type a for the prophylaxis of chronic daily headache: subgroup analysis of patients not receiving other prophylactic medications: a randomized double-blind, placebo-controlled study. *Headache.* 2005;45: 315–324.
47. Freitag FG, Diamond S, Diamond M, Urban G. Botulinum toxin type A in the treatment of chronic migraine without medication overuse. *Headache.* 2008; 48:201–209.
48. Mathew NT, Frishberg BM, Gawel M, Dimitrova R, Gibson J, Turkel C. Botulinum toxin type A (BOTOX) for the prophylactic treatment of chronic daily headache: a randomized, double-blind, placebo-controlled trial. *Headache.* 2005;45:293–307.
49. Ondo WG, Vuong KD, Derman HS. Botulinum toxin A for chronic daily headache: a randomized, placebo-controlled, parallel design study. *Cephalalgia.* 2004;24:60–65.
50. Silberstein SD, Stark SR, Lucas SM, Christie SN, Degryse RE, Turkel CC. Botulinum toxin type A for the prophylactic treatment of chronic daily headache: a randomized, double-blind, placebo-controlled trial. *Mayo Clin Proc.* 2005;80:1126–1137.
51. Naumann M, So Y, Argoff CE, et al. Assessment: Botulinum neurotoxin in the treatment of autonomic disorders and pain (an evidence-based review): report of the Therapeutics and Technology Assessment Subcommittee of the American Academy of Neurology. *Neurology.* 2008;70:1707–1714.
52. Brin MF. Botulinum toxin: chemistry, pharmacology, toxicity, and immunology. *Muscle Nerve.* 1997;20:S146–S168.
53. Scott AB. Antitoxin reduces botulinum side effects. *Eye.* 1988;2:29–32.
54. Souayah N, Karim H, Kamin SS, McArdle J, Marcus S. Severe botulism after focal injection of botulinum toxin. *Neurology.* 2006;67:1855–1856.
55. Tepper SJ, Bigal ME, Sheftell FD, Rapoport AM. Botulinum neurotoxin type A in the preventive treatment of refractory headache: a review of 100 consecutive cases. *Headache.* 2004;44:794–800.

56. Eross EJ, Gladstone JP, Lewis S, Rogers R, Dodick DW. Duration of migraine is a predictor for response to botulinum toxin type A. *Headache.* 2005;45:308–314.
57. Jakubowski M, McAllister PJ, Bajwa ZH, Ward TN, Smith P, Burstein R. Exploding vs. imploding headache in migraine prophylaxis with Botulinum toxin A. *Pain.* 2006;24:1872–6623.

17

Physical Therapies for Refractory Migraine

Temporomandibular and Cervical Spine Disorders

Steven Graff-Radford, DDS, and Phuu Pwint Han, DDS, PhD

Introduction

Migraine is generally regarded as a genetic disorder wherein the headache is precipitated by external stimuli and/or systemic or central nervous system changes. This suggests that the migraine patient is constantly at risk for triggering a headache. The risk may be genetic or related to external or internal triggers. The current opinion is that genetics alone cannot explain migraine and most likely it is a multifactorial disorder. The migraine diagnosis remains a clinical description and not a genotype.[1] Effective treatment of migraine requires the patient and physician identify and control the triggering and perpetuating factors for headache, including diet and nutrition, environmental and weather changes, and emotional changes and to relieve symptoms created by other structures around the head, such as facial muscles, cervical muscles, jaws and teeth, etc., that may be contributing to the problem. In preventing and controlling these triggering factors, the patient and the treating physician will be able to decrease the headache frequency and severity to manageable levels by standard pharmacological, behavioral, and physical protocols. Because migraineurs have lower nociceptive thresholds, temporomandibular disorders (TMDs) and cervical spine disorders may be implicated as triggers, and can be significant contributors to refractory migraine in some patients.

Migraine is a public health problem that has an impact on both the individual sufferer and on society. The American Migraine Study II estimates that 28 million Americans are affected by migraine headache, although only 50% are diagnosed as migraine.[2] In the U.S. population, pain in the temporomandibular joint (TMJ) may occur in 10%, and TMD has been reported in 46.1%.[2,3] In a population-based study, Ciancaglini and Radaelli[5] reported that subjects who had TMD pain were more likely to report headache than subjects who did not have TMD pain, 27.4% versus 15.2%. There is a reported relationship between headache frequency and comorbid musculoskeletal symptoms, defined as pain or stiffness in muscles and joints of both cervical spine and jaw.[6] When a population of TMD patients is evaluated, there are significantly more tender points in the cervical muscles and limitations in function of the higher cervical region compared with a non-TMD control group.[7,8] Because migraine,[2] TMD,[3] and cervical dysfunctions[4] are so common in the general population, they may be linked or separate entities in an individual patient. Researchers who conducted systematic reviews of the association between the cervical dysfunction and migrine as well as the cervical dysfunction and temporomandibular disorders could not find any clear cause–effect relationship between these disorders.[9,10] Some reasons for these inconclusive findings include methodological flaws and inconsistencies between different studies, for example, the epidemiological studies have not specifically differentiated headache from facial pain; the broad range of disorders included in the terms cervical dysfunction and TMDs; and the common occurrence of all three disorders (i.e., headache, TMDs, and cervical disorders) in the general population.

However, there are theoretical animal studies and limited clinical evidence that coexisting TMDs and cervical dysfunction can cause worsening of primary headache, and treating them can reduce headache serverity and frequency.[2,10,11] Headache may result from temporomandibular structures,[12] or pain may be referred to the temporomandibular structures and muscles of mastication, secondary to a primary headache diagnosis.[2] This is also true for the case of migraine and cervical dysfunction.[10] These overlaps are related primarily to the anatomy and neural innervations of the head and neck structures. Convergence of nociceptive afferents and sensitization of trigeminocervical neurones with subsequent central sensitization and increased receptive fields are the basic mechanisms that explain the neurophysiological pathways and mechanisms of how migraine, TMDs, and cervical dysfunction can interact each other.[11,13,14] Neurons in the trigeminocervical complex are the major relay for nociceptive afferent input from the meninges, facial structures and TMJ, and the cervical structures.[11,13,14] The cervical dermatomes include the back of the head, parts of the ear, the TMJ, and lower border of the mandible. Rarely, nerve root irritation or entrapment may cause pain to be experienced in these dermatomal projections. The primary afferent nociceptors of the trigeminal nerve synapse in the nucleus caudalis of the spinal trigeminal tract. The nucleus caudalis descends as low as C3–C4 in the spinal cord. Many nociceptors from the deep cervical structures synapse on the same second-order pain transmission neurons as the trigeminal nerve. Bartsch and Goadsby[11] provided a model describing how neural inflammation opens the silent or latent connections between the trigeminal nucleus caudalis and the upper cerivical afferents and increases responses in trigeminocervial nociceptive neurons to cervical input after stimulation of the dura mater.[13] Moreover, the evidence for the referral patterns seen in myofacial pain accounts for why injection of cervical afferents with anesthetic (nerve block of the occipital or cervical afferents) may stop migraine, myofascial pain, and cervical neuropathies. Convergence and central modulation at these locations of nociceptive input, such as that from myofascial trigger points (TrPs), can readily account for these referred pain phenomena.

It is essential not to confuse and suggest a cause-and-effect relationship among headache, TMD, and cervical disorders based on symptoms and/or treatment responses. The frequent coexistence of these clinical disorders suggests a degree of physiological overlap that has not yet been elucidated. It is suggested that all of these factors are separate but may aggravate or perpetuate each other in susceptible patients.[2] Patients with primary headache can see their pain worsened or triggered when there is a coexisting TMD and/or cervical dysfunction. Often, ignoring the TMJ, muscles, and other orofacial or cervical structures as peripheral triggers will result in a poor clinical outcome in managing headache; at the same time, not making the correct diagnosis may lead to unnecessary therapy and poor outcome.[2] TMD and cervical dysfunction can be controlled by noninvasive physical therapy, and all patients with chronic or refractory headache should be examined and treated for these disorders. In this chapter, we will focused on the noninvasive physical therapies for TMDs and cervical disorders.

Definitions

Temporomandibular Disorders

Temporomandibular disorder is a collective term embracing a number of clinical problems that involve the masticatory musculature, the TMJs and associated structures, or both.[15] TMDs are basically subdivided into TMJ disorders (arthrogenous) and masticatory muscle disorders (myogenous). Clinically, the two frequently occur together, but this arbitrary separation facilitates research and discussion (Table 17.1). The diagnostic criteria for headache attributed to TMDs are listed in the diagnostic classification of the International Headache Society (IHS) under the 11th major classification. The three most common TMDs are myofascial pain and dysfunction, disk displacements, and osteoarthrosis. Muscle-related conditions account for at least 50% of TMDs. The three cardinal features of TMD are orofacial pain, joint noise, and restricted jaw function. The most common presenting complaint is pain.[16]

Joint sounds such as clicking and crepitation are very common in TMD patients. Clicking noise may be present in approximately 33% of the

Table 17-1 Classification of Temporomandibular Disorders with Corresponding International Headache Society (HIS) Classification and International Classification of Diseases, Ninth Revision (ICD-9) Codes[15]

A. TMD arthrogenous
   1. Congenital or developmental disorders (IHS 11.1.1.x)
      a. Aplasia (IHS 11.1.1.1; ICD-9 754.0)
      b. Hypoplasia (IHS 11.1.1.2; ICD-9 526.89)
      c. Hyperplasia (IHS 11.1.1.3; ICD-9 526.89)
      d. Dysplasia (IHS 11.1.1.4; ICD-9 526.89)
      e. Neoplasia (IHS 11.1.2.1)
         – Benign (ICD-9 213.1)
         – Malignant (ICD-9 170.1)
   2. Disc derangement disorders (IHS 11.7.1.1.x; ICD-9 524.63)
      a. Disc displacement with reduction (IHS 11.7.1.1.1; ICD-9 524.63)
      b. Disc displacement without reduction (IHS 11.7.1.1.2; ICD-9 524.63)
   3. TMJ dislocation (IHS 11.7.1.2.x; ICD-9 830.0)
   4. Inflammatory disorders (IHS 11.7.1.3.x)
      a. Synovitis and capsulitis (IHS 11.7.1.3.1; ICD-9 524.62 or 726.90 or 716.98)
      b. Polyarthritides (IHS 11.7.1.3.2; ICD-9 714.9)
   5. Non-inflammatory disorders
      a. Primary osteoarthritis (IHS 11.7.1.4.1; ICD-9 715.18)
      b. Secondary osteoarthritis (IHS 11.7.1.4.2; ICD-9 715.28)
   6. Ankylosis (IHS 11.7.1.5; ICD-9 524.61)
   7. Fracture (IHS 11.7.1.6; ICD-9 802.2x closed; ICD-9 802.3x open)
B. TMD myogenous
   1. Local myalgia (IHS 11.7.2.1; ICD-9 729.1)
   2. Myofascial pain (IHS 11.7.2.2; ICD-9 729.1)
   3. Centrally mediated myalgia (IHS 11.7.2.3; ICD-9 729.1)
   4. Myospasm (IHS 11.7.2.4; ICD-9 728.85)
   5. Myositis (IHS 11.7.2.5; ICD-9 728.81)
   6. Myofibrotic contracture (IHS 11.7.2.6; ICD-9 728.9)
   7. Masticatory muscle neoplasia (IHS 11.7.2.4; ICD-9-CM 171.0)

asymptomatic general population. Crepitation noises correlate highly with osteoarthritis, with the sound present in 90%.[16] However, not all patients with TMJ osteoarthritis have symptoms, and the asymptomatic patient rarely needs treatment. Patients with refractory headache who also have TMJ noises and symptoms such as limited opening of the mouth (<40 mm), pain with eating or function, and joint tenderness should be considered for TMD therapy.

The gold standard for diagnosis of TMD is history taking and physical examination. A thorough TMD history should include patient chief complaint(s), and pain should be evaluated for location, onset, quality, duration, and intensity. Modifying factors (aggravating and alleviating factors) and associated symptoms (joint sounds, limitation of oral function, ear ringing, dizziness, relationship to other pain complaints, etc.) supplement the understanding. Clinical examination of a patient with TMD should include cranial nerve examination, upper quarter and cervical spine examination, and muscle palpation examination identifying trigger points (points that when palpated replicate the pain complaint and cause referral in characteristic patterns). The TMJ is evaluated by measuring the interincisal opening, which should be greater than 40 mm, and the lateral movement of the jaw, which should be 8 mm. The evaluation includes palpation over the lateral aspect of the joint to ascertain if there is tenderness, auscultation for joint noise, and finally assessment of the occlusion (how the teeth meet). Computed tomography (CT) and magnetic resonance imaging (MRI) are current standards for hard and soft tissue TMJ imaging, respectively.

Cervical Disorders

The potential for cervical dysfunction to manifest as headache is recognized under the classification of cervicogenic headache, and the pain is typically perceived within the dermatomes of the trigeminal and upper cervical (C2, 3) nerves and the cervical structures within the receptive field of the trigeminocervical complex or nucleus. These structures include the C1–3 nerve roots and their branches; the O–C3 joints; the alar and transverse ligaments; the pre- and postvertebral, trapezius, and sternocleidomastoid muscles; the cervical dura mater; and the vertebral and carotid arteries.[10,14,17,18] (Table 17.2). Cervical spine dysfunction or disorders are manifested by decreased range of motion, pain and stiffness on movement of the neck, crepitations from the cervical spine on function, altered sensation of the arms and hands, pain on palpation of the cervical muscles and the subluxation or hypermobility of atlanto-occipital joint on examination.[9]

The mobility of the neck is examined by asking the patient to do simple neck movements. Lateral rotations of the neck (look over the shoulder) to the left and right side should be 70 degrees each way, flexion movement (chin toward the chest) should be 45 degrees, and extension (look upward as far as

Table 17-2 Structures and Tissues Innervated by the C1, C2, and C3 Spinal Nerves[18]

1. Atlanto-occipital joint
2. Lateral atlantoaxial joint (C1–C2)
3. Ligaments of the median atlantoaxial joint
4. C2–C3 zygapophyseal joint
5. Suboccipital and upper posterior neck muscles
6. Upper prevertebral muscles
7. Upper cervical spinal dura mater
8. Vertebral arteries
9. C2–C3 intervertebral disk
10. Trapezius muscle
11. Sternocleidomastoid muscle

possible) should be 60 degrees. Lateral flexion of the neck (ear to the shoulder) should be 35 to 40 degrees each way. Care should be taken to do the passive movement examination with gentle pressure to avoid trauma and serious complications. Passive upper cervical rotation for detecting subluxation of the atlanto-occipital joint is performed with manual stabilization of the axis by the examiner's hands on the patient's head while the patient's neck is in flexion and guide the patient's head to rotate sideways. The limitation of the accessory joint motion can be accessed by the Maitland mobilization technique. It is performed by applying gentle unilateral posteroanterior pressure on the lateral aspect of C1 and over the spinous process of C2 and C3 through the thumbs of examiners when the patient is in the prone position. Pain and limitation of movements should be recorded and investigated for the source of pain.

Cervical muscles, including the sternocleidomastoid, trapezius, and splenius capitis, are palpated for trigger points and tender points. The areas of the scalp supplied by the greater and lesser occipital nerve are also investigated for signs and symptoms of nerve irritation. If nerve impingement or joint dysfunction of the cervical vertebrae is suspected, proper referral or further imaging studies are indicated. Diagnostic nerve blocks, trigger point injections, and facet blocks might be considered to obtain a definitive diagnosis.

Management

Management of TMDs

The general principles of management in patients with headache and TMD is the same as that of patients with TMD alone (Table 17.3). The aims include pain control or elimination, increased mandibular mobility when necessary, reduced joint loading, and resumption of normal functional activity of the mandible. These goals may be achieved through a structured, time-limited program that addresses the physical disorder and the perpetuating factors. The therapies described here may reduce headache that is aggravated by the coexistence of the TMD.[19] Common etiologic factors for headache associated with TMD include bruxism, trauma, occlusal interferences, and emotional stressors. However, not all people with these etiologic factors have chronic TMD and/or chronic headache. When the exact cause of the problem cannot be identified, the patient and provider have to eliminate all the possible contributing factors and symptomatic treatment has to be provided. Because the signs and symptoms of TMD can be transient and self-limiting, simple and reversible treatments have to be preferred over complicated and irreversible procedure.[2] The most common form of TMD in headache patients is myogenous pain, and noninvasive physical therapies for myofascial pain of the cervical and masticatory muscles are the focus here, and are summarized in Table 17.3.

Table 17-3 Basic Principles of Management of Temporomandibular Disorders

A. Patient education and self-care
B. Cognitive behavioral interventions
C. Pharmacological management (e.g., analgesics, anti-inflammatories, muscle relaxants, sedatives, antidepressants)
D. Physical therapies (e.g., Posture training, stretching exercises, mobilization, trigger point injections, physical modalities, occlusal applicance therapies)
E. Surgery (last resort)

Posture Training

The first step in treating myofascial pain and headache is to identify the perpetuating factors. These may include mechanical factors, systemic disorders, and behavioral factors. Mechanical factors usually are obvious and seem to be very important in assessing long-term outcome. Posture and body mechanics as they relate to working and relaxation should be considered.[20] Patient education for increased posture awarness and training to have correct body posture is very important. The goal of postural training is to prevent untoward activity on the head, neck, and shoulder muscles, as well as the masticatory and tongue muscles. The more anterior the head is relative to the spinal column, the greater is its effective weight, causing strain on the postural muscles. Manitaining orthostatic posture prevents increased cervical and shoulder muscle activity and possible protrusion of the mandible.[20] Except during functional activity (e.g., chewing, swallowing, and speaking), the mandible should be in a relaxed position, with the teeth separated and the tongue gently resting on the roof of the palate (N-position).[15] With the cervical muscle problems, a forward or lateral head posture must be corrected by guiding the chin in (chin tuck) and the head vertex up. The shoulders fall back naturally if the thorax is positioned up and back with proper lumbar support. Patients need to be instructed on the proper posture for each position—sitting, standing, and lying down—as well as in movements that are done repetitively throughout the day, such as lifting or turning the head to the side. Work station modification and ensuring well-adjusted eye wear will prevent anterior head position and eyestrain. Sleeping posture on the side or back is particularly important for patients who wake up with neck pain.[20,21]

Spray and Stretch Exercise

Application of vapocoolant spray such as ethyl cholride spray followed by muscle stretching exercises decreases muscle soreness and tightness, and is thought to inactivate myofascial trigger points and increase range of motion. Different exercises may be recommended to stretch and relax muscles, mobilize and stabilize TMJs, increase muscle strength, and develop normal coordination arthrokinematics to reduce joint clicking.[15] Repetitive exercises like hinge opening of the mandible up to the maximum of 25 mm is recommended to establish coordinated, rhythmic muscle function. Isotonic exercises such as N-stretch exercise suppress muscle tension, and passive stretching helps to increase range of motion while isometric exercises such as muscle contraction against resistance are given to increase muscle strength. These exercises are prescribed to achieve specific goals and are modified as the patient's condition progresses.

While the pain is mostly myogenous in origin, the most important component of a self-applied treatment program for masticatory muscle pain is stretch therapy. Stretch therapy must be done multiple times a day to be effective, and its purpose is not to strengthen or condition muscles but to suppress muscle tension levels. Stretch therapy is critical to treatment of spontaneous muscle pain disorders where the muscles exhibit taut band and stiffness. Daily (every 2 hours) stretch therapy is certainly worthy. The two essential elements of a stretch program for masticatory muscle pain are the N-stretch and chin-chest stretch. The first is done by placing the tip of tongue up against roof of mouth (in the "N" position). Stretch the jaw open in a straight line without dropping the tongue. If the jaw is tight the patient will feel the muscles being stretched so they should hold this open position for about 5 or 6 seconds and repeat the stretch five or six times every 2 hours. Chin-to-chest stretching involves having the patient slowly tilt their chin to their chest. Alternative versions of this stretching exercise would involve a slight turning (approximately 20 degrees) of the head to the side during the chin-to-chest stretch. This allows slightly different and more lateral neck muscles to be stretched.[22]

The exercises may initially increase pain causing patients to avoid complying. It is therefore recommended that a vapocoolant spray be employed to relieve symptoms during exercise. The sudden drop in skin temperature is thought to produce temporary anesthesia and counterstimulation resulting in blocking the spinal stertch reflex and the sensation of pain at a higher center. The decreased pain sensation allows the muscle to be stretched toward a normal length[23] and it must be emphasized to avoid rapid, jerky stretching or overstretching of the muscle to reduce potential injury to the muscle.

The technique involves directing a fine stream of vapocoolant spray from the finely calibrated nozzle toward the skin directly overlying the muscle with the trigger points. A few sweeps of the spray is passed over the trigger points and zone of reference before adding sufficient manual stretch to the muscle to elicit pain and discomfort. The spray is applied in one direction from the TrP toward its reference zone in slow even sweeps, at a rate of 10 cm per second directed at an acute angle from 30 to 50 cm (1–1.5 feet) away. This sequence can be repeated up to four times if the clinician warms the muscle with his or her hand or warm moist packs to prevent overcooling after each sequence.[21]

The goal of stretching exercise is to train the patient to self-manage the pain and dysfunction effectively. However, the spray and stretch treatment requires consistency and patience and the benefits may not be apparent for a few days. The range of passive and active motion can be tested before and after spraying as an indication of responsiveness to therapy. A maintenance level of exercise is recommended to ensure long-term effects even after the patient has achieved normal range of motion.

Mobilization of Temporomandibular Joint

Mobilization of the TMJ is indicated for decreased range of motion and pain due to muscle contracture, disc displacement without reduction and fibrous adhesions of TMJ. Warm and cold compresses, ultrasound or transcutanneous electrical stimulation to the joint and affected muscles in conjuction with joint mobilization will help with muscle relaxation and pain reduction during the process.[15] Mobilization of the joint with disc displacement without reduction may even need local anesthetic injections into the joint space. TMJ mobilization is done by gripping the mandible firmly with the thumb on the occlusal surfaces of the posterior teeth, securely bracing the unaffected side of the head and neck and by applying firm and controlled force to the mandible in a downward, forward and inward direction. The manipulation and mobilization does not produce anatomic reduction of the disc but they increase disc mobilization and thus increase range of motion. Following mobilization, therapy to maintain joint mobility should be considered such as orthopedic appliance therapy, relaxation therapy and stretching exercises.

Trigger Point Injections

Trigger points are discrete, focal, hyperirritable spots located in a taut band of the skeletal muscle. They are painful when a firm pressure is applied over the trigger point and can produce referred pain even to distant sites. Trigger points are the hall marks of myofascial pain syndrome, a common painful muscle disorder. Patients with myofascial pain often report regional, persistent pain that is reproducible and does not follow a dermatomal or nerve root distribution. The pain is usually dull-aching in character, either spontaneous or increased during muscle activity, and results in stiffness and decreased range of motion of the muscle in question.[15,20,22–24] Trigger point injections alone or in conjunction with stretching exercises are considered when patients are in severe pain with active trigger points where spray and stretch therapy cannot be done effectively or when repeated spray and stretch therapy fails to provide the desired result.[21,23]

Trigger point injections are anesthetic injections to the active trigger points that produce a twitch response to pressure and referred pain. The injections can effectively inactivate the trigger points and provide immediate pain relief after injection. It is generally a safe procedure when given by an experienced provider. Trigger point injections are usually done with low concentration local anesthetic (0.5%–1% procaine or lidocaine) without vasoconstrictors into the located and isolated trigger points using sterile needle. The needle is inserted 1 to 2 cm from the trigger point at an acute angle of 30 degrees to the skin and advanced into the stabilized trigger point.

After deposition of a small amount of local anesthetic (0.2 mL), a fan-shaped needling with repeated redirection of the needle and deposition are done for mechanical disruption of the trigger point until the local twitch response is no longer elicited. Dry needling without local anesthesia was reported to be equally effective as trigger point injection,[25] but post-injection soreness resulting from dry needling was more intense and longer duration than that of the trigger point injections with local anesthetic. Increased postinjection soreness was also reported with the use of normal saline. Pressure should be applied to the injected area for 2 minutes to promote hemostasis.[23]

It is recommended that immediate active stretching of the injected muscle should be done at least three times to its full range of motion for better efficacy of trigger point therapy.[24] Concentrated anesthetic solution, local anesthetic with vasoconstrictors and longer acting anesthetic should not be used for trigger point injections because of increased risk of myotoxicity. Several other substances, including diclofenac (Voltren), botulinum toxin type A (Botox) and corticosteroids have been used in trigger point injections but these substances have been associated with significant myotoxicity.[23] A series of three to five treatments to a muscle group initially at weekly intervals might be necessary to gain control of the active trigger points to the point until they can be managed by self-care exercises.[15]

Miscellaneous Physical Therapies

Electrotherapy

Electrotherapy has been applied clinically to reduce or eliminate muscle spasm and soft tissue edema, to increase blood flow to tissues with decreased circulation and for muscle re-education and trigger point therapy. Transcutaneous electrical nerve stimulation (TENS) uses low-voltage, low-amperage, biphasic current of varied frequency and is designed primarily for sensory counter stimulation in painful disorders. Electrogalvanic stimulation (EGS) uses a high-voltage, low-amperage, monophasic current of varied frequency.[15] The use of TENS has been reserved primarily for the treatment of body or extremity pains because of the fear of potential epileptogenic effects of electric current running through the head. With proper placement of electrodes and the use of low-intensity currents, it appears to be safe to apply this technique to the head. However, there is little objective evidence about the efficacy of TENS. Considering the inconvenience and the limited efficacy, this treatment is not recommended as a standard treatment for either headache or TMDs.[26]

Ultrasound

Ultrasound, when transmitted through the tissue with the high-frequency oscillating transducer head, produces heat that can reach a depth of 5 cm. It is a frequently used physical treatment modality for musculoskeletal problems. When it is used to carry medication into the tissue, the process is called phonophoresis, although the mechanism and efficacy of drug delivery are unknown.[15]

Iontophoresis

Iontophoresis is a technique to enhance the transport of drug ions across the skin into the deeper tissue using a weak current. However, recent studies question the efficacy of this modality to provide pain relief.[15]

Laser Treatment

Low level laser therapy has been suggested to have biostimulating and analgesic effects through direct irradiation without causing a thermal response. Several studies investigated the efficacy of laser therapy in TMDs are nonconclusive because of the poor methodology designs, or due to the small sample size. Further research is needed to support the use of low-level laser therapy in TMD treatment.[15]

Occlusal Appliance Therapy for Headache and TMD

The role of TMDs and migraine is still poorly understood although there appears to be a relationship. In patients with migraine, activation or inflammation in the TMJ may increase the headache frequency.[2] It would stand to reason that therapy aimed at reducing the TMD would reduce the migraine frequency. Stabilization appliances are used as an adjunct for managing symptoms associated with myogenous as well as arthrogenous TMDs.

Consideration to occlusal appliance therapy is given to those patients who have painful internal derangements and/or a history indicative of significant parafunction (such as chronic or frequent daytime clenching, nocturnal bruxism, focally painful joints or temples on awakening, or have other abusive oral habits such as gum chewing or finger nail biting), also to those who, on examination, have evidence of notable occlusal wear (such as lock and key patterns of the anterior teeth with excursive movements or flattening of molar cusps) and muscular pain. Loss of occlusal support (missing teeth) in one quadrant of the jaw is another potential factor that may indicate the use of an intraoral appliance, especially if there is symptomatic TMJ disease. The appliance can provide the missing occlusal support until painful symptoms subside enough to allow more permanent prosthodontic reconstruction (crown and bridge or dentures).

There is clinical evidence that splint therapy is useful in reducing pain and dysfunction in the TMJ but the exact mechanism whereby this effect occurs is unknown and the researchers do not agree, how the appliance works or what the most effective occlusal design is.[15,27] Some believe that the pain is directly related to problems with the occlusion. This is refuted by most experts as in placebo controlled trials, modifying the occlusion or doing mock equilibration treatments, are just as effective.[28] In general, it is believed that the mechanism for splint therapy is unrelated to the occlusion and the review studies suggest that occlusal appliances function mainly as behavioral interventions and not as mechanical devices for altering the patients' maxillomandibular relationships.[15,27] Moreover, the meta-analyses on intraoral appliance therapies for temporomandibular disorders and headache concluded that there is insufficient evidence either for or against the use of splints for the treatment of TMD. There is need for further, rigorous randomized controlled trials (RCTs) that consider the method of allocation and outcome assessment, have large sample size, sufficient duration of follow-up, and standardization of the outcomes of the treatment of TMD.[29] Different types of oral appliance have been used and major categories of occlusal appliances are complete-coverage stabilization appliances, partial-coverage appliances, and anterior positioning appliances.

Complete-Coverage Stabilization Appliances

This type of oral appliance is a nonrepositioning, flat surface device that provides complete coverage of all the teeth in either maxillary or mandibular arch with bilateral, even, posterior occlusal contacts for the opposing teeth on closure. It is commonly made with hard acrylic resin and is adjusted to the jaw closure position known as maximum intercuspation or muscular contact position or centric occlusion position.[15,27] When properly adjusted, the stabilization splint delivers a good method of providing centric relation occlusion (the position of the jaw relative to the skull when the muscles are at their most relaxed and least strained position), eliminating posterior interferences (any predominant contacts between the back teeth that interfere with or hinder harmonious jaw movement), provides anterior guidance on anterior teeth (the contact between the anterior teeth without any posterior contact during jaw movements), reducing neuromuscular activity, and obtains stable occlusal relationships with uniform tooth contacts throughout the dental arch.[30]

It has been reported in the literature that the stabilization splints may provide orthopedically stable jaw positions, optimize functional occlusion, prevent tooth wear, reduce masticatory muscle activity, reduce TMJ loading, alter the structural relationship in the TMJ, increase patients' awareness of jaw habits, and position the mandible into a relaxed, open position.[15] However, a Cochrane Review on stabilization splint therapy for temporomandibular pain[29] report no evidence of a statistically significant difference in the effectiveness of stabilization splint therapy in reducing symptoms in patients with TMDs compared with other active treatments although modest active therapeutic effects in reducing TMJD pain was noted compared to a placebo control in patients with severe symptoms.

Stabilization splints are preferably worn during sleep and 1 to 2 hours during the day to allow the patient to practice keeping the teeth apart. It is important to instruct the patient to keep the teeth apart even with the appliance. Patients can reduce the use of appliance after the jaw and facial pain has been relieved .[27] In the case of ongoing nocturnal bruxism with morning pain and tooth wear, continued use at night is appropriate even over a long period of time.[15,27] Patient must be given instruction on the daily cleaning and care of the appliance. The complications that can occur with the excessive or incorrect use of any oral appliance include caries, gingival inflammaion, mouth odors, speech difficulties, occlusal changes, and psychological dependency on the applicance.[15] However, assuming that the device is properly cared and used with regular follow-up, the only long-term consequence is that it may not be as effective as the short-term use. Even with that, changing the occlusal surface of the device every 3 to 6 months, can give back its efficacy.

The use of stabilization appliances made with a soft, resilient thermoplastic material has provided mixed results regarding their effect in reducing nocturnal bruxism and the signs and symptoms of TMDs.[15] The main concern for using these soft appliances is the long-term effect of using these unadjusted appliances on occlusal contacts.[31] Studies compared soft appliances with hard acrylic appliances, and soft appliances, electronic acupuncture and palliative treatments with placebo. In reducing painful symptoms, the resilient splint were equally effective with other treatments compared to no-treatment groups.[15,32,33] However, they are not better than the hard-acrylic stabilization appliance which can be adjusted for proper occlusal contacts and hence decrease the risk of change in occlusion.

Partial Coverage Appliances

A new form of partial-coverage splint therapy has been suggested to manage headache effectively. Shankland et al.[34] suggested an intraoral nociceptive trigeminal inhibition tension suppression system (NTI-tss) device for the reduction of frequency and severity of tension-type and migraine headaches, as compared to the known efficacy of the noncommercially available full-coverage occlusal splint. It was a multicenter open labeled trial to determine the response in migraine. However, a clinical trial by Magnusson et al.[35] comparing the NTI appliance to stabilization splint for TMD symptoms including headache found the stabilization splint to be slightly better than the NTI in improving TMD pain. The difference in the studies may be explained by the higher sample size in the Shankland study,[34] the subject selection of migraine headache versus TMD headache, and the potential bias in both study designs.[34,35]

The NTI-tss is a small intraoral device, which is fitted over the two maxillary central incisors and has a dome-shaped protrusion, which extends lingually. The dome is customized by the provider, to act as a single-point contact at the incisal embrasure of the two mandibular central incisors, thereby preventing posterior or canine tooth contact. With regard to the complications, the working hypothesis was that occlusal forces applied to a few anterior teeth would be lighter than forces applied to a full occlusion. This is a modification of the older concepts in using either anterior bite plane appliances (only anterior teeth have contacts) or posterior bite plane appliances (only posterior teeth are in contact). Whether the appliance provides anterior or posterior coverage only, the studies supporting the efficacy of these partial coverage appliances in TMD symptoms are limited by methodological weakness in the studies. These appliances have the potential to produce malocclusion by either protrusion or retrusion of the teeth or by internal TMJ changes.[15,27] Moreover, there is no evidence that these partial-coverage appliances can more effectively reduce TMD symptoms than full-arch stabilization appliances.

Anterior Repositioning Appliance

The third major group of oral appliances comprise those that are used to deliberately alter the position of maximum intercuspation. This design is aimed at encouraging a more comfortable therapeutic condyle–disc–fossa relationship and can be fabricated for either dental arch. However, the maxillary appliance is usually more effective at guiding the mandible into the protrusive position. The appliance covers all teeth in the arch to provide opposing posterior teeth with occlusal indentations and/or the anterior teeth with a protrusive guidance ramp. These appliances are also known as anterior positioning appliance or mandibular othopedic repositioning appliances (MORAs). Although anterior positioning appliances are suggestively effective to treat all or most TMD problem, the primary inidcation for anterior positioning appliance therapy is acute joint pain associated with TMJ disc displacement with reduction (painful clicking and/or intermittent locking of the joint). By holding the mandibular condyles in a more forward position, the device is believed to recapture the displaced disc.

Anderson et al.[36] compared anterior repositioning appliances to stabilization appliances for management of TMJ pain from disc displacement with reduction. Both appliances were worn 24 hours per day. Repositioning appliances were more effective in reducing joint noises, locking, and pain. Davies and Gray[37] studied effectiveness of anterior repositioning appliances when worn 24 hours per day, only at night, and only during the day. There was greater improvement in joint sounds, reduction in tenderness, and range of motion when appliances were worn 24 hours per day. Since terminating use of the splint did not increase symptoms, the authors suggest there is no need to complete phase II dental treatment to permanently change the occlusion. However, there is the potential for irreversible changes to the occlusion with use of anterior position splints used 24 hours per day, it should be worn only at night. In another study, Tecco et al.[38] compared the effectiveness of the repostitioning appliance, the stabilization appliance, and no treatment in reduction of joint pain and frequency of joint noises. The pain was reduced significantly in the repositioning appliance group but the frequency of joint noises decreased over time in all three groups. Finally, the authors concluded that the repositioning appliance was not better than the stabilisation appliance for treating joint noises.

The difficulty with the use of anterior repositioning appliance is that it requires constant monitoring by the dentist to ensure that the altered jaw position prevents the disc-condyle displacement form recurring and to detect permanent adverse occlusal changes (especially when the patient is instructed to wear it 24 hours a day). Becauses of the potential of a major irreversible change in the patient's occlusion and also because the clicking is not substantially reduced by the repositioning appliances, the use of these appliances is not a logical choice for treating TMJ disc derangement.[27]

Management of Cervical Disorders

Headaches attributed to cervical dysfunction are defined as cervicogenic headaches and considered as secondary headaches. However, the concept of cervicogenic headache is a controversial one. The term cervicogenic headache was coined in 1983 by Sjaastad et al.[39] It implies a peripheral generation of the head pain from the cervial structures. These headaches present as unilateral head pain in the temporal, frontal, and occipital regions and have associated autonomic symptoms. The criteria for cervicogenic headache were proposed by Sjaastad et al. in 1990. Cervicogenic headache is diagnosed if the following three features are present: (1) unilateral headache triggered by neck or head movements or posture; (2) unilateral headache triggered by pressure on the neck; and (3) unilateral headache spreading to the neck and the homolateral shoulder and arm.[40]

Recent IHS criteria for cervicogenic headache[41] include:

A. Pain, referred from a source in the neck and perceived in one or more regions of the head and/or face, fulfilling criteria C and D
B. Clinical, laboratory, and/or imaging evidence of a disorder or lesion within the cervical spine or soft tissues of the neck known to be, or generally accepted as, a valid cause of headache
C. Evidence that the pain can be attributed to the neck disorder or lesion based on at least one of the following:
    1. Demonstration of clinical signs that implicate a source of pain in the neck
    2. Abolition of headache after diagnostic blockade of a cervical structure or its nerve supply using placebo or other adequate controls
D. Pain resolves within 3 months after successful treatment of the causative disorder or lesion

However, if a patient with primary headache disorders has cervical dysfunction, the headache frequency and intensity may improve when the peripheral cervical triggers are blocked by the diagnostic block and it is also very difficult to distinguish the chronic tension type headache, cervicogenic headache and migraine by any means. Leone et al. also pointed out that there are no clear criteria for differentiating cervicogenic headache trigger points from myofascial trigger points. They conclude that neck structures may play a role in some headaches, but clinical patterns indicating a neck–headache relationship have not been sufficiently supported.[42] Although animal and neurophysiological theory studies showed evidence of cervicogenic input as the trigger and perpetuating factors of migraine,[11,13,14] a systematic review[10] evaluating the strength of the evidence for the role of cervical musculoskeletal dysfunction in migraine found that there is currently no convincing evidence to confirm this phenomenon in humans.

Despite the pharmacological treatment and physical treatment including nerve blocks available for headache treatment, the Cochrane Database of Systematic Reviews on noninvasive physical therapy for chronic/recurrent headache concluded that spinal manipulation may be an effective treatment option with a short-term effect similar to that of a commonly used, effective drug (amitriptyline) for the prophylactic treatment of migraine headache. Other possible treatment options with weaker evidence of effectiveness are pulsating electromagnetic fields and a combination of transcutaneous electrical nerve stimulation (TENS) and electrical neurotransmitter modulation.[43,44] For the prophylactic treatment of cervicogenic headache, there is evidence that both neck exercises and spinal manipulation/mobilization are effective in the short and long term when compared to no treatment or spinal manipulation/mobilization alone.[43–47] There is also evidence that spinal manipulation is effective in the short term when compared to massage or placebo spinal manipulation, and weaker evidence when compared to spinal mobilization.

Posture Modification

Posture is defined as "the attitude of the body." Good posture is when the muscles and bones are aligned and work together in harmony, protecting the body from injury or progressive deformity, regardless of attitude. Poor posture is basically a bad but correctable habit resulting in misalignment of various body parts. These body parts are at higher risk for injury or pain due to the increased strain misalignment places on the supporting structures. Body mechanics is defined as "the application of kinesiology to use of the body in daily life activities and to the prevention and correction of problems related to posture." There are many situations that occur on a day- to-day basis that place the body, various joints, and the muscles in positions requiring extra strain and work. Some examples are poor body posture during sitting and studying, holding the phone between the ear and shoulder, sleeping on the stomach, and reading before going to sleep in awkward position.[24]

Detailed history taking with a daily activity diary for a week or 2 weeks and careful initial clinical examination can be extremely useful in terms of identifying poor body mechanics and posture. Patients with an anterior head position should be treated with exercises to achieve good body posture. These exercises target the head and shoulder position and a physical therapist can help train the patient to use the correct neck muscles for achieving good posture. Anterior head positioning with loss of cervical lordosis is the most common cause of cervical myofascial pain. Identifying poor body mechanics in daily activity and modifying them to ergonomic mechanics is also very important.

Mobilization and Manipulation of the Cervical Spine

Several systematic reviews, cases series, and controlled studies that examined the efficacy of cervical manipulative treatment in the management of headache were identified. Mobilization and manipulation are similar terms that frequently are used interchangeably in the literature. Both terms refer to passive movement techniques used to restore normal motion to a joint. Manipulation is defined as a small-amplitude, high-velocity thrust applied at the limit of the available range of motion (ROM). Mobilization implies passive movement, usually rhythmic in nature, which varies in amplitude, but never exceeds the joint's normal range of motion.[46]

A Cochrane Review[43] on the efficacy of cervical spine manipulation in the prevention of migraine concluded that for the prophylactic treatment of migraine headache, there is evidence from a high-quality study that spinal manipulation may be an effective treatment option with a short-term effect similar to that of a commonly used, effective drug (amitriptyline). Combining the two treatments does not seem to offer an advantage. Weaker evidence from a lower-quality study showed that spinal manipulation was ineffective in reducing pain, but was superior to a sham interferential therapy for reducing headache frequency, duration, and medication use. However, other systematic reviews[18,43] as well as the evidence-based guidelines for migraine treatments from The United States Headache Consortium expert consensus[26] stated that there is very little evidence to evaluate cervical manipulation as a preventive or acute treatment for migraine. Neck manipulation or mobilization and PT are most beneficial when combined with an exercise plan (multimodal treatment). Chiropractic manipulation appears to be no more effective than manipulation or mobilization performed by a medical practitioner or a physical therapist.[18] Mobilization of the upper cervical joint with different mobilization techniques seems to be relatively safe and helpful for cervical headache but the small sample size (10 patients) and short-term follow-up (only 4 weeks) are disadvantages of the study.[46]A correct and careful technique is of great importance to prevent aggravation of symptoms or potential injury from the manipulation and mobilization procedures. The patient should be informed of the potential risk for serious complications including vascular injury and overall safety of cervical spine manipulation, especially with a high-velocity thrust like chiropractic manipulation. More than 100 cases of serious complications from chiropractic manipulation have been reported, and it can be assumed that a fairly large number of similar complications go unreported.[48] The rare but potential serious complications are increased risk of vertebral artery dissection and an approximately sixfold increase in stroke or transient ischemic attack. Warnings of these potentially serious complications to patients contemplating chiropractic treatment may be appropriate and reasonable when considering a recommendation for this treatment.

Summary

Treating refractory migraine can be a stressful and frustrating experience for both the treating physician and the patient. Detailed history taking with attention to the other possible contributors of chronic headache, careful examination, and treatment of all the possible contributing factors such as TMDs and cervical dysfunction in conjunction with other standard treatments of migraine can greatly improve the treatment outcome for refractory headaches. Physical therapies for TMDs and cervical dysfunction in migraine patients lack solid scientific evidence and much needs to be learned to identify and understand the pain mechanisms in relation to headache. But this is also true for many drugs that are used for prophylaxis of headaches. We as the clinicians have to be mindful that it is important to understand the mechanisms causing pain. However, when we still are not able to identify the etiologies and mechanisms, our primary goal must be to alleviate head, neck, and facial pain. We therefore are obliged to approach pain management using all the therapies at our disposal, with special care not to worsen the situation. Harmless therapy with potential benefits to patients with coexisting conditions should be worthwhile if it is affordable.

References

1. Nixdorf DR, Velly AM, Alonso AA. Neurovascular pains: implications of migraine for the oral and maxillofacial surgeon. *Oral Maxillofacial Surg Clin North Am.* 2008;20:221–235.
2. Graff-Radford SB. Temporomandibular disorders and headache. *Dent Clin North Am.* 2007;51:124–144.
3. Le Resche L. Epidemiology of temporomandibular disorders: implications for the investigation of etiologic factors. *Crit Rev Oral Biol Med.* 1997;8:291–305.
4. Von Korff M, Crane P, Lane M, Miglioretti DL, Simon G, Saunders K, Stang P, Brandenburg N, Kessler RCP. Chronic spinal pain and physical mental morbidity in the United States: results from the national comorbidity survey replication. *Pain.* 2005;113(3):331–339.
5. Ciancaglini R, Radaelli G. The relationship between headache and symptoms of temporomandibular disorders in the general population. *J Dent.* 2001;29:93–98.
6. Hagen K, Hagen K, Einarsen C, Zwart JA, Svebak S, Bovin GEC. The co-occurrence of headache and musculoskeletal symptoms amongst 51,050 adults in Norway. *Eur J Neurol.* 2002;9(5):527–533.
7. Clark G, Green E, Dornan M, Flack V. Craniocervical dysfunction levels in a patient sample from a temporomandibular joint clinic. *J Am Dent Assoc.* 1987;115:251–256.

8. De Laat A, Meuleman H, Stevens A, Verbeke G. Correlation between cervical spine and temporomandibular disorders. *Clin Oral Invest.* 1998;2(2):54–57.
9. Olivo SA, Olivo SA, Bravo J, Magee DJ, Thie NM, Major PW, Flores Mir CBJ. The association between head and cervical posture and temporomandibular disorders: a systematic review. *J Orofac Pain.* 2006;20(1):9–23.
10. Robertson BA, Morris ME. The role of cervical dysfunction in migraine: a systematic review. *Cephalalgia.* 2008;28:474–483.
11. Bartsch T, Goadsby PJ. The trigeminocervical complex and migraine: current concepts and synthesis. *Curr Pain Headache Rep.* 2003;7(5):371–376.
12. Lupoli TA, Lockey RF. Temporomandibular dysfunction: an often overlooked cause of chronic headaches. *Ann Allergy Asthma Immunol.* 2007;99(4):314–318.
13. Bartsch T, Goadsby PJ. Increased responses in trigeminocervical nociceptive neurons to cervical input after stimulation of the dura mater. *Brain.* 2003;126(8):1801–1813.
14. Bartsch T, Goadsby PJ. Anatomy and physiology of pain referral patterns in primary and cervicogenic headache disorders. *Headache Curr.* 2005;2(2):42–48.
15. De Leeuw R (ed). Temporomandibular disorders. In: Pain TA, *Orofacial Pain: Guidelines for Assessment, Diagnosis and Management*, 4th Ed. Chicago: Quintessence Books;2008:131–132.
16. Kapur N, Kamel IR, Herlich A. Oral and craniofacial pain: diagnosis, pathophysiology and treatment. *Int Anesthesiol Clin.* 2003;41(3):115–150.
17. Bogduk N. Anatomy and physiology of headache. *Biomed Pharmacother.* 1995;49(10):435–445.
18. Biondi DM. Physical treatments for headache: a structured review. *Headache.* 2005;45(6):738–746.
19. Graff-Radford SB, Canavan DW. Headache attributed to orofacial/temporomandibular pathology. In: Olesen J, Tfelt-Hansen P, Goadsby PJ, Welch KM, Ramadan NM (eds), *The Headaches*, 3rd edition. Philadelphia: Lippincott Williams & Wilkins;2005:1029–1034.
20. Graff-Radford SB. Myofascial pain: diagnosis and management. *Curr Pain Headache Rep.* 2004;8:463–467.
21. Fricton J. Myogenous temporomandibular disorders: diagnostic and management considerations. *Dent Clin North Am.* 2007;51:61–83.
22. Clark GT. Classification, causation and treatment of masticatory myogenous pain and dysfunction. *Oral Maxillofacial Surg Clin North Am.* 2008; 20:145–157.
23. Alvarez DJ, Rockwell PG. Trigger points: diagnosis and management. *Am Fam Physician.* 2002;65:653–660.
24. Simons D, Travell J, Simons L. In: *Travell & Simons' Myofascial Pain and Dysfunction: The Trigger Point Manual* Volume 1 (2nd ed.). Philadelphia: Lippincott Williams & Wilkins; 1998:165–182.
25. Hong C. Lidocaine injection versus dry needling to myofascial trigger point. The importance of the local twitch response. *Am J Phys Med Rehabil.* 1994;73(4):256–263.
26. Graff-Radford SB, Mauskop A. In: *National Headache Foundation, Standards of Care for Diagnosis and Treatment of Headache* (4th ed.). National Headache Foundation; 2004:141–149.

27. Clark GT. Oral appliances. In: Laskin DM, Greene CS, Hylander WL (eds.), *Temporomandibular Disorders: An Evidence-Based Approach to Diagnosis and Treatment.* Chicago: Quintessence;2006:377–390.
28. Stohler CS. Management of dental occlusion. In: Laskin DM, Greene CS, & Hylander WL (eds.), *Temporomandibular Disorders: An Evidence-Based Approach to Diagnosis and Treatment.* Chicago: Quintessence; 2006:403–411.
29. Al-Ani M, Davies S, Gray R, Sloan P, Glenny A. Stabilisation splint therapy for temporomandibular pain. *Cochrane Database Syst Rev.* 2004;(1):CD002778.
30. Nelson SJ. Principles of stabilization bite splint therapy. *Dent Clin North Am.* 1995;39(2):403–421.
31. Singh B, Berry D. Occlusal changes following use of soft occlusal splints. *J Prosthet Dent.* 1985;54:711–715.
32. Okeson J. The effects of hard and soft splints on nocturnal bruxism. *J Am Dent Assoc.* 1987;114:788–791.
33. Pettengill C, Growney M, Schoff R, Kenworthy C. A pilot study comparing the efficacy of hard and soft stabilizing appliances in treating patients with temporomandibular disorders. *J Prosthet Dent.* 1998;79:165–168.
34. Shankland W. Nociceptive trigeminal inhibition – tension suppression system: a method of preventing migraine and tension headaches. *Compend Contin Educ Dent.* 2002;23:105–108.
35. Magnusson T, Adiels AM, Nilsson HL, Helkimo M. Treatment effect on signs ans symptoms of temporomandibular disorders – comparison between stabilisation splint and a new type of splint (NTI). A pilot study. *Swed Dent J.* 2004;28:11–20.
36. Anderson G, Schulte J, Goodkind R. Comparative study of two treatment methods for internal derangement of the temporomandibular joint. *J Prosthet Dent.* 1985; 53(3):392–397.
37. Davies S, Gray R. The pattern of splint usage in the management of two common temporomandibular disorders. Part I: The anterior repositioning splint in the treatment of disc displacement with reduction. *Br Dent J.* 1997;183(6):199–203.
38. Tecco S, Festa F, Salini V, Epifania, E., & D'Attilio, M. Treatment of joint pain and joint noises associated with a recent TMJ internal derangement: a comparison of an anterior repositioning splint, a full-arch maxillary stabilization splint, and an untreated control group. *Carnio.* 2004;22:209–219.
39. Sjaastad O., Saunte C, Hovdahl HE. Cervicogenic headache: a hypothesis. *Cephalalgia.* 1983;3(4):249–256.
40. Sjaastad O, Fredriksen T, Pfaffenrath V. Cervicogenic headache: diagnostic criteria. *Headache.* 1990;30(11):725–726.
41. Headache Classification Subcommittee of the International Headache Society. *The International Classification of Headache Disorders,* 2nd ed. *Cephalalgia.* 2004;24: (Suppl)1:9–160.
42. Leone M, D'Amico D, Grazzi LE. Cervicogenic headache: a critical review of the current diagnostic criteria. *Pain.* 1998;78(1):1–5.
43. Brønfort G, Nilsson N, Haas M, Evans R, Goldsmith C, Assendelft W, et al. Non-invasive physical treatments for chronic/recurrent headache. *Cochrane Database Syst Rev.* 2004;(3):CD001878.

44. Brønfort G, Assendelft W, Evans R, Haas M, Bouter L. Efficacy of spinal manipulation for chronic headache: a systematic review. *J Manipulative Physiol.* 2001;24(7):457–466.
45. Gross AR, Hoving JL, Haines TA, Goldsmith CH, Kay T, Aker P, Bronfort G; Cervical Overview Group. A Cochrane Review of manipulation and mobilization for mechanical neck disorders. *Spine.* 2004;29(14):1541–1548.
46. Schoensee S, Jensen G, Nicholson G, Gossman M, Katholi C. The effect of mobilization on cervical headaches. *J Orthop Sports Phys Ther.* 1995;21(4): 184–196.
47. Kay TM, Gross A, Goldsmith C, Santaguida PL, Hoving J, Bronfort G; Cervical Overview Group. Exercises for mechanical neck disorders. *Cochrane Database Syst Rev.* 2005;20 (3), CD004250.
48. Mauskop A. Alternative therapies in headache. Is there a role? *Med Clin North Am.* 2001;85(4):1077–1084.

18

Inpatient Strategies for Refractory Migraine

Joel R. Saper, MD, FACP, FAAN, and Alvin E. Lake III, PhD, BCIAC-SF

Introduction

Migraine falls along a continuum of treatment responsiveness from easy to manage to intractable. It is not always possible to determine in advance which patients with refractory migraine will benefit from outpatient treatment and which will require hospital level care to achieve headache control. Although it is appropriate to admit patients with an acute and prolonged migraine attack to an inpatient setting for a 2- to 3-day intravenous protocol, many of the patients admitted to an inpatient program are those with long duration refractory migraine. They have experienced prolonged and protracted courses of headache, often characterized by continuous, daily or almost daily pain for years at a time. For many, but not all, refractory migraine patients who experience this pattern of pain, the headache disorder is confounded by medication overuse, behavioral disturbances, and sometimes other medical comorbidities. For such headache sufferers, a comprehensive, multidisciplinary inpatient treatment program may be an essential step in the transition from intractability to some level of improvement: in headache control, improved function, and/or enhanced quality of life.[1,2]

Certainly medication overuse headache (MOH) is an important factor in determining whether the treatment venue for a refractory migraine patient should be inpatient or outpatient. It would seem intuitive that patients with simple over-the-counter usage or those with triptan overuse alone could be

Table 18-1 Subclassification of Medication Overuse Headache

Type I (Simple)	Overuse of simple analgesics and/or triptans ***and the absence of severe behavioral disturbances***
Type II (Complex)	Overuse of opioids, opioid-containing analgesics, and/or butalbital-containing analgesics ***and/or*** the presence of strong behavioral disturbances, including but not limited to Axis II disorders

adequately treated in an outpatient setting. In fact, this is often true. But the other factor that may determine the optimal treatment venue is that of behavior. In our most recent published outcome study, 85% of the patients had a primary diagnosis of chronic daily headache (chronic migraine); 59% had MOH, sometimes involving multiple categories of analgesics and abortive medications. Almost half (48%) of all admissions were overusing opioids, and 10% butalbital containing combination analgesics.[1]

Although it is true that not all patients with refractory migraine or severe headaches overuse their medicines, we believe that those who do are often, but not always, behaviorally different than those who don't. There may be many who take medicines as a compensatory response to inadequate treatment efforts, but others overuse their medications because it treats their anxiety, they feel entitled, or because they have addictive tendencies and predispositions. We have recently suggested that MOH is a biobehavioral disorder,[3] a view shared by many other thoughtful clinicians and consistent with accumulating research evidence.[3–8] It is not simply a matter of overuse, but one in which underlying behaviors prompt the overuse or fail to restrain the misuse pattern. More recently, we have proposed a subclassification for MOH patients in which type I and type II MOH would be a helpful categorization that could help determine appropriate care and venue of care.[9,10]

Table 18.1 illustrates this subclassification. Thus, type I MOH would generally be treatable on an outpatient basis because the medications are relatively easy to discontinue and there is an absence of behavioral complexity. Type II MOH would require a more intense venue of treatment because either the medication is more difficult to discontinue or there is the presence of confounding behavioral disturbances.

Criteria for Hospitalization

The following are the criteria justifying admission to the hospital used at the Michigan Head-Pain & Neurological Institute.

1. Moderate to severe intractable headache, failing to respond to appropriate and aggressive outpatient or emergency department services and requiring repetitive, sustained, parenteral treatment

2. The presence of continuing nausea, vomiting, or diarrhea
3. The need to withdraw patients from overused medications and treat toxicity, dependency, or rebound phenomena (MOH) that require parenteral treatment and monitoring services against withdrawal symptoms, including seizures
4. The presence of dehydration, electrolyte imbalance, or prostration requiring parenteral treatment, monitoring, and intravenous fluids
5. Unstable vital signs or electrocardiogram abnormalities related to headache or its treatment
6. The presence of repeated previous emergency department treatments for persisting pain
7. The presence of serious concurrent disease (e.g., subarachnoid hemorrhage, intracranial infection, cerebral ischemia, severe hypertension or hypotension, etc.)
8. To simultaneously develop effective pharmacological prophylaxis in order to sustain improvement achieved by parenteral therapy
9. To acutely address other comorbid conditions contributing to or accompanying the headache, including medical or psychological illness
10. Concurrent medical and/or psychological illness interfering with safe or effective outpatient treatment and requiring monitoring in high-risk situations
11. Patients requiring a pace of treatment, including detoxification, headache interruption, and development of preventive treatment, that would not be possible as an outpatient and would therefore impose the likelihood of failure
12. The presence of such striking behavioral and/or psychological factors enmeshed with the headache disorder that they serve as a barrier to effective treatment, except in an intensive and controlled environment

Principles of Inpatient Care

Hospitalization for acute and prolonged headache is a complex undertaking, because it must address not only the refractoriness of the symptoms, the often present confounding influence of medication overuse headache, but also the behavioral and psychological factors that often influence these dilemmas. Discontinuation of medication and the weaning process cause predictable escalation of headache and the emotional factors that are characteristic of that patient. The principles of hospitalization are listed in Table 18.2.

Hospitalization length of stay varies, depending on a number of factors. These include the intensity and type of medication which is overused and which requires discontinuation; the amount of pain and duration of it during this weaning process; the behavioral issues that emerge; and the confounding factors that are often present in patients with these symptoms. At the time of this writing, the mean length of stay (los) in our comprehensive inpatient unit

Table 18-2 Principles of Inpatient Care

- Interrupt daily/intractable headache pain with parenteral protocols (see text).
- Discontinue offending analgesics or abortives in cases of MOH.
- Implement preventive pharmacotherapy.
- Identify effective abortive therapy.
- Identify and treat behavioral and neuropsychiatric comorbidities.
- Identify and address stressors and life situations that may pose barriers to improvement.
- Teach and reinforce nonpharmacological coping skills.
- Employ interventional modalities when indicated.
- Educate regarding headache, medications, risks of overuse, headache-related behavior.
- Identify and address family issues affecting or related to headache.
- Plan for discharge and outpatient follow-up (medical, nonmedical, behavioral).

was slightly more than 12 days, a reduction of about 1 day from the mean los of 13.0 days in our most recent study.[1] Developing a preventive treatment during this time is difficult, as it takes time for medications to work and because generally patients are in a refractory period that may last up to weeks to months after discontinuation of the offending agents.

Parenteral Regimens

A variety of parenteral agents can be used during hospitalization to control attacks, particularly during withdrawal from overused analgesics and abortives. Table 18.3 lists these.

The literature includes studies and clinical reports on other intravenous protocols not included in the table, but which we no longer use. Metoclopramide has some support as both an antiemetic (e.g., combined with dihydroergotamine[11]) and for pain reduction as a solo medication,[49] but now has a black box warning from the United States Federal Drug Administration because of the risk of tardive dyskinesia. The risk is related to the duration of use and the number of doses taken. Although the risk is probably low when the drug is used intermittently for control of headache, in patients with severe or frequent headaches who need more frequent treatment the risk is higher. Alternative antiemetics are available, including ondancetron, which can be given parenterally, and phenergan. Intravenous lidocaine has only modest evidence for efficacy,[50,51] with potential risk of toxicity, particularly in older patients.[52] Although we have not used it, there are several published case studies on the use of intravenous verapamil for migraine with prolonged aura[53] and hemiplegic migraine.[54–56] A small double-blind outcome study failed to show increased efficacy for IV verapamil over placebo for acute migraine.[57]

Parenteral opioids are conspicuously absent from Table 18.3. We do not use or recommend them, a position shared by most other headache specialists. Despite a very large literature on the use of intravenous opioids for both

Table 18-3 Parenteral Regimens to Treat Intractable Headaches

- Dihydroergotamine (0.25–1 mg IV or IM, t.i.d.)[11–18]
- Diphenhydramine (25–50 mg IV or IM, t.i.d.)[19]
- Various neuroleptics (e.g., chlorpromazine 2.5–10 mg IV, t.i.d.)[19–29]
- Ketorolac (10 mg IV, t.i.d.; 30 mg IM, t.i.d.)[23,25,27,30]
- Valproic acid (250–750 mg IV, t.i.d.)[26,31–37]
- Magnesium sulfate (1 gram IV, b.i.d.)[38–42]
- Intravenous (IV) steroids[43–48]

Table 18-4 Combined Parenteral Regimens to Treat Intractable Headaches

- DHE, with diphenhydramine or neuroleptics or ketorolac or magnesium
- Diphenhydramine, with neuroleptics, DHE, magnesium
- Steroids with any of the above, except ketorolac
- Ketorolac with diphenhydramine, DHE, neuroleptics

acute and chronic noncancer pain, we could find only one report specifically focused on headache patients: a single-blind (patient, but not physician-blinded) placebo-controlled study of IV tramadol for acute migraine, which did show efficacy over placebo.[58]

The initial choice of a protocol may be based on multiple factors, including the patient's past experience of oral medications in the same class, and safety considerations related to medical comorbidities or the patient's age. When there is evidence for efficacy and tolerability of the intravenous medication, the protocol may be continued over 3 days. These protocols can also be used for emergency department treatment of acute episodic migraine.

Several protocols can be administered simultaneously. For example, dihydroergotamine can be used together with various parenteral neuroleptics, diphenhydramine, or ketorolac. Diphenhydramine can be used with the neuroleptics, ketorolac, or magnesium sulfate. Many of these drugs are easily and safely combined with other drugs in the list, as illustrated in Table 18.4.

Detoxification/Transition Options

In general, detoxification/transition options include both outpatient and inpatient options:

- A slow taper
- Abrupt withdrawal with bridging medications
- The use of buprenorphine as a transition drug from mu receptor opioids[59]
- Inpatient detoxification and comprehensive behavioral and pharmacological treatment strategies

Tapering of benzodiazepines must be done carefully,[60] and sometimes treatment with carbamazepine or similar drugs has proven useful.[61] If not managed carefully, barbiturate (e.g., butalbital) withdrawal can lead to seizures, behavioral disturbances, and even psychotic behavior.[62] We usually rely on benzodiazepines for safe and effective cross coverage in cases of barbiturate withdrawal.[63] Loder and others have advocated oral phenobarbital loading as a substitute for butalbital; its long half-life allows for gradual reduction of drug levels and can protect against withdrawal seizures.[64]

In the outpatient setting, oral, rectal, nasal, or parenteral routes of drug administration should be considered. Infusion protocols, such as DHE, valproic acid, chlorpromazine, steroids, and diphenhydramine, among others, are potentially helpful.[65] Drugs that can be used to control pain but are not likely to cause rebound with frequent use are shown in Table 18.5.

Note that the likelihood of a given category of abortive medication causing rebound varies with the class of drug and the individual patient. In some cases, there is conflicting evidence and opinion about which drugs and doses are needed to produce medication overuse headache. NSAIDs alone, without caffeine or acetaminophen, have not been conclusively shown to result in MOH, although in our experience some individuals may show a rebound pattern with high levels of use (escalation of headache with increasing frequency of use, with headache improvement after NSAID withdrawal). Aside from the risk of MOH, some drugs should be limited in their frequency of use over the long term due to adverse effects and safety issues, including gastrointestinal damage,[108,109] renal toxicity,[110] and cardiovascular risks.[109,111]

In our experience, inpatient treatment is much more appropriate for the majority of patients with significant (e.g., type II, complex) MOH. Inpatient strategies center around establishing the correct medical and psychological diagnosis, detoxifying through interruption of rebound, administering the effective dosage of parenteral and oral therapy, the implementation of

Table 18-5 Abortive Medications for Headache with Low Risk of Contributing to Medication Overuse Headache (Outpatient Applicability)

- Hydroxyzine (25–50 mg PO, IM); alone[66,67] or in combination with DHE[68,69] (hydroxyzine has both anti-nauseant and analgesic properties)
- NSAIDS including naproxen,[70–77]> indomethacin (both oral and rectal),[78–80] and ketoralac (IM)[81–86]
- Neuroleptics (IM, po, p.r.n.)[87, 88]
- Baclofen (10–20 mg t.i.d. p.r.n. PO)[89–94]
- Tizanidine (2–6 mg PO t.i.d.)[95–98]
- Diphenhydramine (intramuscular)[99]
- Lidocaine (intranasal)[100–104]
- Steroids, including oral prednisone[105–107]

behavioral and psychological therapy, and establishing a preventive and outpatient treatment program. While it is most desirable to treat patients on an outpatient basis, inevitably many patients require at least a short stay in a hospital in a controlled setting, since support can be essential in getting people through difficult days and nights.

Assistance in helping patients achieve a quality night's rest is important, if not critical. Many patients going through withdrawal report added difficulty sleeping, well beyond that which they generally experience. In our experience, effective headache control is rarely achieved unless we have also established effective sleep control. Boe and colleagues also recently identified poor sleep quality as a negative prognostic indicator for the efficacy of drug withdrawal therapy in MOH.[112] Some patients going through withdrawal experience autonomic disturbances, including hypotension and hypertension, as well as dehydration. Nausea is common. Management of these problems is often suboptimal in an outpatient setting.

Opioid withdrawal poses particularly difficult challenges, both during and after detoxification. The use of an opioid taper to transition from opioids is well established. The use of buprenorphine as a substitute transition drug on an outpatient basis is not well studied in the headache population, but preliminary experience in this center suggests possible value. Refractoriness to effective pain control may last for months or longer after prolonged opioid use and discontinuation.[10,113,114] Patients with opioid-related MOH more often meet criteria for substance dependence than those with MOH related to other medications,[7] and the onset of comorbid psychiatric disorders is significantly more likely to precede the development of MOH than follow it.[8] Relapse rates are significantly higher in MOH related to analgesic overuse (including opioids) than triptans or ergots.[115] The prognosis is also worse; some patients with both opioid-dependent MOH and significant comorbid psychiatric complications can undergo cycles of relapse and recovery over a period of years.[116] Physicians should be very cautious about reintroducing an overused drug, even months after withdrawal: return to overused drugs is a significant negative prognostic factor in maintaining headache control in the year following withdrawal.[117] Characteristics of patients with opioid-related MOH are shown in Table 18.6.

Table 18-6 Characteristics of Patients with Medication Overuse Headache Due to Opioids

- More often meet formal criteria for a substance use disorder than patients who overuse other drugs for headache
- Are more likely to have comorbid psychiatric disorders that precede the development of MOH
- Have a higher relapse rate after drug withdrawal
- Have a worse long-term headache prognosis

Neuroblockade

Approximately 15 years ago, after finding neuroblockade to be helpful in selected patients, the primary author hired the Institute's first anesthesiologist to provide interventional care to difficult cases or where it was obvious that interventional neuroblockade was an appropriate treatment. The presence of an anesthesiologist appears to have made a substantial difference in our ability to alter many cases of intractable head and neck pain, including those with MOH, even when identifiable significant peripheral nerve or cervical pathology was absent.

It is unclear whether it is necessary for identifiable pathology to be present in the cervical region in order for an interventional blockade to reduce pain. *It is the primary author's impression that the C2–3 zone is a "therapeutic window" and that a "block" may induce a pain modulatory stimulus rather than a blockade.* Many of our patients with and without identifiable neck pain benefit from a variety of C2–3 "blocking" procedures, including greater occipital nerve blocks[118–122] and cervical facet blocks.[123–125] Some patients with dramatic pain reduction following a facet block have experienced longer-term improvement from a radiofrequency (RF) denervation procedure.[126–131] As Goadsby and others have shown,[132–136] the cervical region communicates with trigeminal circuits, modulates pain in the dorsal horn, and may well determine threshold firing in the trigeminal system. However, controlled studies of neural blockade in headache patients, with long-term follow-up, are few, and long-term efficacy has yet to be convincingly demonstrated.[137] For example, in a small randomized, sham-controlled, patient- and evaluator-blind study, Stovner found that the RF patients were "somewhat improved" at 3 months, but did not differ from the sham procedure at 6-month and longer follow-up.[138]

Though the pain control from neuroblockade is often temporary, it provides a window of opportunity nonetheless. It instills in the patient hope that more prolonged relief can be found, which is very helpful in gaining the patient's confidence and further interventions. Also, it may provide a biologically significant interruption of pain, which is an opportunity for other treatments to gain effect. Although we can only speculate, downregulation of important neurotransmitter receptors may occur with repetitive injections.

Cognitive–Behavioral Therapy and Its Relevance

Our program includes intensive cognitive–behavioral therapy in both individual and group settings.[1] Patients undergo a formal psychological assessment before admission, and sign a detailed pre-admission agreement in which they agree to the goals of hospitalization (e.g., withdrawal in cases of MOH), full participation in the behavioral components of treatment, and contributing to a positive atmosphere on the unit for the other patients (e.g., controlling inappropriate pain behavior and addressing individual concerns with the staff rather than complaining to other patients). Psychologists assess stressors affecting headache, dysfunctional coping styles, comorbid psychiatric diagnoses (including personality disorders), and behaviors contributing to medication overuse, both with the patient and family. Patients receive structured training in various relaxation and cognitive–behavioral pain management strategies by means of individual instruction, group experiences, and a specialized program on compact disc.

The team provides other group sessions on the role of psychological factors in pain perception and maintenance, medication overuse issues, understanding psychiatric comorbidity and its relevance, personality patterns and pain, sleep management, proactive coping strategies, and the impact of pain on family relationships, among other topics. The group milieu can provide significant support for adaptive coping skills—few patients have previously encountered a group of others with refractory chronic daily headache. At times, however, the team must assertively intervene in cases where a troubled patient begins to intrude on the welfare of others. In addition, the psychologist plays a key role in discharge planning with respect to arranging psychological follow-up for those patients where this may be a critical aspect of their recovery.

Outcome

Long-term outcome varies depending upon the medications a patient is overusing and from center to center, but in 11 of 24 papers reviewed by Silberstein, Lipton, and Saper, the reported rate of improvement after drug withdrawal was 77% or higher.[139] It is likely that outcome results, long-term success, and avoidance of medication misuse after discharge depend in large measure on patient motivation and the follow-up care and attention to continuity of treatment. Behavioral treatment before and during detoxification transition may be critical. Frequent visits are also essential. The headache vulnerability is still present after misuse transition, but if support, frequent visits, behavioral management, and aggressive pharmacological intervention and monitoring are available, desirable long-term results are achievable. It seems clear to those of us who treat many patients with MOH that prognosis will depend on the intensity and effectiveness of treatment following removal of the agents. While different studies show various rates of long-term success, frequent visits, behavioral treatment, and effective intervention for periods of headache worsening seem to be important parameters.

Many patients get better, and some do not. We have published several outcome studies over the years, and the reader is encouraged to review these.[1,140,141] In general, approximately three-quarters of our patients respond to treatment while in the hospital. Long-term benefit is difficult to determine, and since many of our patients return to their local systems of care following discharge, it is difficult to judge matters of compliance, the quality of care, and the other variables necessary to assure long-term control once established. In our first prospective study (published in 1993) we followed patients for a mean of 8.3 months after discharge. The mean number of days of severe to incapacitating headache in a 2-week interval of time dropped by 64% compared to prehospital admission status (6.29–2.26 days), with a corresponding increase in pain-free days (1.03–5.40). The frequency of severe headaches was reduced by at least 50% for 75% of the patients. The mean subjective rating of overall improvement as estimated by patients was 74%.[140]

Over the past two decades, patients admitted to our inpatient program have become increasingly complex, having failed to respond significantly to advances in both abortive (e.g., the triptans) and prophylactic pharmacotherapies in the intervening years. With increasing advocacy for sustained-release opioids for the management of chronic noncancer pain, we have also seen an increasing frequency of patients with refractory migraine and opioid-related MOH. Our most recent outcome paper (published 2009) reviewed the response to treatment at discharge of 276 consecutively discharged patients.[1] The study demonstrated that more than three-quarters of patients reported moderate to significant improvement across a range of dimensions (pain, mood, function, and behavior) at the time of discharge. Most patients (90%) had at least two significant medical comorbidities, including one-third (36%) with non-headache painful disorders in additions to their headaches. All met criteria for at least one psychiatric comorbidity, including stress-related physiological response affecting headache (82%), mood disorders (70%), and anxiety disorders (49%). Personality disorders (PD) were diagnosed in one-fourth of the sample (26%). The most common PDs in the sample fell into cluster B (borderline, histrionic, narcissistic, antisocial): 61% of those with a PD, and 16% of this consecutive series of admissions.

Among the most interesting findings was that the most responsive cases were suffering MOH from the overuse of either simple analgesics or triptans (the few patients who overused ergotamine tartrate also had a good response at discharge): more than 97% of the patients with triptan-dependent MOH were at least moderately improved at discharge, compared to about 81% of the opioid-dependent and 79% of the butalbital compound-dependent patients – a statistically significant difference. The least likely patients to benefit were those with a PD ***not accompanied*** by medication overuse: only about half of this group (52.9%) reached at least moderate improvement. Of interest, even those with a PD but who had medication overuse had a reasonably good response to treatment (73% at least moderately improved).

Equally interesting was the observation that patients with Axis II personality disorders, such as borderline or narcissistic personality, seemed to have a predilection to overuse opioids when compared to those with no PD (62% vs. 38%). Although the data underscore the importance of biobehavioral factors in MOH—opioid-related MOH in particular—the reason for this remains a matter of speculation. We believe that there are neurobiological factors that might explain this observation.[8,142–144] Moreover, we believe that these patients are most likely to impose upon their physicians a pressure that results in acquiescence to the demand of the patient rather than to the physician's best clinical judgment. Length of stay was longer for those patients with opioid dependency. The reader is referred to our most recent publication for further details.[1]

Selected Recommendations on Treating Hospitalized Patients (Based on Our 30 Years of Treating Patients Hospitalized for Headache)

Over the years, our program has treated more than 15,000 hospitalized patients for headache. The following are selected thoughts and suggestions (some would call them pearls) that have been gleaned from the inpatient care of many patients over many years.[145] Almost all admitted patients experienced daily or almost daily pain, most but not all had medication overuse, and many (but certainly not most) were afflicted by significant behavioral and/or major psychiatric disturbances, either primary to the headache problem or secondary to it.

1. Integrate Expert Behavioral Therapists into the Treatment System for Difficult Headache Cases

Pain affects behavior, and behavioral disturbances and personality influence the reports and expressions of pain and suffering. Whether neurobiologically related or otherwise, both the behavioral and psychological disturbances of patients with chronic headache, as well as the pain itself, must be treated simultaneously. Both influence the other: a synergism is likely. Early aggressive behavioral assessment and treatment are often essential tools. This fundamental element of the chronic pain patient must be addressed.

2. Don't Rest Until You Test

Primary headaches may begin early in one's life, but this fact does not exclude the development of superimposed secondary headache conditions. *Don't assume that a migraineur will suffer only migraine headaches during the course of his/her life. Be alert to the possibility that current headache patterns represent a new, serious secondary condition.*

Careful physical examination, including a neurological exam, must be performed. Blood studies must include standard metabolic and laboratory profiles, in addition to inflammatory marker tests, endocrinological studies, and general chemistry and hematology. Cervical and cranial imaging must be current and competently interpreted. Such imaging must include at least an MRI and possibly an MR or CT angiogram and/or an MR or CT venogram; the latter is particularly important when intracranial pressure disturbances are suspected or likely.

A careful review of head, neck, nasal, and dental structures is important. Patients with possible disturbances of CSF pressure must have an LP or when there is a suspicion of inflammatory mechanisms, including infection. Chronic (fungal, etc.) meningitis can at times only be identified with examination of the spinal fluid pressure. Special tests for Lyme disease, West Nile virus, and other infections are appropriate when cases are refractory or there are reasons to believe that such could be present. Numerous other neurological and non-neurological tests must be performed when appropriate. Is there a trauma history? Could carotid or vertebral dissection mimic migraine? Could sphenoid sinusitis, a serious and potentially fatal disorder, be mimicking trigeminal neuralgia, migraine, or cluster headache? Ample use of consultants to aid in the diagnosis of other disorders should be undertaken liberally.

Recently we have become impressed with the possible association of pituitary, sphenoid, or parapituitary pathology in association with either cluster headaches or cluster-like syndromes. Careful testing is essential to identify some of these syndromes.

3. Identify the Problem Patient Early

Don't miss the signals and signs (red flags) of the problem patient.[146] While most patients who would submit to treatment in an inpatient program are committed to improving their lives and complying with treatment expectations, there is nonetheless a subset of patients whose lives and emotional profiles are so complex and conflicted that they are unable, unwilling, or simply will not benefit from care. This patient must be distinguished from the patient whose headache condition defies, on a biological basis, current therapeutic response to treatment efforts. Some patients will obstruct efforts to help them and even disrupt the delivery of care to others.

Expressions of pain and suffering are powerful communicators. They can communicate when words fail. Thus, *pain can control others; pain can punish. Pain can prevent abandonment* and can protect from obligation and expectation. *Pain pays* – both in the abstract and in terms of actual payments for disability or suffering. Pain and suffering for some have become a part of their nature and personality and influence the way they relate to others. *Pain defines them.* Unfortunately, for these individuals *the cost of getting better has become higher than the cost of remaining ill.* Ironically, for them there is a "value added" to chronic illness.

The problem patient is often characterized by drug misuse, various forms of noncompliance, somatization, family dysfunction, enmeshment, anger (overt or disguised), and what we refer to as "*pain theater.*" *Pain theater* is a behavioral display that takes on various characteristics in which suffering or symbols of illness or debilitation are exhibited. These range from the inappropriate use of wheelchairs, canes, walkers, service dogs, costumes (glasses, hats, etc.), and other occasionally dramatic displays of suffering.

Table 18-7 Signs or Signals of the Problem Patient

- Blameful behavior
- Oversolicitous behavior
- Ongoing disagreement with diagnostic or treatment recommendations
- Anger (overt or subtle)
- Overly patronizing and and excessive support to other patients
- Selective forgetfulness
- Incongruity between complaint of pain and social function
- Enmeshment and codependency of the patient with significant others (overinvolvement that keeps everyone focused on the negative, with reinforcement of maladaptive pain-related behavior)
- The presence of "others" accompanying the patient, who needlessly speak for or interpret for the patient
- The patient who is surrounded by many family members in attendance, as though he or she were terminal

Because headache is a subjective illness, it is necessary that we make decisions, sometimes very serious or costly ones, based upon symptoms that are neither provable nor disprovable. Thus the clinician must rely on experience-based judgments using behavioral cues and clues. Signals and signs are important. Be alert to the patient who demonstrates the following signs or signals. Table 18.7 lists some of these.

Recently we have become increasingly sensitive to the partner or family member whose life has seemingly merged with that of the patient. He/she often speaks in collective pronouns, such as "***Our*** headaches have gotten very bad," "***We*** had a bad experience with that doctor."

4. Identify Medication Misuse AND the Behavior that Underlies It

Not everyone with severe headaches overuses medicines for the same reason. Some do it for practical reasons; others have underlying behavioral dynamics that make overuse a part of a deeper neurobehavioral disorder. Some patients overuse their medications because their medical care has not adequately controlled their pain. To function they compensate by overusing medications, attempting to maintain responsibility to their families and their vocation. This patient is not a "drug addict." The motive is simple: to carry on in the absence of an adequately effective treatment. One marker of such a patient is that despite the overuse and pain, the individual maintains function despite the pain.

Some patients overuse medication because they cannot tolerate pain, while others will take the drugs to control anxiety. Some overuse medications as part of a broader obsessive drug-taking dynamic. Some patients take drugs to hide from life while others take drugs to cope with life (Herbert Malinoff, personal communication). Some patients are fearful of pain, a phenomenon called *cephalgiaphobia*, a term coined by Dr. Harvey Featherstone in the mid-1980s,[113,146] that has received recent attention in the research literature.[147]

Table 18-8 Drug Misuse and Abuse

- Diagnose and constructively confront.
- Educate.
- Insist on the development of coping skills and restraint.
- Make a therapeutic referral with mandatory compliance and continued care.
- Establish firm limits.
  1. Restrictive treatments
  2. Frequent visits
  3. Limited, calculated quantity of meds for each visit
  4. Short intervals between visits; frequent visits
- Monitor compliance, including prescription records.
- Regular contact with family physicians, NPs/PAs, pharmacists, therapists.
- Urinary drug screens when appropriate.
- Obtain pharmacy and insurance records.
- Execute a treatment contract.

Others use drugs excessively because they feel entitled to be pain free and to reject limit setting on their behavior, which includes the amount of drugs they can take. Others overuse their medications as a reflection of true addictive disorders and predisposition.

Table 18.8 identifies a general approach to patients who misuse or abuse medications.

The following message might be appropriate:

> These medications have become part of the problem. Your pattern of usage reflects not simply the presence of pain but behaviors that contribute to your problem. Effectively helping you discontinue the meds will require you to address these behaviors and control them.

5. Approaching the Cluster B Personality Disorder Patient

Of the problem patients, the borderline personality disorder patient stands above most. Patients with cluster B personality disorders, such as borderline and narcissistic disorders, are among the most challenging in the headache field. They generally have difficult-to-control pain problems as well as personalities and behaviors that obstruct effective treatment efforts, not infrequently rejecting or defying physician therapeutic or diagnostic attempts. They require a comprehensive treatment approach and firm limit setting. Such patients are frequently characterized by behaviors that include splitting and triangulation, challenging the tolerance of the professionals who are attempting to provide care, testing of limits that have been set, seductive behaviors toward team members, and often a significant battle for control of care. They may reject certain staff members in favor of others and, as we have seen frequently, display enabling or disruptive influences on other patients. Patients with Axis II cluster B disorders often prompt the doctor to act impulsively, sometimes out of anger, or to make unwise and expedient decisions. ***"Anything to move on."***

Such patients require a firm, no-nonsense approach tha is based on frank talk and expectation. While compassion and reasonable flexibility must underlie the effort, the patient is after all troubled. Compliance must be demanded. Firm, clear, and direct encounters assist in maintaining a suitable therapeutic relationship.

We have found discussions such as this to be helpful with some of our patients:

> "Your behavior is part of the problem." (Give examples). "It is a barrier to effective therapy. You reject our recommendations and battle us for control. This behavior is counterproductive and undermines the basic trust that is required in order to help you. Medical care is voluntary on both sides. Quite frankly, I don't have to be your physician if this unpleasant behavior continues, and you don't have to be my patient if you don't choose to be. If we can't agree that I am in charge of your case and you will be respectful, communicative, and compliant, I will discontinue care."

6. The Rhythm and Pace of Care Must Be Adequate

Because time in the hospital is limited, the pace and choice of treatments must be strategically sensible. As mentioned earlier, in our program we begin with identification of problem patients, medication overuse, and the early implementation of IV protocols to address the pain. Discontinuation of offending drugs begins immediately and is carried out either rapidly over 2-3 days or in a somewhat more protracted course, particularly when opioids are involved. The day-to-day details of this process are beyond the scope of this chapter, but we have outlined the basic principles of such process. Table 18.3 identifies the parenteral protocols that are used. Several are used concurrently. These might include magnesium and diphenhydramine, which together can be used with valproic acid, and/or ketorolac. Ketorolac can be used with a variety of the other parenteral agents. DHE combines well with neuroleptics, ketorolac, and diphenhydramine, among others. A firm knowledge of these drugs, their pharmacokinetic features, their contraindications, and adverse effects is necessary to combine these drugs safely.

7. Trial a Wide Variety of "p.r.n." Medications that Will Not Cause MOH if Overused

Because desperate people sometimes use drugs in desperate ways and without restraint in their pursuit of pain control, it is best to try to find p.r.n. or "as needed" medication that, if moderately overused, will at least not contribute to serious risk or the likelihood of MOH. Table 18.5 identifies several of the drugs that we use alone or in combination in the inpatient program. The reader should be reminded that all drugs when overused can be harmful and potentially fatal, but some are more troubling than others, and at least in moderate overuse, the drugs listed earlier are not likely to cause serious problems or prompt the development of MOH.

8. If the Patient Doesn't Sleep Well, Headaches Won't Be Controlled

It is very important to induce a normal or near normal sleeping pattern. Many intractable pain patients have abnormal sleep patterns. Consider inducing a normal sleep cycle by pharmacological or other means. In our experience, this is a necessary step in gaining headache control. Pharmacological choices include sedating tricyclic antidepressants, benzodiazepines, trazodone, melatonin, and hydroxyzine, among others. Obstructive sleep apnea may cause headaches and a sleep study to evaluate this possibility can be considered on an outpatient basis.

References

1. Lake AE, 3rd, Saper JR, Hamel RL. Comprehensive inpatient treatment of refractory chronic daily headache. *Headache.* 2009;49(4):555–562.
2. Freitag FG, Lake A, 3rd, Lipton R, Cady R, Diamond S, Silberstein S. Inpatient treatment of headache: an evidence-based assessment. *Headache.* 2004;44(4):342–360.
3. Saper JR, Hamel RL, Lake AE, 3rd. Medication overuse headache (MOH) is a biobehavioural disorder. *Cephalalgia.* 2005;25(7):545–546.
4. Andrasik F, Buse DC, Grazzi L. Behavioral medicine for migraine and medication overuse headache. *Curr Pain Headache Rep.* 2009;13(3): 241–248.
5. Boes CJ, Black DF, Dodick DW. Pathophysiology and management of transformed migraine and medication overuse headache. *Semin Neurol.* 2006;26(2):232–241.
6. Pakalnis A, Butz C, Splaingard D, Kring D, Fong J. Emotional problems and prevalence of medication overuse in pediatric chronic daily headache. *J Child Neurol.* 2007;22(12):1356–1359.
7. Radat F, Creac'h C, Guegan-Massardier E, et al. Behavioral dependence in patients with medication overuse headache: a cross-sectional study in consulting patients using the DSM-IV criteria. *Headache.* 2008;48(7): 1026–1036.
8. Radat F, Creac'h C, Swendsen JD, et al. Psychiatric comorbidity in the evolution from migraine to medication overuse headache. *Cephalalgia.* 2005;25(7):519–522.
9. Saper JR, Lake AE, 3rd. Medication overuse headache: type I and type II. *Cephalalgia.* 2006;26(10):1262.
10. Lake AE, 3rd. Medication overuse headache: biobehavioral issues and solutions. *Headache.* 2006;46(Suppl 3):S88–97.

11. Colman I, Brown MD, Innes GD, Grafstein E, Roberts TE, Rowe BH. Parenteral dihydroergotamine for acute migraine headache: a systematic review of the literature. *Ann Emerg Med.* 2005;45(4):393–401.
12. Ford RG, Ford KT. Continuous intravenous dihydroergotamine in the treatment of intractable headache. *Headache.* 1997;37(3):129–136.
13. Mathew NT. Dosing and administration of ergotamine tartrate and dihydroergotamine. *Headache.* 1997;37(Suppl 1):S26–32.
14. Raskin NH. Repetitive intravenous dihydroergotamine as therapy for intractable migraine. *Neurology.* 1986;36(7):995–997.
15. Robbins L, Remmes A. Outpatient repetitive intravenous dihydroergotamine. *Headache.* 1992;32(9):455–458.
16. Saper JR, Silberstein S. Pharmacology of dihydroergotamine and evidence for efficacy and safety in migraine. *Headache.* 2006;46(Suppl 4):S171–181.
17. Silberstein SD, Silberstein JR. Chronic daily headache: long-term prognosis following inpatient treatment with repetitive IV DHE. *Headache.* 1992;32(9): 439–445.
18. Stein M. IV dihydroergotamine therapy for migraine treatment. *Ann Emerg Med.* 1988;17(7):764.
19. Swidan SZ, Lake AE, 3rd, Saper JR. Efficacy of intravenous diphenhydramine versus intravenous DHE-45 in the treatment of severe migraine headache. *Curr Pain Headache Rep.* 2005;9(1):65–70.
20. Fisher H. A new approach to emergency department therapy of migraine headache with intravenous haloperidol: a case series. *J Emerg Med.* 1995;13(1):119–122.
21. Honkaniemi J, Liimatainen S, Rainesalo S, Sulavuori S. Haloperidol in the acute treatment of migraine: A randomized, double-blind, placebo-controlled study. *Headache.* 2006;46(5):781–787.
22. Lane PL, Ross R. Intravenous chlorpromazine—preliminary results in acute migraine. *Headache.* 1985;25(6):302–304.
23. Larkin G. Intravenous ketorolac vs intravenous prochlorperazine for the treatment of migraine headaches. *Acad Emerg Med.* 1999;6(6):668–670.
24. Rothrock JF. Treatment of acute migraine with intravenous droperidol. *Headache.* 1997;37(4):256–257.
25. Seim MB, March JA, Dunn KA. Intravenous ketorolac vs intravenous prochlorperazine for the treatment of migraine headaches. *Acad Emerg Med.* 1998;5(6):573–576.
26. Tanen DA, Miller S, French T, Riffenburgh RH. Intravenous sodium valproate versus prochlorperazine for the emergency department treatment of acute migraine headaches: a prospective, randomized, double-blind trial. *Ann Emerg Med.* 2003;41(6):847–853.
27. Vinson DR. Treatment patterns of isolated benign headache in US emergency departments. *Ann Emerg Med.* 2002;39(3):215–222.
28. Wang SJ, Silberstein SD, Young WB. Droperidol treatment of status migrainosus and refractory migraine. *Headache.* 1997;37(6): 377–382.
29. Trottier ED, Bailey B, Dauphin-Pierre S, Gravel J. Clinical outcomes of children treated with intravenous prochlorperazine for migraine in a pediatric emergency department. *J Emerg Med.* Jan 14, 2009.

30. Jakubowski M, Levy D, Goor-Aryeh I, Collins B, Bajwa Z, Burstein R. Terminating migraine with allodynia and ongoing central sensitization using parenteral administration of COX1/COX2 inhibitors. *Headache.* 2005;45(7):850–861.
31. Edwards KR, Norton J, Behnke M. Comparison of intravenous valproate versus intramuscular dihydroergotamine and metoclopramide for acute treatment of migraine headache. *Headache.* 2001;41(10):976–980.
32. Frazee LA, Foraker KC. Use of intravenous valproic acid for acute migraine. *Ann Pharmacother.* 2008;42(3):403–407.
33. Leniger T, Pageler L, Stude P, Diener HC, Limmroth V. Comparison of intravenous valproate with intravenous lysine-acetylsalicylic acid in acute migraine attacks. *Headache.* 2005;45(1):42–46.
34. Mathew NT, Kailasam J, Meadors L, Chernyschev O, Gentry P. Intravenous valproate sodium (Depacon) aborts migraine rapidly: a preliminary report. *Headache.* 2000;40(9):720–723.
35. Reiter PD, Nickisch J, Merritt G. Efficacy and tolerability of intravenous valproic acid in acute adolescent migraine. *Headache.* 2005;45(7):899–903.
36. Thomaides T, Karapanayiotides T, Kerezoudi E, et al. Intravenous valproate aborts glyceryl trinitrate-induced migraine attacks: a clinical and quantitative EEG study. *Cephalalgia.* 2008;28(3):250–256.
37. Waberzinek G, Markova J, Mastik J. Safety and efficacy of intravenous sodium valproate in the treatment of acute migraine. *Neuro Endocrinol Lett.* 2007;28(1):59–64.
38. Bigal ME, Bordini CA, Tepper SJ, Speciali JG. Intravenous magnesium sulphate in the acute treatment of migraine without aura and migraine with aura. A randomized, double-blind, placebo-controlled study. *Cephalalgia.* 2002;22(5):345–353.
39. Cete Y, Dora B, Ertan C, Ozdemir C, Oktay C. A randomized prospective placebo-controlled study of intravenous magnesium sulphate vs. metoclopramide in the management of acute migraine attacks in the Emergency Department. *Cephalalgia.* 2005;25(3):199–204.
40. Corbo J, Esses D, Bijur PE, Iannaccone R, Gallagher EJ. Randomized clinical trial of intravenous magnesium sulfate as an adjunctive medication for emergency department treatment of migraine headache. *Ann Emerg Med.* 2001;38(6):621–627.
41. Demirkaya S, Vural O, Dora B, Topcuoglu MA. Efficacy of intravenous magnesium sulfate in the treatment of acute migraine attacks. *Headache.* 2001;41(2):171–177.
42. Mauskop A, Altura BT, Cracco RQ, Altura BM. Intravenous magnesium sulphate relieves migraine attacks in patients with low serum ionized magnesium levels: a pilot study. *Clin Sci (Lond).* 1995;89(6):633–636.
43. Colman I, Friedman BW, Brown MD, et al. Parenteral dexamethasone for acute severe migraine headache: meta-analysis of randomised controlled trials for preventing recurrence. *BMJ.* 14 2008;336(7657):1359–1361.
44. Evers S, Afra J, Frese A, et al. EFNS guideline on the drug treatment of migraine - report of an EFNS task force. *Eur J Neurol.* 2006;13(6):560–572.
45. Noyan Ashraf MA, Sadeghi A, Azarbakht Z, Salehi S, Hamediseresht E. Evaluation of intravenous hydrocortisone in reducing headache after spinal

anesthesia: a double blind controlled clinical study [corrected]. *Middle East J Anesthesiol.* 2007;19(2):415–422.
46. Prakash S, Brahmbhatt KJ, Chawda NT, Tandon N. Hemicrania continua responsive to intravenous methyl prednisolone. *Headache.* 2009;49(4): 604–607.
47. Prakash S, Shah ND. Migrainous vertigo responsive to intravenous methylprednisolone: case reports. *Headache.* 22 2009.
48. Rowe BH, Colman I, Edmonds ML, Blitz S, Walker A, Wiens S. Randomized controlled trial of intravenous dexamethasone to prevent relapse in acute migraine headache. *Headache.* 2008;48(3):333–340.
49. Colman I, Brown MD, Innes GD, Grafstein E, Roberts TE, Rowe BH. Parenteral metoclopramide for acute migraine: meta-analysis of randomised controlled trials. *BMJ.* 2004;329(7479):1369–1373.
50. Reutens DC, Fatovich DM, Stewart-Wynne EG, Prentice DA. Is intravenous lidocaine clinically effective in acute migraine? *Cephalalgia.* 1991;11(6): 245–247.
51. Schere D, Silberstein SD. Intravenous lidocaine infusion for the treatment of post-acoustic neuroma resection headache: a case report. *Headache.* 2009;49(2):302–303.
52. Pfeifer HJ, Greenblatt DJ, Koch-Weser J. Clinical use and toxicity of intravenous lidocaine. A report from the Boston Collaborative Drug Surveillance Program. *Am Heart J.* Aug 1976;92(2):168–173.
53. Mariani C, Farina E, Scarlato G. Intravenous verapamil in acute migraine with prolonged aura. *Eur J Med.* 1992;1(5):319.
54. Hsu DA, Stafstrom CE, Rowley HA, Kiff JE, Dulli DA. Hemiplegic migraine: hyperperfusion and abortive therapy with intravenous verapamil. *Brain Dev.* 2008;30(1):86–90.
55. Ng TM, Kohli A, Fagan SC, Mohamed AE, Geiszt G. The effect of intravenous verapamil on cerebral hemodynamics in a migraine patient with hemiplegia. *Ann Pharmacother.* 2000;34(1):39–43.
56. Yu W, Horowitz SH. Familial hemiplegic migraine and its abortive therapy with intravenous verapamil. *Neurology.* 2001;57(9):1732–1733.
57. Molaie M, Olson CM, Koch J. The effect of intravenous verapamil on acute migraine headache. *Headache.* 1987;27(1):51–53.
58. Alemdar M, Pekdemir M, Selekler HM. Single-dose intravenous tramadol for acute migraine pain in adults: a single-blind, prospective, randomized, placebo-controlled clinical trial. *Clin Ther.* 2007;29(7):1441–1447.
59. Gowing L, Ali R, White JM. Buprenorphine for the management of opioid withdrawal. *Cochrane Database Syst Rev.* 2009(3):CD002025.
60. Ashton H. The diagnosis and management of benzodiazepine dependence. *Curr Opin Psychiatry.* 2005;18(3):249–255.
61. Rickels K, DeMartinis N, Rynn M, Mandos L. Pharmacologic strategies for discontinuing benzodiazepine treatment. *J Clin Psychopharmacol.* 1999;19 (6 Suppl 2):12S-16S.
62. Raja M, Altavista MC, Azzoni A, Albanese A. Severe barbiturate withdrawal syndrome in migrainous patients. *Headache.* 1996;36(2):119–121.
63. Sellers EM. Alcohol, barbiturate and benzodiazepine withdrawal syndromes: clinical management. *CMAJ.* 1988;139(2):113–120.

64. Loder E, Biondi D. Oral phenobarbital loading: a safe and effective method of withdrawing patients with headache from butalbital compounds. *Headache.* 2003;43(8):904–909.
65. Krymchantowski AV, Moreira PF. Out-patient detoxification in chronic migraine: comparison of strategies. *Cephalalgia.* 2003;23(10):982–993.
66. Bellville JW, Dorey F, Capparell D, Knox V, Bauer RO. Analgesic effects of hydroxyzine compared to morphine in man. *J Clin Pharmacol.* 1979;19(5–6): 290–296.
67. Stambaugh JE, Jr., Lane C. Analgesic efficacy and pharmacokinetic evaluation of meperidine and hydroxyzine, alone and in combination. *Cancer Invest.* 1983;1(2):111–117.
68. Carleton SC, Shesser RF, Pietrzak MP, et al. Double-blind, multicenter trial to compare the efficacy of intramuscular dihydroergotamine plus hydroxyzine versus intramuscular meperidine plus hydroxyzine for the emergency department treatment of acute migraine headache. *Ann Emerg Med.* 1998;32(2):129–138.
69. Charles JA, Jotkowitz S. Observations of the "carry-over effect" following successful termination of chronic migraine in the adolescent with short-term dihydroergotamine, dexamethasone and hydroxyzine: a pilot study. *J Headache Pain.* 2005;6(1):51–54.
70. Allais G, Bussone G, De Lorenzo C, et al. Naproxen sodium in short-term prophylaxis of pure menstrual migraine: pathophysiological and clinical considerations. *Neurol Sci.* 2007;28 Suppl 2:S225–228.
71. Andersson PG, Hinge HH, Johansen O, Andersen CU, Lademann A, Gotzsche PC. Double-blind study of naproxen vs placebo in the treatment of acute migraine attacks. *Cephalalgia.* 1989;9(1):29–32.
72. Bellavance AJ, Meloche JP. A comparative study of naproxen sodium, pizotyline and placebo in migraine prophylaxis. *Headache.* 1990;30(11):710–715.
73. Krymchantowski AV, Peixoto P, Higashi R, Silva A, Jr., Schutz V. Lysine clonixinate vs naproxen sodium for the acute treatment of migraine: a double-blind, randomized, crossover study. *Med Gen Med.* 2005;7(4):69.
74. Nestvold K. Naproxen and naproxen sodium in acute migraine attacks. *Cephalalgia.* 1986;6 Suppl 4:81–84.
75. Sances G, Martignoni E, Fioroni L, Blandini F, Facchinetti F, Nappi G. Naproxen sodium in menstrual migraine prophylaxis: a double-blind placebo controlled study. *Headache.* 1990;30(11):705–709.
76. Stronks DL, Tulen JH, Bussmann HB, Mulder LJ, Passchier J. Effects of naratriptan versus naproxen on daily functioning in the acute treatment of migraine: a randomized, double-blind, double-dummy, crossover study. *Headache.* 2003;43(8):845–852.
77. Welch KM. Naproxen sodium in the treatment of migraine. *Cephalalgia.* 1986;6 Suppl 4:85–92.
78. Anthony M, Lance JW. Indomethacin in migraine. *Med J Aust.* 1968;1(2):56–57.
79. Galeotti N, Ghelardini C, Grazioli I, Uslenghi C. Indomethacin, caffeine and prochlorperazine alone and combined revert hyperalgesia in in vivo models of migraine. *Pharmacol Res.* 2002;46(3):245–250.
80. Ghelardini C, Galeotti N, Grazioli I, Uslenghi C. Indomethacin, alone and combined with prochlorperazine and caffeine, but not sumatriptan,

abolishes peripheral and central sensitization in in vivo models of migraine. *J Pain.* 2004;5(8):413–419.

81. Davis CP, Torre PR, Schafer NC, Dave B, Bass B, Jr. Ketorolac as a rapid and effective treatment of migraine headache: evaluations by patients. *Am J Emerg Med.* 1993;11(6):573–575.
82. Davis CP, Torre PR, Williams C, et al. Ketorolac versus meperidine-plus-promethazine treatment of migraine headache: evaluations by patients. *Am J Emerg Med.* 1995;13(2):146–150.
83. Duarte C, Dunaway F, Turner L, Aldag J, Frederick R. Ketorolac versus meperidine and hydroxyzine in the treatment of acute migraine headache: a randomized, prospective, double-blind trial. *Ann Emerg Med.* 1992;21(9): 1116–1121.
84. Klapper JA, Stanton JS. Ketorolac versus DHE and metoclopramide in the treatment of migraine headaches. *Headache.* 1991;31(8):523–524.
85. Larkin GL, Prescott JE. A randomized, double-blind, comparative study of the efficacy of ketorolac tromethamine versus meperidine in the treatment of severe migraine. *Ann Emerg Med.* 1992;21(8):919–924.
86. Shrestha M, Singh R, Moreden J, Hayes JE. Ketorolac vs chlorpromazine in the treatment of acute migraine without aura. A prospective, randomized, double-blind trial. *Arch Intern Med.* 2–1996;156(15):1725–1728.
87. Ashkenazi A, Silberstein SD. The evolving management of migraine. *Curr Opin Neurol.* 2003;16(3):341–345.
88. Silberstein SD, Peres MF, Hopkins MM, Shechter AL, Young WB, Rozen TD. Olanzapine in the treatment of refractory migraine and chronic daily headache. *Headache.* 2002;42(6):515–518.
89. Freitag FG. Preventative treatment for migraine and tension-type headaches: do drugs having effects on muscle spasm and tone have a role? *CNS Drugs.* 2003;17(6):373–381.
90. Fromm GH. Baclofen as an adjuvant analgesic. *J Pain Symptom Manage.* 1994;9(8):500–509.
91. Hering-Hanit R. Baclofen for prevention of migraine. *Cephalalgia.* 1999;19(6):589–591.
92. Panerai AE, Massei R, de Silva E, Sacerdote P, Monza G, Mantegazza P. Baclofen prolongs the analgesic effect of fentanyl in man. *Br J Anaesth.* 1985;57(10):954–955.
93. Terrence CF, Fromm GH, Tenicela R. Baclofen as an analgesic in chronic peripheral nerve disease. *Eur Neurol.* 1985;24(6):380–385.
94. Yomiya K, Matsuo N, Tomiyasu S, et al. Baclofen as an adjuvant analgesic for cancer pain. *Am J Hosp Palliat Care.* 2009;26(2):112–118.
95. Lake AE, 3rd, Saper JR. Chronic headache: new advances in treatment strategies. *Neurology.* 2002;59(5 Suppl 2):S8–13.
96. Saper JR, Lake AE, 3rd, Cantrell DT, Winner PK, White JR. Chronic daily headache prophylaxis with tizanidine: a double-blind, placebo-controlled, multicenter outcome study. *Headache.* 2002;42(6):470–482.
97. Saper JR, Winner PK, Lake AE, 3rd. An open-label dose-titration study of the efficacy and tolerability of tizanidine hydrochloride tablets in the prophylaxis of chronic daily headache. *Headache.* 2001;41(4): 357–368.

98. Smith TR. Low-dose tizanidine with nonsteroidal anti-inflammatory drugs for detoxification from analgesic rebound headache. *Headache.* 2002;42(3): 175–177.
99. Friedman BW, Hochberg M, Esses D, et al. A clinical trial of trimethobenzamide/diphenhydramine versus sumatriptan for acute migraines. *Headache.* 2006;46(6):934–941.
100. Kudrow L, Kudrow DB, Sandweiss JH. Rapid and sustained relief of migraine attacks with intranasal lidocaine: preliminary findings. *Headache.* 1995;35(2):79–82.
101. Maizels M. Intranasal lidocaine to prevent headache following migraine aura. *Headache.* 1999;39(6):439–442.
102. Maizels M, Geiger AM. Intranasal lidocaine for migraine: a randomized trial and open-label follow-up. *Headache.* 1999;39(8):543–551.
103. Maizels M, Scott B, Cohen W, Chen W. Intranasal lidocaine for treatment of migraine: a randomized, double-blind, controlled trial. *JAMA.* 4–1996;276(4): 319–321.
104. Mills TM, Scoggin JA. Intranasal lidocaine for migraine and cluster headaches. *Ann Pharmacother.* 1997;31(7–8):914–915.
105. Krymchantowski AV, Barbosa JS. Prednisone as initial treatment of analgesic-induced daily headache. *Cephalalgia.* 2000;20(2):107–113.
106. Pageler L, Katsarava Z, Diener HC, Limmroth V. Prednisone vs. placebo in withdrawal therapy following medication overuse headache. *Cephalalgia.* 2008;28(2):152–156.
107. Smith CD, Reeves AG. Amelioration of ophthalmoplegic migraine by prednisone: a case report. *Headache.* 1986;26(2):93–94.
108. Lane ME, Kim MJ. Assessment and prevention of gastrointestinal toxicity of non-steroidal anti-inflammatory drugs. *J Pharm Pharmacol.* 2006;58(10):1295–1304.
109. van der Linden MW, van der Bij S, Welsing P, Kuipers EJ, Herings RM. The balance between severe cardiovascular and gastrointestinal events among users of selective and non-selective non-steroidal anti-inflammatory drugs. *Ann Rheum Dis.* 2009;68(5):668–673.
110. John R, Herzenberg AM. Renal toxicity of therapeutic drugs. *J Clin Pathol.* 2009;62(6):505–515.
111. Farkouh ME, Greenberg BP. An evidence-based review of the cardiovascular risks of nonsteroidal anti-inflammatory drugs. *Am J Cardiol.* 2009;103(9): 1227–1237.
112. Boe MG, Salvesen R, Mygland A. Chronic daily headache with medication overuse: predictors of outcome 1 year after withdrawal therapy. *Eur J Neurol.* 2009;16(6):705–712.
113. Saper JR, Silberstein JR, Gordon DG, Hamel RL. *Handbook of Headache Management: A Practical Guide to Diagnosis and Treatment of Head, Neck, and Facial Pain*, 2nd ed. Philadelphia: Williams & Wilkins; 1999.
114. Warner JS. Prolonged recovery from rebound headaches. *Headache.* 2001;41(8):817–822.
115. Katsarava Z, Muessig M, Dzagnidze A, Fritsche G, Diener HC, Limmroth V. Medication overuse headache: rates and predictors for relapse in a 4-year prospective study. *Cephalalgia.* 2005;25(1):12–15.

116. Lake AE, 3rd. Screening and behavioral management: medication overuse headache–the complex case. *Headache.* 2008;48(1):26–31.
117. Sances G, Ghiotto N, Galli F, et al. Risk factors in medication-overuse headache: a 1–year follow-up study (care II protocol). *Cephalalgia.* 2009; 30(3):329–336.
118. Afridi SK, Shields KG, Bhola R, Goadsby PJ. Greater occipital nerve injection in primary headache syndromes–prolonged effects from a single injection. *Pain.* 2006;122(1–2):126–129.
119. Akin Takmaz S, Inan N, Ucler S, Yazar MA, Inan L, Basar H. Greater occipital nerve block in migraine headache: Preliminary results of 10 patients. *Agri.* 2008;20(1):47–50.
120. Ashkenazi A, Levin M. Greater occipital nerve block for migraine and other headaches: is it useful? *Curr Pain Headache Rep.* 2007;11(3):231–235.
121. Ashkenazi A, Young WB. The effects of greater occipital nerve block and trigger point injection on brush allodynia and pain in migraine. *Headache.* 2005;45(4):350–354.
122. Vincent MB, Luna RA, Scandiuzzi D, Novis SA. Greater occipital nerve blockade in cervicogenic headache. *Arq Neuropsiquiatr.* 1998;56(4): 720–725.
123. Bovim G, Berg R, Dale LG. Cervicogenic headache: anesthetic blockades of cervical nerves (C2–C5) and facet joint (C2/C3). *Pain.* 1992;49(3): 315–320.
124. Inan N, Ceyhan A, Inan L, Kavaklioglu O, Alptekin A, Unal N. C2/C3 nerve blocks and greater occipital nerve block in cervicogenic headache treatment. *Funct Neurol.* 2001;16(3):239–243.
125. Manchikanti L. Neural blockade in cervical pain syndromes. *Pain Physician.* 1999;2(3):65–84.
126. Blume HG. Cervicogenic headaches: radiofrequency neurotomy and the cervical disc and fusion. *Clin Exp Rheumatol.* 2000;18(2 Suppl 19):S53–58.
127. Bogduk N. Role of anesthesiologic blockade in headache management. *Curr Pain Headache Rep.* 2004;8(5):399–403.
128. Lee JB, Park JY, Park J, Lim DJ, Kim SD, Chung HS. Clinical efficacy of radiofrequency cervical zygapophyseal neurotomy in patients with chronic cervicogenic headache. *J Korean Med Sci.* 2007;22(2):326–329.
129. Sjaastad O, Stolt-Nielsen A, Blume H, Zwart JA, Fredriksen TA. Cervicogenic headache. Long-term results of radiofrequency treatment of the planum nuchale. *Funct Neurol.* 1995;10(6):265–271.
130. van Kleef M, van Suijlekom JA. Treatment of chronic cervical pain, brachialgia, and cervicogenic headache by means of radiofrequency procedures. *Pain Pract.* 2002;2(3):214–223.
131. van Suijlekom HA, Weber WE, van Kleef M, Barendse GA, Sluijter ME. Radiofrequency cervical zygapophyseal joint neurotomy for cervicogenic headache: a short term follow-up study. *Funct Neurol.* 1998;13(1):82–83.
132. Bartsch T, Goadsby PJ. Stimulation of the greater occipital nerve induces increased central excitability of dural afferent input. *Brain.* 2002;125(Pt 7): 1496–1509.
133. Bartsch T, Goadsby PJ. The trigeminocervical complex and migraine: current concepts and synthesis. *Curr Pain Headache Rep.* 2003;7(5):371–376.

134. Bartsch T, Goadsby PJ. Increased responses in trigeminocervical nociceptive neurons to cervical input after stimulation of the dura mater. *Brain.* 2003; 126(Pt 8):1801–1813.
135. Goadsby PJ, Hoskin KL. The distribution of trigeminovascular afferents in the nonhuman primate brain Macaca nemestrina: a c-fos immunocytochemical study. *J Anat.* 1997;190 (Pt 3):367–375.
136. Goadsby PJ, Zagami AS, Lambert GA. Neural processing of craniovascular pain: a synthesis of the central structures involved in migraine. *Headache.* 1991;31(6):365–371.
137. van Boxem K, van Eerd M, Brinkhuize T, Patijn J, van Kleef M, van Zundert J. Radiofrequency and pulsed radiofrequency treatment of chronic pain syndromes: the available evidence. *Pain Pract.* 2008;8(5):385–393.
138. Stovner LJ, Kolstad F, Helde G. Radiofrequency denervation of facet joints C2–C6 in cervicogenic headache: a randomized, double-blind, sham-controlled study. *Cephalalgia.* 2004;24(10):821–830.
139. Silberstein SD, Lipton RB, Saper JR. Chronic daily headache including transformed migraine, chronic tension-type headache, and medication overuse headache. In: Silberstein SD, Lipton RB, Dodick DW, eds. *Wolff's Headache and Other Head Pain*, 8th ed. New York: Oxford University Press; 2008:315–377.
140. Lake AE, 3rd, Saper JR, Madden SF, Kreeger C. Comprehensive inpatient treatment for intractable migraine: a prospective long-term outcome study. *Headache.* 1993;33(2):55–62.
141. Saper JR, Lake AE, 3rd, Madden SF, Kreeger C. Comprehensive/tertiary care for headache: a 6–month outcome study. *Headache.* 1999;39(4):249–263.
142. Bohus M, Limberger M, Ebner U, et al. Pain perception during self-reported distress and calmness in patients with borderline personality disorder and self-mutilating behavior. *Psychiatry Res.* 2000;95(3):251–260.
143. Rothrock J, Lopez I, Zweilfer R, Andress-Rothrock D, Drinkard R, Walters N. Borderline personality disorder and migraine. *Headache.* 2007;47(1):22–26.
144. Saper JR, Lake AE, 3rd. Borderline personality disorder and the chronic headache patient: review and management recommendations. *Headache.* 2002;42(7):663–674.
145. Saper JR. Pearls from an inpatient headache unit. *Headache.* 2008;48(6): 820–827.
146. Lake AE, 3rd. Behavioral medicine for chronic headache: overview and practical tools for the practicing physician. *Continuum.* 2006;12(6):235–258.
147. Peres MF, Mercante JP, Guendler VZ, et al. Cephalalgiaphobia: a possible specific phobia of illness. *J Headache Pain.* 2007;8(1):56–59.

Section III

Special Topics in Refractory Migraine

19

Creating a Foundation for Successful Treatment

Improving Adherence and Fostering a Therapeutic Relationship

Roger K. Cady, MD, Kathleen Farmer, PsyD,
Jeanetta C. Rains, PhD, and Donald B. Penzien, PhD

Introduction

One of the more sobering moments for a healthcare professional and patient with headache is the realization that the migraine is refractory to treatment. Scientifically defining refractory migraine (RM) is a work in progress yet clinically it is a concept intuitively understood and encountered by most clinicians. Salient features of RM are diagnosis of ICDH-II migraine or chronic migraine; failure to respond to multiple acute and preventive medications despite modifications of triggering factors and lifestyle; and significant disability. In addition, the presence or absence of medication overuse is considered a modifier. In many instances, the most important asset a clinician has to offer is a therapeutic alliance directed at care rather than pharmacological control.

The diagnosis of RM evolves over time and is diagnosed only after repeated failure of adequate and appropriate treatment. Both biomedical and psychosocial consequences play a role. For example, early in the process of RM, doubts linger about the diagnosis often leading to multiple tests that inevitably fail to yield a diagnosis and sometimes lead to invasive procedures that likewise are not fruitful. There are repeated attempts at pharmacological therapy, which are by definition in this syndrome ineffective. The patient's lifestyle and motivation to improve typically undergo scrutiny in an effort to explain the patient's unresponsiveness to treatment. As time goes on and resignation sets in, the motivation to continue medical care lessens and eventually deteriorates. All too often, the end result is a breakdown of the provider/patient relationship into what has been termed the "heartsink" patient.[1] Because of repeated treatment failures, they produce a feeling of dread and despair in the clinician.

From the patient's perspective, in addition to unremitting headaches, there often are undesirable side effects from therapy such as weight gain, fatigue, and cognitive impairment, and there is persistent and often progressive disruption in nearly all domains of life. There is doubt from friends, family, medical providers, and even oneself. In the end, and as it becomes apparent the migraine is refractory, the patient rather than the headache often becomes labeled as refractory. The medical provider also may experience doubt and frustration, questioning: Why were the prescribed and usually efficacious treatments ineffective in this case? What more could have been done? What should not have been done? Often there remains an enduring sense of failure and inadequacy for both patient and provider.

With this backdrop, it is valuable for healthcare professionals to respect the limits of medical science and to appreciate the value of the clinical relationship in management of the patient with RM. Over the last 25 years, medical advancements in the field of migraine have been dramatic. Yet it is humbling to realize how little medical science actually understands about the disease of migraine or its treatment. Our understanding of migraine pathophysiology has changed radically from an episodic vascular disorder to a potentially chronic neurobiological disease. Despite advances, many of the scientific nuances underlying this change remain unknown. One can only imagine how migraine will be understood 25 years from now. Likewise, we are only beginning to explore the pathology and neurobiology that leads to migraine chronification. Beyond migraine with or without aura, there is little scientific knowledge of the subtypes of migraine or other primary headaches.

The pharmacological mechanisms by which preventive medications work essentially are unknown; only a few mechanisms are understood by which acute medications abort or terminate a migraine attack. Curiously, even medications with considerable scientific evidence do not work for every patient or every attack of migraine despite a homogeneous clinical diagnosis. The impact of comorbidities on treatment and clinical outcome is largely unknown. Given this stark assessment one could argue that it is remarkable that the majority of migraineurs do improve and indeed it is the minority of cases that become refractory to usual care.

From the patient's perspective, living with migraine is complicated. Particularly as headache becomes more chronic and severe, management requires the patient to engage in significant behavioral changes not only in response to headache but also on symptom-free days. Remembering to take daily medication, having acute medication readily available for the episode of migraine, keeping daily diaries and medication logs, being wary of migraine triggers and vigilant of healthy behaviors are just a few of the many complexities in the life of a migraineur. Perhaps not surprising, it is the rule rather than the exception for patients to be nonadherent to their often complex treatment plans.

To date, there has been little formal scientific study of patients with RM. Most of the medical understanding of this condition is extrapolated from less severe forms of the disease (if it is indeed the same disease). This is true for the use of pharmacological intervention as well as lifestyle and behavioral intervention. This chapter is an effort to put into perspective the role of healthcare professionals in managing the patient with RM. For the healthcare provider, it is switching expectations from control of disease to care of the patient. For patients, it is learning to define success by incremental improvement and solving the complexities of their RM by unraveling pieces of the puzzle rather than seeking a "cure." Despite the limits of the medical provider and patient in stopping RM, the value of a healthy long-term therapeutic relationship cannot be overstated.

Developing a therapeutic relationship requires a patient-centered approach. There is no evidence-based approach to management of RM. Because no two patients are exactly alike, the approach needs to be individualized to fit the patient rather than the disease process. In this chapter, there is a review of the scientific literature on adherence and motivation of behavioral change. In addition, two patient case studies are provided to underscore provider/patient issues common in the medical relationship between clinician and patient with RM and illustrate some of the therapeutic dynamics useful to patient care.

Adherence

Nonadherence represents a threat to the effectiveness of treatment, potentially undermines the therapeutic alliance, and warrants specific attention with the refractory headache sufferer. Low adherence to prescribed medications is almost invariably associated with poorer outcomes across a wide range of disorders.[2] Adherence encompasses the degree to which the patient carries out a recommended treatment plan such as medication regimen, behavioral or lifestyle change, referral, and appointment-keeping. Treatment plans are typically developed to maximize effectiveness of treatment and minimize risk for complications. Misuse and overuse of symptomatic medications is a well-recognized contributor to RM and as described below has been shown to contribute to treatment failure. Nonadherence undermines the effectiveness of pharmacological and behavioral treatments. Identified risk factors for nonadherence include the complexity of the treatment regimen, psychiatric comorbidity, psychological factors, and characteristics of the clinic or provider. Barriers to adherence can be identified and intervention tailored to facilitate adherence and the patient's 'readiness for change.' Although adherence issues almost always can be identified in patients with RM, there undoubtedly is a biological basis for RM. In short, nonadherence alone does not account for refractoriness among headache patients.

Exploring Nonadherence in the Patient with RM

Headache management is greatly hindered by nonadherence. In the headache arena, nonadherence takes the form of failure to initially fill prescriptions, suboptimal application of treatments (both pharmacological and behavioral), and missed appointments. A recent review of headache literature concluded: 11% of all headache prescriptions were never filled; 25% to 50% of patients are nonadherent with various prophylactic medications (adherence declines as the number of doses increases); up to 70% of patients did not use abortive medications optimally; and 40% of patients did not return for recommended follow up after initial consultation.[3] Adherence with headache-related behavioral and lifestyle recommendations (e.g., diet, exercise, sleep) was similarly poor ranging from 22% to 85%.[4] Likewise, misuse or overuse of triptans and other symptomatic medication can seriously aggravate primary headache disorders and has been associated with treatment failure.[5,6] It is therefore paramount that patients with RM be evaluated thoroughly as to adherence with therapeutic recommendations.

Patients' reported reasons for nonadherence include cost, complexity and side effects of the medication regimen, fear of medication overuse or addiction, and characteristics of provider or clinical operation.[3] For example, a prospective observational study examining a large sample of pharmacist-identified migraineurs who were prescribed rizatriptan or nontriptan oral medications (e.g., nonsteroidal anti-inflammatory drug [NSAID], analgesic-sedative combination with or without narcotic, isometheptene mucate or ergot derivative) found 49% of patients avoided or delayed taking acute medications even though the majority described their migraines as severe (lasting on average 20+ hours per attack).[7] Self-reported reasons for delaying or avoiding treatment included: waiting to see if headache was migraine (68.7%) or severe migraine (46.2%), concerns about side effects (37.2%), concerns about drug effectiveness if taken too frequently (34.3%), concerns about dependency or addiction (28.7%), limits imposed by insurance (15.1%), and cost (8.9%, although 96% of patients had at least some insurance coverage for prescription medication), and a small number instructed by prescriber not to take right away (2.4%).

The first paper on early intervention was published in 2000 and was an ad hoc analysis of a small number of protocol violators who treated when their headache was mild rather than moderate to severe as was instructed in the protocol.[8] The observation of benefit with early treatment was initially met with considerable and appropriate skepticism by the headache community. It was not for several more years that this early intervention paradigm became widely accepted in clinical practice and even today early intervention is debated and being redefined. Paradoxes such as this underscore the complexity of provider/patient interactions when information as clinical guidance changes and evolves over time.

Regarding appointment-keeping, Spierings and colleagues[9] reported that 40.5% of patients did not comply with the provider's recommendation for a follow-up appointment after initial consultation. Patients' stated reasons (not mutually exclusive) for not returning were categorized as: (1) administrative (e.g., fee burdensome, lengthy wait time in office, dissatisfaction with staff interactions, calls not returned, insurance not filed), (2) dissatisfaction with clinician's skills and/or personal character, (3) change in headache/illness status (e.g., headache improved, sufficient care received elsewhere, decreased life stress,), or (4) problems associated with recommended treatment regimen (e.g., disagreement or difficulty with regimen, adverse effects). Discussing these difficulties openly with patients usually leads to a mutual understanding and ultimately to correcting the underlying problem.

Barriers to Adherence

Although barriers to adherence have not been fully elucidated in migraine, risk factors including the regimen variables, psychiatric comorbidity, psychological factors and patient-provider relationship are well established across chronic medical conditions and are consistent with the available evidence in migraine.

Medication Regimen

Medication regimen variables represent the most extensively and objectively studied risk factors to date. Not surprisingly, adherence declines with multiple medications, more frequent or complex medication dosing regimens, higher medication costs, and side effects; these findings are consistent across various acute and chronic medical conditions with the poorest adherence noted for chronic illnesses.[3] Gallagher and Kunkel[10] surveyed headache sufferers and found two-thirds of 1160 migraineurs delayed or avoided taking their prescribed medications because of side effects. The complaints were chiefly sleepiness/tiredness (58%) and difficulty in thinking clearly (30%).

Adherence measurement warrants some attention insofar as subjective reports are known not only to overestimate but also to be discordant with more objective measures. Meta-analysis across various medical conditions has demonstrated that the least reliable measurement strategy (and most widely used) for compliance is retrospective self report via the face-to-face interview, followed by daily diaries and questionnaires, with the most accurate information obtained by objective monitoring (e.g., electronic tracking, pill counts, plasma levels, insurance claims data).[11] In migraine, Mulleners and colleagues[12] collected objective compliance data using an electronic covert tracking devices in pill bottles (Medication Event Monitoring System [MEMS]) as well as pill counts for patients prescribed common prophylactic headache medications requiring various dosing regimens (propranolol LA, atenolol, pizotifen, methysergide); overall compliance based on pill count over the 8-week trial was 91% compared to MEMS 66% with a linear trend toward poorer compliance with multiple daily dosing regimens (once < twice < three times per day dosing). Results confirmed in migraine two well documented findings from the broader medical literature—adherence declines with multiple dosing schedules and subjective measures overestimate adherence relative to objective measures. Frequently the source providers use to establish nonresponse to a medication is a patient's self report or a previous physician's statement of nonresponse, again based on a patient's self report. Where adherence is not well documented, it is reasonable to question the validity of nonresponsiveness and ask that patients try again a pharmacological intervention.

Psychiatric Comorbidity

Psychiatric comorbidity is a negative prognostic indicator for patient adherence across a wide variety of medical conditions and this is probably true for headache. Radat and colleagues[13] have reported increased risk for mood disorders, anxiety, and psychoactive substance use disorders (other than analgesics) among patients with medication overuse headache, and noted that the psychiatric disorders occurred significantly more often before transformation from migraine into medication overuse headache than after. Similarly, Saper and colleagues[14] observed suggested psychological states and behaviors (e.g., fear of headache, anticipatory anxiety, obsessional drug-taking behaviors, psychological drug dependence) may play a key role in the overuse of headache medication. Likewise, they have acknowledged that individuals with personality disorders (e.g., antisocial, borderline, histrionic, narcissistic) are likely to exhibit behavior patterns that substantially contribute to nonadherence such as defiance of limits regarding medication usage, battles of control over treatment, and attitudes of entitlement regarding pain control. It is critical to provide these patients with a complete psychiatric and psychological evaluation and treat comorbidities appropriately.

Patient–Provider Relationship

In headache care, the quality of the provider/patient relationship has been demonstrated to contribute to nonadherence at least with respect to persistence in treatment.[9] Unfortunately, patients' basic priorities and expectations for headache treatment may be incongruent with those of the provider and hinder the therapeutic alliance. For example, a survey of patients and providers found patients most often desired that a headache specialist be willing to answer questions whereas physicians believed medical expertise to be the single most important physician attribute.[15] The broader adherence literature documents that adherence may be diminished when there is discordance between the patient's beliefs and those of the provider; conversely, adherence is increased after an encounter of longer duration, more frequent communication and the patient's perception of a personal relationship with her healthcare provider.[3] This underscores the importance of listening to the patient and using communication strategies to define goals and expectations that can be mutually agreed upon. In the American Migraine Communication Study, an accurate exchange of critical historical information was obtained when a provider asked open-ended questions and communicated with the patient using the "ask-tell-ask method." In this model, providers restated what they understood from the patient's dialogue and specifically asked if their understanding was accurate. This method also provided an opportunity for providers to educate patients about myths and misconceptions.[16]

Essential Elements for Adherence

Virtually all pharmacological and behavioral treatments require some degree of active participation and behavior change on the part of the patient relating to adherence (e.g., appointment-keeping, filling prescriptions, administering medications as prescribed, reporting outcomes, side effects, and deviations from prescription, lifestyle changes, behavioral skills training, headache diary, homework). Such health behavior change requires three essential elements: patient's readiness for change, perceived importance of change, and confidence in one's ability to change (*self-efficacy*)—simply, patients must be at once *ready, willing, and able* to change some aspect of behavior.[17]

Refractory headache sufferers, by definition, have experienced treatment failure that is likely to undermine confidence and participation in future treatment. Self-efficacy (confidence in one's ability to perform an action) and outcome-efficacy (expectations that the behavior will lead to a desirable result) have received considerable attention in the adherence literature and are generally known to be powerful predictors of adherence.[3] Simply possessing the skills needed to carry out a treatment plan is not sufficient to ensure that those skills will be performed. Rather, patients must believe they possess the requisite skills *and* that these behaviors will achieve the desired outcome. Self-efficacy and outcome-efficacy are considered critical components of adherence because they determine the degree of effort and persistence a patient will put forth in the face of challenges.

Adherence also appears to hinge on patients' "readiness for change." The transtheoretical model[18] arguably is the prevailing model of health behavior change and useful guide in patient care.[19] The model holds that change does not necessarily proceed in a linear fashion, but instead that patients cycle through "stages of change." These stages are: precontemplation (not thinking about changing behavior), contemplation (actively thinking about changing behavior but not trying to change), preparation (beginning to make changes slowly), action (actively engaged in regular behavior change), and maintenance (maintaining changes). In the maintenance stage, behaviors are performed habitually and automatically and require little thought. Relapse is considered to be movement from one stage back to a prior stage.

Various refractory headache patients can be grouped into any one of the five stages of change. Despite prior treatment, patients may remain in the stage of "precontemplation" and have devoted little or no consideration to altering relevant behaviors (e.g., daily use of over-the-counter analgesics, depression, stress). Here, education linking headache with precipitants is likely to be more a fundamental component of intervention than prescription for prophylaxis. Patients in the 'contemplation' stage of change likewise warrant education about treatment options and also may benefit from social support and encouragement. Those in 'preparation' for change stage warrant clear step-by-step behavioral instruction, modeling, discussion of barriers, and close follow up. The "action" stage is the stage in which specific behavioral and pharmacological treatments are best utilized. Action stage also warrants the closest adherence assessment and reinforcement to maintain the behavior through barriers until the benefits of treatment (i.e., headache and functional improvement) can emerge to maintain the behavior. 'Maintenance' of treatment gains would include continued enhancement of self-efficacy and relapse prevention. Although no published studies to date have been reported with headache patients, interventions directed at each of these processes have proven effective in improving adherence among wide-ranging chronic illnesses and warrant application to headache.

Adherence Facilitation

Risks for nonadherence should be considered in headache treatment planning and adherence evaluated specifically over time as a treatment variable. Patient–provider collaboration in treatment planning tends to increase the patient's investment in a positive outcome, and results in a plan that is more realistic to the patient's particular circumstance. Generally, a collaborative alliance with a negotiated rather than dictated plan is associated with greater adherence. Patients should be encouraged to articulate potential barriers such as cost, side effects, etc., which then can be taken into account. A simple four-item questionnaire was effective in assessing and predicting adherence in patients being treated for hypertension and likewise may prove helpful in assessing adherence in patients with headache.[20] The questions asked were: (1) Do you ever forget to take your medication? (2) Are you careless at times about taking medication? (3] When you feel better, do you sometimes stop taking your medications?; and (4) Sometimes, when you feel worse, do you stop taking your medications? Asking treatment nonresponders about their adherence will detect more than 50% of those with low adherence, with a specificity of 87%.[20]

Particularly with refractory cases, strategies and formal tools to facilitate adherence may be warranted.[21] Written treatment plans provide a reference for patients after they leave the office. Medication contracts may be utilized that specify behavioral expectations on the part of patient and provider. Patients should be encouraged to self-monitor medication use along with headache parameters. Review of self-monitoring by the healthcare provider enables opportunities for feedback and reinforcement for successful adherence. The presence of comorbid psychiatric disorders is known to undermine adherence and thus screening and treating comorbid depression and anxiety is strongly encouraged (see Chapter 7).

Clinic Structure

Failed appointment-keeping is significant in headache care and acts as a ceiling on all future treatment and adherence efforts. With 40% of headache patients failing to return for treatment after consultation,[9] this would appear to be the single greatest opportunity to improve adherence. Calling patients to remind them of appointments and recalling those who miss a scheduled appointment are fundamentally the most cost-effective adherence-enhancing strategies. Although not studied among headache patients, additional simple strategies have been shown across other chronic disorders to improve appointment keeping including reminders (mail, telephone), clinic orientations, and contracting with patients.[22]

Treatment Regimen

Simplified treatment regimens are associated with higher rates of adherence. Once-a-day regimens taken at bedtime or on awakening are associated with the highest levels of adherence, and adherence diminishes with each successive dosing. Behavioral and social learning principles may enhance basic medication prescribing practices with: use of simplified regimens, fixed-dose combinations, or unit-of-use packaging when possible; stimulus control strategies (e.g., day-of-the-week pill box, electronic calendars/palm pilots/cell phones, environmental cues like meals, personalized internal cues for abortive medications); communication skills such as active listening, enlisting patient in treatment planning process, soliciting/trouble-shooting potential barriers to adherence, supplementing verbal instructions with written materials, requesting patients restate recommendations back to the provider; and medication contracts.

Self-management

Shared collaboration between patients and healthcare providers, utilizing self-management strategies, may improve adherence with prescribed medications.[27] For example, use of abortive medication and headache outcomes improved in patients who participated in a half-hour education session on recognition of migraine and use of abortive medication along with three brief phone calls to identify and remedy problems with medication use. Patients also received a self-management workbook to assist the patient in monitoring and identifying adherence problems, improve decision-making, and correct adherence problems.[23] The brief intervention resulted in significant improvement in adherence that resulted in improved headache outcome.

Motivational Interviewing

Motivational interviewing (MI) is a specific patient-centered counseling approach for development of self-efficacy and behavior change, which has been shown to improve adherence in variety of medical and psychological disorders.[24] MI involves structuring the therapeutic encounter to enable patients to see for themselves a discrepancy between their current state and their desired outcome. Motivation to change is believed to increase when patients, rather than the healthcare providers, examine the pros and cons of change and then make decisions for themselves. Thus, the healthcare provider's role involves motivating rather than directing patients for behavior change. MI involves four key principles: (1) Express empathy—actively listening without judgment and accurately reflecting patients' ambivalence about change; (2) Develop discrepancy—assist patients in identifying the discrepancy between their ultimate goals and their present behavior; (3) Role with resistance—reflect resistance with empathy, recognizing that arguing with patients is counterproductive; and (4) Support self-efficacy—encourage confidence and reinforce small steps toward change.

Summary

Low rates of appointment-keeping, nonadherence to treatment recommendations, attrition from treatment, and relapse pose significant problems for patients and practitioners. Evidence suggests most patients do not fully comply with treatment as recommended and nonadherence is recognized as an important and potentially modifiable factor in treatment failure. All patients are candidates for adherence facilitation as a mode of practice, and this is likely to be particularly important in cases of refractory headache. Strategies are available to the provider that promise to facilitate adherence. It can be helpful to match treatment to patient's current readiness for change and establish a mode of practice that facilitates adherence. There are many tools to help us including enhancing clinic structure, behavioral prompts and our own communication styles. It should be recognized, headache by its very nature tends to vary in frequency and severity. Likewise, patient's priorities and competing demands may change over time. Thus, it is important to recognize that our patient's individual cost-benefit analysis for treatment can vary over time. Finally, it should be noted that there is no cure for low adherence. Adherence facilitation efforts must be maintained as long as treatment is needed.

Principles for Fostering a Therapeutic Relationship

Although there is no formula for managing patients with RM, the guiding principle for developing a therapeutic relationship is collaborative care, where instead of merely prescribing care, the physician develops a treatment plan with participation of the patient.[25] Over time, through this relationship, the patient is encouraged to develop and implement self-management skills.

Evaluation

A useful perspective for providers includes recognition that the patient is an expert with regard to her own pain. Even though she seeks medical guidance and consultation, she appreciates being listened to and relies on the provider's scientific and clinical understanding of headache to help her. The provider is not, however, the expert of this patient's headache—she is. This is particularly true when there are no clearly defined evidence-based treatment guidelines or medical dictates to follow. Additionally it is important to begin the initial encounter with the understanding that important management issues can be targeted that positively impact clinical outcome even when the headache itself is not completely resolved.

Trust

A critical and sometimes most difficult step in managing a patient with RM is to develop a relationship based on trust and mutual respect. By creating an environment of encouragement, the stage is set for the patient to agree to enter into this relationship. Those with RM often have been through a litany of failed medical promises and sometimes have experienced conflict with medical providers. Refractory patients frequently view the medical profession with skepticism, sometimes justifiably so. Early in the therapeutic relationship, it may be useful to acknowledge the patient's frustration and fear over trying another treatment program. Likewise the healthcare professional may want to voice concerns and expectations in initiating a therapeutic relationship. The patient can benefit from reassurance that she will neither be blamed nor abandoned if her migraines persist. The doctor will be evaluating, "what are we missing," rather than "what are you doing wrong." In this way, trust is built and the pursuit of wellness is shared by the partners.

A pitfall for the physician can be overly emphasizing that a "new" treatment will be effective when from the patient's viewpoint many "new" treatments already have proven ineffective. Indeed this is a slippery slope because the clinician wants to convey hope and optimism. But with each subsequent failure, there looms an increasing likelihood of diminishing return from future interventions. A more effective approach might be to prescribe a new therapy as a component of a larger care plan and to acknowledge the patient's frustration without blame for past treatment failures. Also this is a good time to begin exploring how (and if) the patient might define success if the headache cannot be stopped, such as pursuing functional improvements despite headache and limiting disability.

Setting Goals

Goal setting is paramount. Goals need to be obtainable and ethically agreeable to you as well as the patient. The refractory patient often has learned to live with two goals, the pain is either better or it is worse but it never goes away. To turn around this self-defeating dynamic, the focus is not on pain but on behaviors. What would the migraineur like to accomplish? The goals need to be measurable and obtainable. Perhaps the individual wants to be able to sleep more than four hours a night. Management would revolve around helping her develop skills to attain that goal.

The disconnect between goals of the provider and the patient with RM often occur because of divergent expectations. A healthcare provider is trained to prioritize the patient's complaints based on their seriousness and treatability. But with refractory pain both of these factors may come into question. Motivational guidance may have little direct relationship to the medical condition but instead provides a behavioral option at which the patient can readily succeed. For example, it is tempting to focus on a patient's need for weight loss, smoking cessation, or a structured exercise program. However, these large (albeit important) goals may need to be deferred initially to avoid yet another failure for the patient. The initial behavioral prescription may be as simple as drinking three 8-ounce glasses of water a day to rehydrate. After keeping a diary for 2 weeks, indicating to the doctor that indeed she was able to accomplish drinking more water, she may be ready to tackle a more complex goal, such as walking to the mailbox to get her mail. Pride in accomplishing small goals often sets the stage for improved self-efficacy and adherence over time and change the medical dynamic from facing failure to charting success. Ideally, goals need objective endpoints and to be assessed repeatedly over time (even after success is achieved).

Another subtle inroad toward health is to focus on the positive. Ask the patient to keep a diary recording days she feels normal, instead of those she has a headache, and to measure her comfort level, rather than pain intensity, on a scale of 1 to 10. During future appointments, the doctor makes a point of reviewing in detail the diary, asking for clarification about why she felt more comfortable one day but much less comfortable the next. Helping the person link behaviors with comfort reinterprets for her the actions she can perform to lessen the intensity of the headache.

Setting Boundaries

Physicians are not necessarily trained to trust patients. They have been trained to believe that information from a patient must be filtered through them to reach the truth. There also is an inherent fear of being "tricked" by an unscrupulous patient. Although no clear assurance exists for detecting a person intent on dishonesty, engaging the relationship in small steps with an open mind and the goal of success is a good beginning. Reassurance can be gained through use of tools such as a written contract, providing clear rules of your practice, or providing quantities of medication that last only for a week rather than 3 months. A key to successful implementation is that when you provide these guidelines, be certain that you and your staff adhere to them.

Biopsychosocial Model

The biopsychosocial model explains disease as a complex interaction between biology and the environment, both internal and external.[26] In the context of migraine, even though there is a biological basis for the disease, the attack is believed to occur with triggering events that interact with a person's biology. In episodic migraine, triggering events appear to be relatively discrete and linked by a short interval of time to the event of migraine. With chronification of migraine, the ability to define discrete triggers may not be possible. What does become apparent is that RM produces life consequences of living with a chronic pain condition. There is disruption in nearly all domains of an individual's function, biological, behavioral, psychological, and social.

In management of patients with RM, the biopsychosocial model becomes a useful clinical tool for allowing patients and providers to define interactions between biology and environment and to develop management strategies beyond the headache itself. This model can provide an understandable avenue to explore, define, and work with the patient to ameliorate psychosocial factors while still confirming a biological basis for migraine. This can improve a patient's quality of life and may improve the underlying headache pattern. Utilizing this model evolves over time and readies the patient for change. Ideally most components will be addressed as part of the treatment plan.

This model also helps explain the value of interdisciplinary care to patients. It readily allows integration of psychologists, physical therapists, and other healthcare providers while assuring that the medical nature of the RM will be addressed. Treatment plans eventually can expand to address important biological factors such as sleep and diet, behavioral factors such as taking on too many responsibilities or believing anything less than perfection is failure, and social factors such as fear of being alone or losing a job.

Finally, it is valuable to impress upon the patient that RM did not develop in a day and that recovery likewise will take time. Intensity of treatment needs to be matched with the patient's intensity of need. Ultimately, healthcare professionals and patients benefit from energy and ingenuity.

Case Study 19-1

Donna is a 34-year-old Caucasian female who has suffered headache and insomnia since childhood. She first sought treatment in her early 20s and was diagnosed with migraine. Headache initially improved with abortive treatment. However, after the birth of her second child her migraine frequency increased from one or two to three or four attacks per month and her response to abortive treatment deteriorated. She was started on a prophylactic tricyclic antidepressant which improved sleep but did not significantly alter the frequency of migraine. She was referred for neurological consultation and had a normal magnetic resonance imaging (MRI) scan with and without contrast. The tricyclic was replaced with topiramate, the dosage eventually increased to 200 mg per day. There was no improvement in migraine frequency and she required at least nine doses of a triptan per month (headache and medication use confirmed by diary).

Migraine continued to increase in frequency and became chronic about 6 years ago during a time her husband threatened divorce. She was referred to a headache specialist who repeated an MRI and performed a spinal tap. Both were normal. She was diagnosed with migraine without aura and medication overuse headache. The topiramate was discontinued. She was started on propanolol and referred to a psychologist. She gained 20 pounds and became depressed over the subsequent 9 months. The propanolol was discontinued and she was prescribed an antidepressant and calcium channel blocker. She used the emergency department on occasion and made several unscheduled office visits per month to her primary care physician asking for a "shot." Approximately 2 years ago, her primary care physician and neurologist advised her there was nothing more they could do for her and she should find another doctor. The psychologist reported that primary issues in Donna's marriage have been her husband's lackadaisical attitude and his acceptance of her only if she put on a "happy face." For example, he forgot their 8th wedding anniversary but when she expressed her hurt over this, he refused to talk to her for 3 weeks. She keeps a headache diary faithfully, and her diaries confirm adherence to physician recommendations, failure at multiple acute and preventive pharmacological interventions, failure of dietary recommendations and prescribed exercise and weight loss program.

Last year she was hospitalized with intractable migraine and suicidal ideation. She was treated with repetitive doses of dihydroergotamine, intravenous valproic acid, and an increase of her antidepressant. Posthospitalization use of abortive medication was discontinued for 12 weeks which was monitored and confirmed by random drug testing and her diary. Through this time period her headache pattern worsened, and she was eventually placed on a medical leave of absence from her employment. Since then her abortive medication was restarted with a nine-tablet limit of triptan per month and additional naproxen as needed; her preventive treatment was a selective serotonin reuptake inhibitor (SSRI) to treat depression, which she reports has improved. She has been able to return to work but continues with nearly daily migraine.

For 20 years she worked for a federal agency and has reached the position of supervisor. But in her office, "I can't complete a thought without someone popping in asking for help. I'm worn down. I can't take it anymore." She was referred for long term management with a diagnosis of RM. After complete evaluation of the patient and her medical record, the diagnosis of RM was confirmed. She has insurance and a pharmacy benefit plan but frequently has been denied specific medications or had quantity limits placed on their use.

The first issue to understand and build on is the motivation of the patient in seeking further medical consultation. In the case presented here, Donna wanted the headaches to go away. Without headaches, she believed that other areas of her life such as her marriage, employment, and family would improve. She was frustrated by the repeated empty promises of previous providers that a "pill" will resolve her headaches. When the pill didn't work, she felt as if it was her fault, somehow associated with a failing marriage or depression or not trying hard enough to get better. "What a Catch 22," she stated. She reported feeling angry and hurt that her primary care physician discharged her from care and implied she was simply seeking drugs to avoid her marriage problems. She insisted she only wanted relief from a headache so severe that she "couldn't take it anymore."

Barriers to a Therapeutic Relationship

This case produces a quandary for the healthcare professional because the diagnosis is straightforward but the management issues are complex. In order for the clinician to construct a plan for management with the patient, various prognostic indicators and barriers to management need to be assessed. These include questions about the patient's medication usage, adherence with treatment plans, the presence of a personality disorder, potential secondary gain from pain, and readiness for change. Highlights in this early clinical assessment were:

I. Medication Usage and Drug Seeking?

Despite Donna's overuse of prescription medication, it appears that she takes medicine in an effort to help her function and find relief rather than to alter her consciousness. In fact, she seems to be overly conscientious about medication usage rather than demanding more. She endured 12 weeks without acute treatment believing her headache pattern might improve.

(continued)

II. Noncompliant?

Adherence was assessed and managed through regular collection and review of the headache and medication diary, objective drug testing, and dose limits imposed by insurance. Donna very much wants help. She feels as if she's falling apart and knows something has to change. She cannot relax because her mind races. In fact, trying to relax actually increases her anxiety. She considers relaxation a waste of time and engaging in it will only further subtract from her already meager list of daily accomplishments. She needs training in biofeedback but readiness for this intervention will require time and reorientation.

III. Personality Disorder?

An individual with a personality disorder projects blame onto those around her and assumes no responsibility for her behaviors. With this perception, alterations in coping mechanisms would be unlikely because such a person feels victimized and unable to grasp control of what happens to her. Donna, by contrast, is highly responsible to the point where she internalizes others' negative feelings and tries to solve people's problems for them as noted in her discussion in her home and work environment.

IV. Secondary Gain from Pain?

Do frequent headaches provide Donna with extra attention or an excuse for not reaching her goals? Although history included a medical leave from work, Donna was able to return to work. There is little evidence on the surface that this is true as she rarely misses work or draws attention from her husband because of the headaches. One could argue that she finds solace in pain but there is little objective evidence of secondary gain garnered from her clinical presentation.

V. Readiness to Change?

As discussed earlier, change is a process. There are stages that can be defined for readiness to consciously engage the change process that are useful in motivating and assisting patients to succeed. However, change is only rarely linear; more often it is a process characterized by stutters and falters. It is important to prepare the patient for the "ride" of change. She appears to be in the precontemplative state of the readiness for change model.

In this case, Donna certainly has low self-efficacy for change and appeared initially to be resistant to change. She could not see an opportunity to change her circumstance until her headache was resolved. To welcome change to her was to admit defeat which is unacceptable. She has not yet made a definite commitment to change. This black and white thinking will need to be modulated and reinterpreted over time. She will undoubtedly require psychological intervention.

VI. Donna's Outcome

Donna's clinical course was one of slow but progressive improvement over a 9-month period. Today, she continues with frequent migraine but the impact of the RM has decreased significantly and her utilization of healthcare resources has lessened dramatically. She has integrated many behavioral strategies into her daily life that allow her to enjoy and participate with activities of importance to her. She continues with regular medical follow up as well as with her psychologist. She and her husband are in relationship counseling and both feel this has had a positive effect on their marriage and ability to enjoy one another. Like all patients with RM, there is hope of a future where better understandings and therapeutics might someday control her migraines.

Case Study 19-2

Christy is a 13-year-old Caucasian female 8th grader. She has two older half-siblings who attend college away from home. During the last month of 7th grade, Christy's migraine increased in frequency and intensity, forcing her to miss 3 to 4 school days per week. She underwent multiple exhaustive medical evaluations with normal neurological examinations and imaging studies. Despite various trials of preventive and acute pharmacology, her underlying migraine pattern remained unchanged. She continued with significant school absenteeism. When at home with a migraine, she and her mother would watch soap operas or play cards or she would withdraw and sleep in her room. On weekends when she traveled with her parents or during the summer vacation, her migraine frequency diminished to once or twice a month. A psychological evaluation suggested she was using headaches to avoid school and separation from her mother.

On entering junior high school, after migraines became refractory to abortive and preventive treatment, she was referred to an interdisciplinary headache center. Medical and neurological re-examinations were normal. She was tried on repetitive dihydroergotamine (DHE) and IV valproic acid without benefit. During her psychological evaluation, it was noted that her mother answered all the questions for Christy. The psychologist separated Christy from her mother for future medical and psychological appointments and used biofeedback to aid her in developing a sense of physical and psychological self-awareness. Consultation was arranged for the parents with a family therapist who was familiar with the interdisciplinary model used by the clinic.

(continued)

Barriers to the Therapeutic Relationship

This case presents the difficulty of treating a child when a parent's behavior is an integral component of the problem. The same list of prognostic indicators and barriers to a therapeutic relationship were assessed.

I. Medication Usage and Drug Seeking?

There is no evidence that Christy is seeking drugs. She is not engaged in drug seeking behavior and on the contrary understands that medication doesn't help her headaches.

II. Noncompliant?

Christy's stance is passive. She misses her friends at school and realizes she is falling behind in her schoolwork. Repeatedly however, she takes the path of least resistance by staying home with her mother whom she sees as alone and in need of support. Psychologically, theirs is a codependent relationship, lacking a healthy boundary between parent and child.

III. Personality Disorder?

A personality disorder cannot be diagnosed until the individual is 15 years of age. However, without changing her behavior, she's on her way to developing symptoms of a dependent personality disorder.

IV. Secondary Gain from Pain?

Christy is receiving secondary gain though the biology of her disease should not be discounted in the presence of a psychological diagnosis. She does receive extra attention for suffering from migraine from parents, teachers, friends, and the medical professionals. Her parents plan special weekend escapes with her, knowing that her headaches improve with these excursions. Last fall she was put into a special class for students with medical problems and discovered, much to her surprise, that she wasn't as "bad off" as those with head injury, heart problems, cancer, or other diseases. The next semester she chose to return to her regular classroom. Exposure of an individual to the reality of her situation often begins a process of normalization and is valuable in defining a pathway to success.

V. Readiness to Change?

Why should she? Other than the headaches, she likes the arrangement. There is obvious reinforcement for illness in this case. Likely, Christy would be classified as in a "precontemplative" phase and not thinking about changing her behavior. Both Christy and her parents need to be guided into establishing consequences to her missing school, and understand that staying at home is not allowing her the normal growth and development for an adolescent. This can assist both parent and child to accept needed change. The problem involves the family system and will benefit from family therapy.

The physician plays a major role in regular follow-up appointments to reevaluate Christy's status and to emphasize to Christy and her parents the importance of attending school regularly, socializing with friends, and continuing with a family therapist.

Summary

The person with RM is a challenge because she often is desperate to find relief yet feels hopeless of finding an end to her pain. She may have experienced repeated failures and has lost confidence in herself and the medical system. But the therapeutic relationship offers an atmosphere of trust and an expectation that the problem is a puzzle that may be solved one piece at a time. The endpoint is overall improvement, not necessarily a cure. Goal setting becomes designing an individualized clinical study with an *N* of 1 that objectively tests the effectiveness of therapeutic interventions and monitors the patient's motivation and adherence to agreed upon goals of therapy.

Key Points

Barrier to Adherence

1. Complex treatment regime
2. Psychiatric comorbidity
3. Psychological factors
4. Characteristics of clinic or relationship with clinician

Patient's Health Behaviors Change When:

1. Ready for change
2. Change judged as important
3. Confident in ability to change (self-efficacy)

Stages of Change

1. Precontemplation: Not thinking about changing behavior
2. Contemplation: Thinking about changing behavior
3. Preparation: Beginning to make changes slowly

(continued)

4. Action: Actively engaged in change
5. Maintenance: Maintaining change

Motivational Interviewing

1. Express empathy.
2. Identify discrepancy between patient's behavior and goal.
3. Empathize with resistance of patient.
4. Support self-efficacy.

Expectations of RM Patient

1. I will be listened to.
2. I will get answers.
3. I can trust my clinician.
4. I want to return to normal.

Prognostic Indicators

1. Medication usage and drug seeking
2. Nonadherent
3. Personality disorder
4. Secondary gain from pain
5. Readiness to change

References

1. O'Dowd T. Five years of heart sink patients in general practice. *BMJ.* 1988; 297:528–530.
2. Haynes RB, McDonald H, Garg AX, Montague P. Interventions for helping patients to follow prescriptions for medications. *Cochran.* 2002;3:1–55.
3. Rains JC, Lipchik GA, Penzien DB. Behavioral facilitation of medical treatment for headache—Part I: Review of headache treatment compliance. *Headache.* 2006;46(9):1387–1394.
4. Hoodin F, Brines BJ, Lake AE 3rd, Wilson J, Saper JR. Behavioral self-management in an inpatient headache treatment unit: increasing adherence and relationship to changes in affective distress. *Headache.* 2000;40(5): 377–383.
5. Ottervanger JP, Valkenburg HA, Grobbee DE, Stricker BH. Pattern of sumatriptan use and overuse in general practice. *Eur J Clin Pharmacol.* 1996;50(5):353–355.
6. Cupini LM, Calabresi P. Medication-overuse headache: pathophysiological insights. *J Headache Pain.* 2005;6(4):199–202.
7. Foleyw KA, Cady R, Martin V, Adelman J, Diamond M, Bell CF, Dayno JM, Hu XH. Treating early versus treating mild: timing of migraine prescription medications among patients with diagnosed migraine. *Headache.* 2005;45(5):538–545.

8. Cady RK, Lipton RB, Hall C, Stewart WF, O'Quinn S, Gutterman D. Treatment of mild headache in disabled sufferers: results of the Spectrum Study. *Headache.* 2000;40:792–797.
9. Spierings EL, Miree LF. Non-compliance with follow-up and improvement after treatment at a headache center. *Headache.* 1993;33(4):205–209.
10. Gallagher RM, Kunkel R. Migraine medication attributes important for patient compliance: Concerns about side effects may delay treatment. *Headache.* 2003;43:36–43.
11. Garber MC, Nau DP, Erickson SR, Aikens JE, Lawrence JB. The concordance of self report with other measures of medication adherence: a summary of the literature. *Med Care.* 2004;42(7):649–652.
12. Mulleners WM, Whitmarsh TE, Steiner TJ. Noncompliance may render migraine prophylaxis useless, but once-daily regimens are better. *Cephalalgia.* 1998;18(1):52–56.
13. Radat F, Creac'h C, Swendsen JD, Lafittau M., Irachabal S, Dousset V, Henry P. Psychiatric comorbidity in the evolution from migraine to medication overuse headache. *Cephalalgia.* 2005;25:519–522.
14. Saper JR, Hamel RL, Lake AE. Medication overuse headache (MOH) is a biobehavioural disorder. *Cephalalgia.* 2005;25:545–546.
15. Lipton RB, Stewart WF. Acute migraine therapy: Do doctors understand what patients with migraine want from therapy? *Headache.* 1999; 39(Suppl 2):S20–S26.
16. Lipton RB, Hahn SR, Cady RK, et al. In-office discussions of migraine: results from the American Migraine Communication Study. *J Gen Intern Med.* 2008;23:1145–1151.
17. Miller W R, Rollnick S. *Motivational Interviewing: Preparing People for Change,* 2nd ed. New York: Guilford;2002.
18. Prochaska JO, DiClemente CC. Towards a comprehensive, transtheoretical model of change: states of change and addictive behaviors. In: Miller WR, Heather N, eds. *Applied Clinical Psychology,* 2nd ed. *Treating Addictive Behaviors.* New York: Plenum Press;1998:3–24.
19. Prochaska JO. Decision making in the transtheoretical model of behavior change. *Med Decis Making.* 2008;28:845–849.
20. Stephenson BJ, Rowe BH, Haynes RB, et al. Is this patient taking the treatment as prescribed? *JAMA.* 1993;269:2779–2781.
21. Rains JC, Penzien DB, Lipchik GA. Behavioral facilitation of medical treatment for headache—Part II: Theoretical models and behavioral strategies for improving adherence. *Headache.* 2006;46(9):1395–1403.
22. Macharia WM, Leon G, Rowe BH, Stephenson BJ, Haynes RB. An overview of interventions to improve compliance with appointment keeping for medical services. *JAMA.* 1992;267(13):1813–1817.
23. Holroyd KA, Cordingley GE, Pingel JD, Jerome A, Theofanous AG, Jackson DK, Leard L. Enhancing the effectiveness of abortive therapy: a controlled evaluation of self-management training. *Headache.* 1989;29(3):148–153.
24. Rollnick S, Miller WR, Butler CC. *Motivational Interviewing in Health Care: Helping Patients Change Behavior.* New York: Guilford Press;2008.
25. Lipton RB, Cady RK, Farmer K, Bigal ME. *Managing Migraine: A Healthcare Professional's Guide to Collaborative Migraine Care.* Hamilton, Canada: Baxter Publishing; 2008.

26. Andrasik F, Flor H, Turk DC. An expanded view of psychological aspects in head pain: the biopsychosocial model. *Neurol Sci.* 2005;26:S87–S91.
27. Penzien DB, Rains JC, Lipchik GL, Creer TL. Behavioral interventions for tension-type headache: overview of current therapies and recommendation for a self-management model for chronic headache. *Curr Pain Headache Rep.* 2004;8(6):489–499.

20

Emerging Therapies in Refractory Headache

Nabih M. Ramadan, MD, MBA, FAAN, FAHS

Introduction

Effective therapies for illnesses and disorders are discovered by serendipity or through targeted drug development programs. The latter assumes (1) an accepted and operational definition of the disorder when based on a constellation of symptoms-complex and in the absence of psychometric robust surrogates or biomarkers; and (2) distinct understanding of illness mechanisms and means of modeling the illness, its symptoms or its biological basis in the laboratory (clinical, basic or both). Unfortunately, both prerequisites are lacking in this disorder. Indeed, a recent study highlighted the absence of a widely recognized definition or criteria for refractory migraine (RM), as well as the disagreement on a proposed definition.[1] The authors found that failure of response to optimal and therapeutic doses of two or more preventative therapies was not accepted universally. Others argued similarly and defined intractability when patients failed adequate doses of "all drugs considered as first line therapy for episodic migraine by International guidelines.[2] Further, the mechanisms of RM remain elusive, particularly when there is little understanding of the process of chronification or the etiologies that underlie refractoriness to medical management. To this end, Goadsby and Hargreaves attempted to dissect the mechanisms of RM by providing answers to (1) a genetic basis; (2) structural underpinning; (3) CNS physiological dysfunction; and (4) a pharmacological derangement.[3] The authors acknowledged that answers to these questions are not available. Until then, emerging therapeutics for refractory or intractable migraine are advanced on the basis of our understanding of (1) episodic migraine mechanisms; (2) theories of refractoriness that are borrowed from the chronic pain fields; and (3) clinical observations based on level III studies (e.g., case reports, retrospective analysis). Consequently, proposed therapies for RM that are discussed in this chapter are largely based on level III evidence, and are not based on rigorous clinical trials or pivotal studies that form the basis for United States Food and Drug Administration (FDA) drug approval for the stated indication. Also, it should be noted that publication bias against negative trials and reporting failed interventions[4] perhaps are more pronounced when nonrandomized controlled studies (RCT) are conducted. Therefore, this chapter provides an overview of published interventions for RM, which at best should be hypothesis generators for further studies. Further, the chapter concerns resistance or refractoriness to preventive therapy, which forms the basis of intractability. The treatment of acute migraine attacks that prove resistant to conventional abortive agents is covered elsewhere. Lastly, only pharmacological approaches are discussed because neurostimulation techniques and invasive procedures such as closure of patent foramen ovale (PFO) are highlighted briefly and the readers are referred to other chapters of this book for details.

Underpinning of Refractoriness: A Difficult Road Ahead in Search of Best Practice

Merriam-Webster online defines refractory as "resistant to treatment or cure." This simple definition is conceivable easily, at least relatively, in oncological medicine when tumor load cannot be reduced adequately with chemotherapeutic agents. This situation is similar in infectious diseases when resistant or refractory refers to a therapeutically relevant bactericidal concentration that cannot be achieved in killing bacterial cells. Illnesses that are defined only by symptoms, symptoms-complex, or operational criteria that are based on clinical observations, and in the absence of replicable and valid biomarkers or surrogates, pose a much more difficult challenge. Unfortunately, migraine is a disorder that falls under the latter category, that is, it is defined on operational criteria and lacks valid and reliable biological markers. Consequently, the underpinning of refractoriness is not discernable with certainty.

Several factors contribute to medical refractoriness. Readers are referred to earlier chapters in this book for a broader discussion of this subject but some highlights are worth noting. Causes of refractoriness include, but are not limited to:

- Biological changes that render an otherwise effective drug ineffective for a particular patient or group of patients, i.e., pharmacological resistance
- Genetic alterations that result in treatment resistance

- Iatrogenic factors wherein the effect of a drug or intervention is minimized or eliminated by concomitant therapies
- Environmental factors that alter the biological response to a previously demonstrated effective treatment
- Erratic adherence to treatment recommendations, i.e., noncompliance.,
- Dynamic nature of an illness. Migraine is not a static disorder, although we often assume it is, and therefore response to treatment varies throughout the course of the disorder
- Individualized responses to the administration of a drug, i.e., individual pharmacokinetics (PK)

Evidence-based medicine (EBM) teaches us that a particular therapeutic intervention could be generalized to a patient population with rigorously conducted RCTs when individual heterogeneities are minimized. I posit that such a strategy is quite tasking in RM. Therefore, guidelines based on scientifically robust studies (e.g., RCT), which form the basis of EBM, can be forthcoming only when valid biological markers are identified for a cohort of migraineurs with similar profiles to refractoriness. To this end, suggested steps in the direction of finding effective treatment for RM are:

- Identification of surrogates or biomarkers that diagnose migraine and RM. It is to note that multiple profiles may be discovered during this quest
- Modeling of the surrogates in animal research
- Surrogate-based or biomarker-based targeted preclinical drug or device discovery
- Controlled clinical trials in a homogeneous RM population with similar biomarkers
- Avoidance of generalization from specific, typically phase 2 clinical trials in a homogenous population, to large phase 3 trials that introduce marked heterogeneity that result in wide variability and a great potential for a dilutional effect. In other words, drug development for RM may require alterations in conventional strategies of clinical drug development[5]
- N-of-1 randomized clinical trials

It is gleaned from the aforementioned discussion that treatment of RM should conform to the principles of EBM. However, the author of this chapter, who is a student of EBM, recognizes that EBM should guide, and not dictate, *individualized* therapy, a concept which is particularly relevant in RM.

Pharmacological Approach to RM

This section highlights published studies that detail RM treatment. Such studies were identified on a Pub-Med Search with "refractory" or "resistant" or "intractable" and "migraine" as MeSH. Further, the clinical experience of the author is mentioned occasionally in the absence of rigorously conducted RCTs.

Targets at Reducing Long-Term Potentiation

Glutamate Modulators

Migraine is posited as a state of neuronal hyperexcitability, which becomes more pronounced in chronic states.[6] Consequently, targets at blocking excitation may have relevance in RM.

Glutamate is the main excitatory amino-acid neurotransmitter in the mammalian central nervous system (CNS). Glutamate binds to diverse receptors (GluR) that are distributed diffusely in the CNS. These include ligand-gated ion channels (ionotropic or iGluR) and G-protein coupled receptors (GPCR- metabotropic or mGluR).[7,8] The classical iGluR is the *N*-methyl-D-aspartate receptor (NMDAR), which exists in different subtypes (NR1, NR2A-D, NR3). α-Amino-3-hydroxy-5-methyl-4-isoxazolepropionic acid (AMPA) and kainate (KA) are the other iGluR subtype proteins.

NMDAR antagonists have been used widely in diverse CNS diseases and illnesses, notably in chronic pain. Memantine is a nonselective NMDAR with proven efficacy in neuropathic pain and in Alzheimer's disease (primary indication in the United States). A role for memantine in refractory migraine is increasingly investigated. Charles et al. retrospectively surveyed patients with frequent migraine who received 5 to 20 mg of memantine for at least 2 months and observed greater than 60% improvement in headache-related disability.[9] The findings from this retrospective study were duplicated in a pilot prospective study of 28 patients with refractory migraine whose mean disability scores were significantly improved 3-month post-treatment with 10 to 20 mg of memantine.[10] The author of this chapter has experienced mixed successes with memantine in patients with chronic and refractory migrainous headaches. Notwithstanding, the case of a 28-year-old patient is worth highlighting.

Case Study

A 28-year-old Caucasian woman presented to a headache specialty clinic with symptoms of severe migrainous headaches and vertigo that were most pronounced during menstruation and which have been resistant to a multitude of conventional migraine preventative drugs and at adequate doses. The patient observed that rubbing the skin just anterior to the left auricular tragus would exacerbate her symptoms, particularly the vertiginous feeling. On the assumption that the symptoms-complex represents (1) peripheral hypersensitivity of the cutaneous branch of the vagal nerve (Arnold nerve), which terminates in the nucleus of the spinal trigeminal tract; (2) activity-dependent and -independent central sensitization of the trigeminal nucleus caudalis (TNC); and (3) existence of TNC-vestibular nucleus connections that lead to ipsilateral vestibular activation with subsequent sensation of vertigo, the patient was treated with the application of topical 5% lidocaine (peripheral sensitization blocker) over the course of the Arnold nerve along with daily memantine 10 mg orally (central sensitization blocker). Several months after treatment with this combination, the patient reported a subjective 70% improvement in overall function.

Targets at Enhancing Long-Term Depression

GABA Enhancers

Sensory input into the dorsal horn and the trigeminal system is associated with collateral activation of inhibitory neurons that release γ-aminobutyric acid (GABA) into the synaptic cleft with the resultant recurrent inhibition of postsynaptic second order cells (chloride-induced hyperpolarization via $GABA_A$ receptors; potassium-mediated hyperpolarization by acting on $GABA_B$ receptors). Valproic acid, which indirectly increases GABA activity, is a well established drug for episodic migraine prevention.[11] Its GABA-enhancing role is thought to be related to a presynaptic inhibition of GABA aminotransferase and an increased response to GABA postsynaptically.

The role of valproate in refractory migraine was suggested in a small open-label trial with a response rate (reduction in headache frequency) of greater than 60%.[12] Its combination with other anti-migraine agents such as non-steroidal anti-inflammatory drugs (NSAIDs), tricyclic antidepressants or β-adrenergic blockers may be considered but it is likely that such a polytherapeutic approach will be associated with untoward side effects.

Targets at Restoring Anti-nociceptive Mechanisms

Dopamine Antagonists

Atypical antipsychotics such as quetiapine and olanzapine possess some pharmacological properties that may be operant in nociception and hyperalgesia (e.g., D1 and D2 receptors). A retrospective chart review of 50 patients with chronic headaches who have failed at least four standard preventative drugs indicated that daily 2.5 to 35 mg of olanzapine may be effective in improving headache days and daily pain scores.[13] Side effects, particularly weight gain, were common. The author of this chapter has used the combination of olanzapine 10 mg and topiramate 200 mg in one male patient with chronic refractory migraine; success has been limited.

Recently, results of an open-label study of quetiapine were published.[14] Patients ($n = 34$) who failed atenolol (60 mg/day), nortriptyline (25 mg/day), and flunarizine (3 mg/day) in combination were placed on a titrating regimen of quetiapine (up to 75 mg) and prospectively studied. Ten weeks post treatment, 22/29 reported marked improvement in headache frequency and almost one third of patients had adverse events.

Ion-Channel Modulators (e.g., Nav and Cav)

Gabapentinoids

Gabapentin, pregabalin, and XP13512—a gabapentin prodrug in clinical development for migraine prevention) regulate intracellular calcium influx by modulation of the non-pore- forming a2d subunit of the P/Q type calcium channel,[15] which results in reduced extracellular release of glutamate and blunted activation of AMPA receptors on noradrenergic nerve terminals.[16] The proof of effectiveness of gabapentinoids in episodic migraine is limited and only anecdotal use in combination with other treatments is suggested in patients with RM.

Mexiletine

Mexiletine is a class I anti-arrhythmic oral analogue of lidocaine with some evidence for efficacy in chronic pain states.[17] The anti-nociceptive mechanism of mexiletine is thought to be use-dependent blockade of voltage-gated Na^+ neuronal channels.[18] A recent clinic-based study of nine patients with chronic refractory headaches including migraine indicated that daily 600 to 1500 mg mexiletine offers an alternative therapeutic approach to more conventional anti-migraine agents.[19] The author of this chapter has used up to 600 mg oral mexiletine as a short-term (up to 2 weeks) bridge therapy in patients with chronic RM while being withdrawn from medication overuse.

Cinnarizine

Cinnarizine is a wide-spectrum calcium entry blocker – with activities at N-, P, Q- and L-channels–, a histamine type-1 (H1) receptor antagonist, and a dopamine type-2 (D2) antagonist that is commonly used for motion sickness outside of the United States. Following open-label studies, investigators evaluated the role of cinnarizine in patients with chronic and refractory migraine.[20] More than 100 patients who were "refractory" to propranolol and various antidepressants were randomized to receive either cinnarizine or valproate for 8 to 12 weeks. Results of the trial indicated that both medications were comparable in efficacy. Also, the authors reported an acceptable tolerability profile. Sedation and extrapyramidal adverse effects are encountered while using drugs of this category (e.g., flunarizine, dotarizine).

Drugs with Multiple Pharmacological Activities

Topiramate

Topiramate is an antiepileptic drug (AED) with diverse neuromodulatory functions including (1) inhibition of AMPA/KA receptors; (2) potentiation of GABA activity; and (3) blockade of voltage-dependent Na-channels, as well as L- and N-calcium channels.[21] Topiramate has demonstrated efficacy in episodic[22,23] and in chronic migraine.[24] However, the role of topiramate in chronic and refractory migraine patients remains elusive. Pascual et al. reported data on an open label study of topiramate in patients who have failed, or have not tolerated, at least one conventional migraine preventive drug.[25] At a median dose of 100 mg, approximately 60% reported a favorable outcome. The absence of relevant study details, particularly with respect to the number of patients who have failed multiple treatments at adequate doses, and the open nature of the trial are factors that would not allow us to draw firm conclusions. The author of this chapter often uses topiramate in refractory migraine but not as a monotherapeutic agent; it is combined with other conventional anti-migraine preventive drugs, particularly propranolol.

Zonisamide

Zonisamide is a sulfonamide broad spectrum AED with similar pharmacological activities to topiramate. Recently, it has been suggested that zonisamide may be effective in refractory migraine when topiramate is ineffective.[26] The authors reported that zonisamide reduces headache frequency, pain severity, and use of acute migraine medication in a cohort of more than 60 patients who were refractory to topiramate. Doses of up to 400 mg were used in this open label and uncontrolled trial. Similar conclusions have been drawn when other small uncontrolled trials were conducted.[27] Expert opinion with zonisamide in refractory migraine is limited because this AED remains relatively new on the market.

Devices and Invasive Procedures

Several nonpharmacological approaches to the treatment of RM have been suggested (Table 20.1). The level of evidence supporting the use of such interventions in refractory migraine is marginal except for closure of patent foramen ovale where there is good evidence for the lack of efficacy of PFO closure in refractory migraine.

Table 20-1 Devices/interventions and preventive migraine therapy

Procedure	Level of evidence[a]
NTI-tss	Level V. One RCT, J adad score of 1
VNS	Level V. No controlled trails
PFO	Level II.evidence of lack of efficacy
ONS	Level IV.One RCT (reported As Abstract)

[a]Level I = Conclusive; Level II = strong; Level III = moderate; Level IV = limited; Level V = indeteminate (Manchikanti et al., 2007). NTI-tss = nociceptive trigeminal inhibition, tensor suppression system, VNS = vagal nerve stimulation, PFO = patent foramen ovale, ONS = occipital nerve stimulation.

Future Directions

Refractory migraine is a condition that is receiving more due attention in recent years, partly because of its marked individual and societal impacts. Attempts at defining the different phenotypic expressions of this condition are first steps towards finding effective therapies. Perhaps, it is simplistic to assume homogeneity among patients with refractory migraine and therefore clinical trials in this condition should stratify patients by similar phenotypic profiles and more importantly by genotype, if available. Concurrently, biomarkers should be advanced in an effort to define RM better. Once these clinical trial development strategies are in place, therapeutic options should be tested using standard and scientifically sound methods (e.g., RCT). The approach to clinical trials with single agent trials, although relevant in episodic and some forms of chronic migraine, is probably futile in refractory migraine. Combination therapies using drugs acting at different targets of the migraine mechanisms spectrum[28] should be explored as early as it is possible.

Chapter Highlights

- Refractory migraine is a heterogeneous condition in search of a unified taxonomy.
- Rational polypharmacy is a recommended approach to managing patients with refractory migraine.
- Neuromodulators such as the newer antiepileptic drugs and N-methyl D-aspartate glutamate receptor blockers are options for refractory migraine; they have shown promise in uncontrolled trials.
- Atypical antipsychotics may have a role in refractory migraine but limited evidence combined with frequent adverse events mitigate against recommending such agents except when all else fails.

References

1. Schulman EA, Peterlin BL, Lake AE III, Lipton RB, Hanlon A, Siegel S, Levin M, Goadsby PJ, Markley HG. Defining refractory migraine: results of the RHSIS Survey of American Headache Society members. *Headache.* 2009;49:509.

2. D'Amico D. Leone M, Grazzi L, Bussone G. When should "chronic migraine" patients be considered "refractory" to pharmacological prophylaxis? *J Neurol Sci.* 2008 May;29 Suppl 1:S55-8.
3. Goadsby PJ, Hargreaves R. Refractory migraine and chronic migraine: pathophysiological mechanisms. *Headache.* 2008;48:1399–1405.
4. Olson CM, Rennie D, Cook D, Dickersin K, Flanagin A, Hogan JW, Zhu Q, Reiling J, Pace B. Publication bias in editorial decision making. *JAMA.* 2002; 287:2825–2828.
5. Sheiner LB. Learning versus confirming in clinical drug development. *Clin Phamacol Ther.* 1997;61:275–291.
6. Welch KM. Brain hyperexcitability: the basis for antiepileptic drugs in migraine prevention. *Headache.* 2005;45(Suppl 1):S25–32.
7. Ramadan, NM. The link between glutamate and migraine. *CNS Spectr* 2003;8:446–449.
8. Vikelis M, Mitsikostas DD. The role of glutamate and its receptors in migraine. *CNS Neurol Disord Drug Targets.* 2007;6:251–257.
9. Charles A, Flippen C, Romero Reyes M, Brennan KC. Memantine for prevention of migraine: a retrospective study of 60 cases. *J Headache Pain.* 2007;8:248–250.
10. Bigal M, Rapoport A, Sheftell F, Tepper D, Tepper S. Memantine in the preventive treatment of refractory migraine. *Headache* 2008;48:1337–1342.
11. Ramadan NM, Silberstein SD, Freitag FG, Gilbert TT, Frishberg BM. Evidence-based guidelines for migraine headache in the primary care setting: pharmacological management for prevention of migraine. April, 2000. Available at http://www.aan.com/professionals/practice/pdfs/gl0090.pdf (accessed 7/12/09)
12. Erdemoglu AK, Ozbakir S. Valproic acid in prophylaxis of refractory migraine. *Acta Neurol Scand.* 2000;102:354–358.
13. Silberstein SD, Peres MF, Hopkins MM, Shechter AL, Young WB, Rozen TD. Olanzapine in the treatment of refractory migraine and chronic daily headache. *Headache.* 2002;42:515–518.
14. Krymchantowski AV, Jevoux C. Quetiapine for the prevention of migraine refractory to the combination of atenolol + nortriptyline + flunarizine: an open pilot study. *Arq Neuropsiquiatr.* 2008;66:615–618.
15. Brown JP, Dissanayake VU, Briggs AR, Milic MR, Gee NS. Isolation of the [^{3}H]gabapentin-binding protein/alpha 2 delta Ca^{2+} channel subunit from porcine brain: development of a radioligand binding assay for alpha 2 delta subunits using [3H]leucine. *Ann Biochem.* 1998;255:236–243.
16. Fink K, Dooley DJ, Meder WP, Suman-Chauhan N, Duffy S, Clusmann H, Gothert M. Inhibition of neuronal Ca^{2+} influx by gabapentin and pregabalin in the human neocortex. *Neuropharmacology.* 2002;42:229–236.
17. Tremont-Lukats IW, Challapalli V, McNicol ED, Lau J, Carr DB. Systemic administration of local anesthetics to relieve neuropathic pain: a systematic review and meta-analysis. *Anesth Analg.* 2005;101:1738–1749.
18. Fozzard HA, Lee PJ, Lipkind GM. Mechanism of local anesthetic drug action on voltage-gated sodium channels. *Curr Pharm Des.* 2005;11: 2671–2686.
19. Marmura MJ, Passero FC Jr, Young WB. Mexiletine for refractory chronic daily headache: a report of nine cases. *Headache.* 2008;48:1506–1510.

20. Togha M, Rahmat Jirde M, Nilavari K, Ashrafian H, Razeghi S, Kohan L. Cinnarizine in refractory migraine prophylaxis: efficacy and tolerability. A comparison with sodium valproate. *J Headache Pain.* 2008;9:77–82.
21. Shank RP, Gardocki JF, Streeter AJ, Maryanoff BE. An overview of the preclinical aspects of topiramate: pharmacology, pharmacokinetics, and mechanism of action. *Epilepsia.* 2000;41(Suppl 1):S3–9.
22. Brandes JL, Saper JR, Diamond M, Couch JR, Lewis DW, Schmitt J, Neto W, Schwabe S, Jacobs D. Topiramate for migraine prevention: a randomized controlled trial. *JAMA.* 2004;291:965–973.
23. Silberstein SD, Neto W, Schmitt J, Jacobs D. MIGR-001 Study Group. Topiramate in migraine prevention: results of a large controlled trial. *Arch Neurol.* 2004;61:490–495.
24. Silberstein SD, Lipton RB, Dodick DW, Freitag FG, Ramadan N, Mathew N, Brandes JL, Bigal M, Saper J, Ascher S, Jordan DM, Greenberg SJ, Hulihan J; Topiramate Chronic Migraine Study Group. Efficacy and safety of topiramate for the treatment of chronic migraine: a randomized, double-blind, placebo-controlled trial. *Headache* 2007;47:170–180.
25. Pascual J, Sánchez del Rio M, Mateos V, Láinez JM, Hernández-Gallego J, Leira R, Jiménez MD. Topiramate for patients with refractory migraine: an observational, multicenter study in Spain. *Neurologia.* 2003;18:364–367.
26. Bermejo PE, Dorado R. Zonisamide for migraine prophylaxis in patients refractory to topiramate. in *Neuropharmacol* 2009;32:103–106.
27. Ashkenazi A, Benlifer A, Korenblit J, Silberstein SD. Zonisamide for migraine prophylaxis in refractory patients. *Cephalalgia.* 2006;26:1199–1202.
28. Pascual J, Rivas MT, Leira R. Testing the combination beta-blocker plus topiramate in refractory migraine. *Acta Neurol Scand.* 2007;115:81–83.
29. Manchikanti L, Boswell MV, Giordano J. Evidence-based interventional pain management: principles, problems, potential and applications. *Pain Physician* 2007;10:329–356.

21

Other Refractory Headaches

Chronic Tension-Type Headache, New Daily Persistent Headache, Cluster Headache and Other Trigeminal Autonomic Cephalalgias, and Posttraumatic Headache

Rigmor Jensen, MD, and Jes Olesen, MD

Introduction

Patients referred to headache clinics, in most cases, have failed to benefit from or tolerate numerous previous treatment strategies. They may also complain of a long history of misunderstanding by the health care system, and a trial and error approach in their past pain-management history. The patients may be absolutely right: some physicians regard headache sufferers as problematic patients and do not have a dedicated interest in or knowledge about headache. In other cases, the diagnosis is incorrect and the patient has received an inappropriate palette of treatment strategies. And last but not least, their headaches may actually be absolutely refractory and unresponsive to standard treatments.

As in all other medical disciplines, a very systematic approach and a proper diagnosis are mandatory for a good outcome, and these headache patients require exactly the same approach. In fact, in a recent report from The Danish Headache Center where the outcome of 1326 consecutive patients with so-called refractory headaches were analyzed, the number of headache days per month were reduced by 45% and their absence rate by 60% (Jensen et al., personal communication). In our clinical practice, we regard refractory headache patients with scientific interest as a complex but also as a very rewarding diagnostic and therapeutic challenge. This chapter focuses on refractory headaches other than migraine, namely chronic tension-type headache, cluster headache and other trigeminal autonomic cephalalgias (TACs), new daily persistent headache, and posttraumatic headache; describes their clinical features, and evaluates present management strategies.

Chronic Tension-Type Headache

Tension-type headache (TTH) is the most prevalent and costly headache.[1] Chronic TTH (CTTH) occurs 15 days or more per month for at least 3 months, affects 3% to 4% of the adult population,[2] and is very often considered as a refractory and complex disorder. Patients usually presents in their second decade with episodic, bilateral headaches of pressing quality, mild to moderate in intensity and not aggravated by physical activity, and according to the *International Classification of Headache Disorders*, 2nd edition (ICHD-II) criteria, only one associated symptom with photo- or phonophobia or nausea is allowed.[3] Over a period of 5 to 10 years, maybe longer, the headache may increase in frequency without any external triggers and becomes chronic with a near daily, daily, constant occurrence.[4] A range of heterogeneous mechanisms is likely to play a role. In contrast to the episodic forms, increased sensitivity of the central nervous system,[5,6] as well as psychological mechanisms often complicate the treatment. It is therefore important to consider which mechanisms may be important for the individual patient, to tailor the treatment accordingly and adjust the patient's expectations.

Obviously, a correct diagnosis should be assured by means of a headache diary[7] recorded over at least 4 weeks. The diagnostic problem most often encountered is to discriminate between TTH, migraines, and medication-overuse headache (MOH). The general term chronic daily headache is therefore frequently used as a diagnostic short cut. The diary is also extremely important to reveal triggers and medication overuse, and it will establish the baseline against which to measure the efficacy of treatments. Identification of a high intake of analgesics is essential as other treatment modalities are largely ineffective in the presence of medication overuse.[8] Significant comorbidity, for example, anxiety or depression, should be also identified and treated concomitantly, as discussed in other chapters in this book.

It should be explained to the patients that CTTH can be difficult to manage but a meaningful improvement can be obtained with the combination of nonpharmacological and pharmacological treatments. In most cases, these strategies are recommended to go hand in hand but described separately in the following text.

Nonpharmacological Management

Information, reassurance, and identification of trigger factors are the mainstay in the general nonpharmacological management of refractory headache patients. Nondrug management should also be considered for all CTTH patients and is very widely used as pharmacological treatment is unspecific or ineffective. However, the scientific evidence for efficacy of most treatment modalities in CTTH is sparse. The very fact that the physician takes the problem seriously may have a therapeutic effect, particularly if the patient is concerned about serious disease, and can be reassured by thorough examination.

A detailed analysis of trigger factors should be performed, but in CTTH patients where their headaches have lasted for years, trigger factors may only play a minor role. The most frequently reported triggers for TTH are stress (mental or physical), irregular or inappropriate meals, high intake of coffee and other caffeine containing drinks, dehydration, sleep disorders, too much or too little sleep, reduced or inappropriate physical exercise, psychological problems as well as variations during the female menstrual cycle and hormonal substitution.[9,10] Most of triggers are self-reported and so far none of the triggers have been systematically tested.

Information about the nature of the disease is important. It can be explained that muscle pain can lead to a disturbance of the brain's pain-modulating mechanisms so that normally innocuous stimuli are perceived as painful,[4,11] with a secondary perpetuation of a normal muscle pain and risk of secondary anxiety and depression. Moreover, it should be explained to the patient that the prognosis in the longer run is favorable, since 45% with frequent or chronic TTH had remission of their headaches in a 12-year epidemiological follow-up study.[12] Poor outcome was, however, associated with baseline chronic tension-type headache, coexisting migraine, not being married and sleeping problems.[12] The individual role of these predictive factors remains, however, to be elucidated but they may help the physician to give the patients a realistic prognosis.

Psychological Treatments

A large number of psychological treatment strategies have been used to treat TTH. Three strategies have reached reasonable scientific support for effectiveness[13] and are described.

Relaxation Training

The goal of relaxation training is to help the patient to recognize and control tension as it arises in the course of daily activities. During the training, the patient sequentially tenses and then releases specific groups of muscles throughout the body. Later stages involve relaxation by recall, association of relaxation with a cue word, and maintaining relaxation in muscles not needed for current activities.[13]

Electromyographic (EMG) Biofeedback

The aim of EMG biofeedback is to help the patient to recognize and control muscle tension by providing continuous feedback about muscle activity recorded from surface electrodes. Sessions typically include an adaptation phase, baseline phase, training phase where feedback is provided, and a self-control phase where the patient practices controlling muscle tension without the aid of feedback.[13]

Cognitive–Behavioral Therapy

The aim of cognitive–behavioral therapy (CBT) is to teach the patient to identify thoughts and beliefs that generate stress and aggravate headaches.[14] These thoughts are then challenged, and alternative adaptive coping self-instructions are considered. A variety of exercises may be used to challenge thoughts and beliefs, including experimenting with adoption of another person's view of the situation, actively generating other possible views of a situation, and devising a behavioral experiment to test the validity of a particular belief.

Meta-analyses have concluded that the treatments described in the preceding text reduce headache frequency or intensity by 37% to 50% with no significant difference among treatments.[15] However, the exact degree of effect is difficult to estimate because of methodological difficulties of designing appropriate placebo procedures. The most useful information on efficacy derives from a study by Holroyd et al. comparing outcomes for patients with CTTH after stress management therapy (relaxation training plus CBT), tricyclic antidepressants, and a combination of the two.[16] Both the behavioral and pharmacological treatment strategies reduced headache index by approximately 35% versus 29% for placebo medication at an 8 month follow-up. Patients who received the combination of the two treatments were more likely to show substantial reductions in headache activity than patients who received either treatment alone, with a 64% reduction in the headache index.[16]

Although the psychological treatments seem to have similar efficacy in controlled trials, they place more demands on the individual patient. Psychological treatments can be relatively more time-consuming, and require a certain level of patient motivation. On the other hand, some patients have difficulty tolerating medications. Unfortunately there are no documented guidelines for which psychological treatment(s) to choose for the individual patient. Therefore, until scientific evidence is provided common sense must be used. For example, it appears most likely that CBT will be most beneficial for the patient where psychological problems or affective distress play a major role, while biofeedback or relaxation training may be preferable for the patient who mainly experience increased muscle tension.

Physical Therapy

Physical therapy is the most frequently used nonpharmacological treatment for TTH and includes the improvement of posture, relaxation, exercise programs, hot and cold packs, ultrasound and electrical stimulation, but the majority of these modalities have not been properly evaluated.[17] Active treatment strategies are generally recommended.[17] A controlled study[18] combined various techniques such as massage, relaxation, and home-based exercises and found a modest effect. It was recently reported that adding craniocervical training to classical physiotherapy was better than physiotherapy alone[19] but there are no confirmatory studies. A recent study found no significant long lasting differences in efficacy among relaxation training, physical training, and acupuncture[20] and spinal manipulation has no effect for the treatment of episodic TTH.[21] Oromandibular treatment with occlusal splints is often recommended but the evidence is lacking and cannot be recommended in general.[22] It can be concluded that there is a huge contrast between the widespread use of physical therapies and the scientific evidence for efficacy of these therapies, and that further studies of improved quality are necessary to either support or refute the effectiveness of physical modalities in TTH.[23,24]

Acupuncture and Nerve Block

There are conflicting results regarding the efficacy of acupuncture for the treatment of TTH. A recent large trial found acupuncture better than no treatment but not superior to minimal sham like acupuncture,[25] while another recent trial[26] found no significant effect of traditional Chinese acupuncture over sham puncture on the primary efficacy parameter, while secondary efficacy parameters indicated a modest effect of traditional acupuncture. Laser acupuncture has recently been reported effective,[27] while acupuncture-like electrical stimulation was not effective.[28] A recent study reported no effect of greater occipital nerve block in patients with CTTH.[29]

Acute Pharmacological Management

Acute drug therapy refers to the treatment of individual attacks of headache in patients with episodic and chronic TTH. The efficacy of the simple analgesics tends to decrease with increasing frequency of the headaches and in patients with CTTH, simple analgesics are usually ineffective and should be used with caution because of the risk of MOH at a regular intake of simple analgesics above 14 days a month or combination analgesics above 9 days a month (ICHD-II). Other interventions such as non-drug treatments and prophylactic pharmacotherapy should therefore be applied.

Prophylactic Pharmacological Treatment

Prophylactic pharmacotherapy should be considered in CTTH patients. For many years the tricyclic antidepressant amitriptyline has been used. More lately other antidepressants, nonsteroidal anti-inflammatory drugs (NSAIDs), muscle relaxants, anticonvulsants, and botulinum toxin have been tested in CTTH.

Amitriptyline

The tricyclic antidepressant amitriptyline is the only drug that has proven to be effective in several controlled trials in TTH. Thus, five out of six placebo-controlled studies found a significant effect of amitriptyline.[30] One large study of properly classified CTTH patients reported that amitriptyline 75 mg/day reduced headache index (duration × intensity) with 30% compared with placebo.[31] The effect was long-lasting (at least 6 months) and not related to the presence of depression. It is important that patients are informed that this is an antidepressant agent but has an independent action on pain. Amitriptyline should be started at low dosages (10 mg/day) and titrated by 10 mg weekly until the patient has either good therapeutic effect or side effects are encountered. The maintenance dose is usually 30 to 70–75 mg daily administered 1 to 2 hours before bedtime to help to circumvent any sedative adverse effects. A significant effect of amitriptyline may be observed already in the first week on the therapeutic dose.[32] It is therefore advisable to change to other prophylactic therapy, if the patient does not respond after 3 to 4 weeks on maintenance dose. The side effects of amitriptyline include dry mouth, drowsiness, dizziness, constipation, and weight gain. Dry mouth was observed in 75% and drowsiness in 53% of CTTH patients.[32] Discontinuation should be attempted every 6 to 12 months.

Other Antidepressants

The tricyclic antidepressant clomipramine and the tetracyclic antidepressants maprotiline and mianserin have been reported more effective than placebo, while the selective serotonin reuptake inhibitors (SSRIs) have not been found effective.[30] Interestingly, antidepressants with action on both serotonin and noradrenalin seem to be as effective as amitriptyline with the advantage that they are tolerated in doses needed for the treatment of a concomitant depression. Thus, the noradrenergic and specific serotonergic antidepressant mirtazapine 30 mg/day reduced headache index by 34% more than placebo in difficult to treat patients including patients who had not responded to amitriptyline.[33] The serotonin and noradrenalin reuptake inhibitor venlafaxine 150 mg/day[34] reduced headache days from 15 to 12 per month. However, the latter study is difficult to compare with the other studies mentioned, because it was a small parallel group study performed in patients with frequent episodic, not chronic, TTH. A recent study demonstrated that low dose mirtazapine 4.5 mg/day alone or in combination with ibuprofen 400 mg/day was not effective in CTTH. Interestingly, ibuprofen alone increased headache indicating a possible early onset of MOH.[35]

Miscellaneous Agents

A recent open study reported an effect of the anti-convulsant topiramate 100 mg/day.[36] Tizanidine, botulinum toxin, propranolol or valproic acid are tested in randomized controlled trials (RCTs), all with negative results and can therefore not be recommended for the prophylactic treatment of CTTH.[30]

In general, the initial approach to prophylactic therapy of CTTH is elimination of medication overuse and a nonpharmacological management strategy with detailed information, reassurance, relaxation (with CBT for selected patients) and through the use of amitriptyline.

Concomitant use of daily analgesics should be avoided. If the patient does not respond to amitriptyline, mirtazapine could be attempted. Venlafaxine or SSRIs could be considered in patients with concomitant depression, if tricyclics or mirtazapine are not tolerated. The physician and the patients should keep in mind that the efficacy of preventive drug therapy in CTTH is often modest, and that the efficacy should outweigh the side effects. More efficient prophylactic drugs with fewer side effects are urgently needed for the preventive treatment of CTTH.

As neither nonpharmacological nor pharmacological treatment alone is highly effective it is usually recommended to combine multiple strategies. It is therefore reassuring that the first study that has evaluated the efficacy of a multidisciplinary headache clinic reports positive results.[37] Treatment results for all patients discharged within one year were evaluated. Patients with episodic TTH demonstrated a 50% reduction in frequency, 75% reduction in intensity, and 33% in absence rate, whereas chronic TTH patients responded with 32%, 30%, and 40% reductions, respectively.[37]

Summary and Perspectives on CTTH

Tension-type headache is the most common primary headache with tremendous socioeconomic impact and the chronic forms are often difficult to treat. Establishment of an accurate diagnosis and exclusion of medication overuse is of utmost importance before initiation of any treatment. Nondrug treatment is the mainstay. Information, reassurance, and identification of trigger factors may be rewarding. Psychological treatments with scientific evidence for efficacy include relaxation training, EMG biofeedback, and CBT. Physical therapy and acupuncture are widely used, but the scientific evidence for efficacy is sparse. Analgesics play only a minor role as most patients actually report lack of effect and are at risk of MOH. The tricyclic antidepressant amitriptyline is still the drug of first choice for CTTH. The efficacy is modest and treatment is often hampered by side effects. Thus, treatment of CTTH is often difficult and multidisciplinary treatment strategies can be useful. The development of specific nondrug and drug treatments for TTH with higher efficacy and fewer side effects is urgently needed. The relative efficacy of the various treatment modalities, for example, psychological, physical, and pharmacological are not yet clarified and treatment programs should be optimized to best suit the individual patient.

Cluster and Other Trigeminal Autonomic Cephalalgias

Cluster Headache

Cluster headache is the most spectacular primary headache characterized by recurrent, severe, short lasting headaches associated with autonomic features, occurring in episodic and chronic subforms. Cluster headache is relatively rare compared to other primary headaches with an estimated prevalence around 1 per 1000. It has a clear male preponderance with a male: female ratio of 4-5:1.[38] Despite the characteristic and stereotypical presentation, there is significant diagnostic delay up to 9 years from the first attack of an episodic cluster headache until a proper diagnosis and treatment plan is acquired.[38] The chronic cluster headache (CCH) subform, which affects 10% to 15% of the cluster headache population, presents with daily and recurrent intense pain attacks, is hopefully recognized earlier in the health care system as they represent the most debilitated patients due to their excruciating and recurrent pain attacks.

The ICHD-II criteria of cluster headache and other TACs are listed in Table 21.1. Patients who suffer from cluster and other TACs often present to the physician in a highly anxious and agitated state, and may live in mortal fear of recurrence of an attack. The doctor's duty (after confirming or

Table 21-1 Comparison of Trigemino-autonomic Headache Syndromes According to ICHD-II[3] with Variations in Attack Duration and Frequency as the Most Significant Differences (marked with bold)

	Cluster Headache	Paroxysmal Hemicrania	SUNCT Syndrome
Attack duration	**15–180 minutes**	**2–30 minutes**	**5–240 seconds**
Attack frequency	**1–8/day**	**5–50/day**	**3–200/day**
Pain quality	Pungent	Twinging	Stabbing or pulsating
Pain intensity	Extremely high	High	Moderate to high
Localization	Peri- or retroorbital	Temporal or orbital	Temporal or orbital
Autonomic symptoms	+++	++	++
Circadian rhythmicity	+++	+	–
Therapy acute	Oxygen 100%, sumatriptan SC	None	None
Therapy preventive	Verapamil, lithium carbonate, corticosteroids, topiramate, methysergide	Indomethacin	Lamotrigin

SUNCT = short–lasting unilateral neuralgiform pain with conjunctival injection and tearing
Modified from ref. 55.

ascertaining the diagnosis) is to reassure the patient that the condition is benign and provide accurate information about it. It is important to advise the patient to avoid triggering factors as alcohol consumption, afternoon naps, and changes in sleep/wake rhythms that can provoke an attack during, but not outside, a bout of cluster headache.

Unfortunately, up to 10% of CCH patients seems drug-resistant to all pharmacological treatments, making daily living miserable and forcing some to consider suicide. Goadsby initially proposed guidelines for defining intractable headache, with the suggested definition of intractable cluster headache shown in Table 21.2.[39] The term drug-resistant CCH (drCCH) is also frequently used indicating failure of medical drug treatment, though not necessarily meaning intractable to other treatment modalities.

Acute Pharmacological Treatment of Cluster Headache

There are two pharmacological approaches to the treatment of cluster headache: acute and prophylactic treatment. To resolve an ongoing cluster headache attack the first choice medication is the selective 5-$HT_{1B/1D}$ receptor agonist sumatriptan. Given subcutaneously, sumatriptan is effective in a few minutes. It is also available as suppositories, nasal spray, and 50- or 100-mg tablets. Since the aim is to intervene rapidly, subcutaneous administration

Table 21-2 Suggested Criteria for Intractable Chronic Cluster Headache [39]

Intractable headache
Failed an *adequate trial* of regulatory approved and conventional treatments according to local national guidelines
Adequate trial
Appropriate dose
Appropriate length of time
Consideration of medication overuse
Failed
No therapeutic or unsatisfactory effect
Intolerable side-effects
Contraindications to use
In cluster headache, failure of at least four classes, where two should come from 1–3
1. Verapamil 2. Lithium 3. Methysergide 4. Melatonin 5. Topiramate 6. Gabapentin

is preferred. However, nasal spray may usually provide relief within an acceptably short period. Zolmitriptan nasal spray is also effective but somewhat less so than sumatriptan.[39]

Inhaled oxygen via a nonrebreathing facial mask with a flow rate of at least 7 to 12 L/min for about 15 minutes is effective for most attacks but most patients report that the inhalation should be initiated as early as possible in the attack to be effective. Detailed insights of mechanisms, and evidence of optimal flow rates and type of masks are needed and most treatment recommendations are based on patient reports.

Prophylactic Pharmacotherapy of Cluster Headache

The aim of prophylaxis is to reduce the frequency and the intensity of the attacks and to revert the chronic to episodic presentation. In patients with episodic cluster headache prophylaxis should be administered only during a cluster period. The older practice of continuing with prophylactic medication after a cluster period should be abandoned. The next cluster period may recur many months, or even longer after the previous one and preventive medication – which is not without side-effects – is totally unnecessary during remission.

There are various factors to weigh in the decision to begin prophylactic treatment in a patient with cluster headache, including the frequency, duration, and severity of the attacks, patient age, and the presence of comorbidities. One should also bear in mind that the chronic and episodic forms of cluster headache may respond differently to a given prophylactic. Prophylactic medications are indicated in most patients with chronic cluster headache unless the attacks are infrequent or very short lasting. The aim of prophylaxis is to bring about rapid disappearance of the attacks and to maintain an attack-free state, with minimal side effects, and preferably to reverse the chronic form to an episodic form. The choice of prophylactic drug is influenced by previous response, previous side effects, contraindications, the duration of the cluster period, comorbidities, and the age and lifestyle of the patient. A combination of two or even more drugs may be necessary to terminate the attacks.

Verapamil

Calcium antagonists, and in particular verapamil, have become established for the prophylaxis of both episodic and chronic cluster headache. Verapamil is now considered the first choice drug for cluster headache prophylaxis worldwide, although it is associated with the side effects of constipation and sometimes hypotension. Before administering and during treatment with verapamil the patient should undergo an electrocardiogram to rule out severe atrioventricular conduction effects.[39] In a trial of verapamil 360 mg/t.i.d. against lithium carbonate at 900 mg/day in patients with chronic cluster headache, verapamil had an efficacy superior to 75% in 80% of the patients.[44]

It was also more rapidly effective than lithium in that, in the first week of treatment, 50% of patients on verapamil improved against 37% on lithium.[40,41] Higher doses, up to 960 mg daily, rarely greater, may be necessary, with regular ECG monitoring before every dose step.

Lithium

Lithium at 600 to 1500 mg/day or 6 to 12 mmol/day, first choice medication before the advent of verapamil, remains a valid alternative particularly for chronic cluster headache.[41,42] Before giving lithium, kidney and thyroid should be checked, and during administration blood lithium should be kept below 1.2 mmol/l to avoid side effects such as polyuria, tremor, vomiting, diarrhea, edema and somnolence.[41,43] Plasma levels of lithium sufficient to stop cluster headaches are generally below those giving rise to side effects but both plasma levels of lithium and thyroid function are recommended to be controlled on a regular basis.

Corticosteroids

Prednisone is effective against cluster headache, particularly the chronic form, but is usually only employed in selected patients who have proved resistant to other drugs. Prednisone can be associated with lithium or verapamil, but because of its side effects is contraindicated for prolonged treatment. In chronic cluster patients, therefore, cycles lasting 2 weeks are recommended beginning at 50 to 60 mg/day orally and tapering slowly to zero.[44] Use of intravenous cortisone should be restricted to patients refractory to all other medications and who experience daily attacks. Such patients should be hospitalized to monitor the treatment efficacy and side effects. More prolonged steroid administration may be necessary in particularly refractory cases although one should be aware of the possible long-term (in some cases irreversible) consequences of such treatments.

Methysergide

Methysergide at 4 to 12 mg/day is particularly effective against episodic cluster headache in young patients. Because this drug is an ergotamine derivative (with major vasoconstrictive effects) the patient must be advised that it should never be taken at the same time as sumatriptan, in view of a possible synergic effect on vasospasm.[44] The most serious side effect of ergotamine derivatives is retroperitoneal, pleural and heart valve fibrosis. The risk of such effects is low if doses are kept low, but after the 4-6 months of treatment, the patient should be recommended 1 to 2 months drug-holiday and a regular examination for renal function and cardiac disease. Blood samples, abdominal and cardiac ultrasound, thoracic radiograph, and magnetic resonance imaging (MRI) should be considered.[45] Methysergide is not currently available in the United States from corporate pharmaceutical sources, but can be obtained from selected local compounding pharmacies.

Melatonin

In a double-blind small study against placebo, melatonin 10 mg/day showed some efficacy against episodic cluster headache. Of the 10 patients treated, five experienced a clear reduction in attacks.[45] The rationale for the use of melatonin in cluster headache derives from the fact that nocturnal levels of this substance are low in the cluster period. It is unclear, however, whether the beneficial effect is due to the fact that melatonin can improve the quality of sleep. Melatonin is perhaps best considered as an add-on therapy.

Antiepileptics

Valproate was reported to be effective against cluster headache, although only very few studies have been performed. A double-blind placebo-controlled group study of sodium valproate (1000–2000 mg/day) in cluster headache prevention found however no significant difference between the patients and the placebo group.[46] Interest in the use of this antiepileptic in the prophylaxis of cluster headache had recently been re-kindled by the finding in animals that valproate prevents plasma protein extravasation from the trigeminovascular system—an effect also exercised by sumatriptan and other triptans.

Topiramate was also expected to be useful in preventing cluster headache attacks but in an open study on 36 patients with episodic and chronic cluster headache, only seven patients responded; six of these had an episodic form and one chronic.[47] Six of these responders received 100 mg/day and one received 150 mg/day during the treatment period. The results did not support initial expectations of efficacy, and topiramate appears of little use as a cluster headache prophylactic.

Surgical Treatment of Drug-Resistant Chronic Cluster Headache

Up to 10% of patients with chronic cluster headache do not respond, or have major contraindications, to prophylactic treatments. To relieve these drug-resistant CCH patients their torments, various primarily destructive surgical procedures have been tried aiming at trigeminal and parasympathetic pathways thought to be responsible for the pain and autonomic symptoms. Surgical procedures among others include partial or complete surgical sectioning of the trigeminal root, radiofrequency trigeminal gangliorhizolysis, and microvascular decompression of the trigeminal nerve, though effect is often sparse, and side effects can be devastating.

Such patients may be candidates for surgical approaches but as surgery is the very last option it is only indicated in patients who have been shown unresponsive to all appropriate pharmaceutical treatments. Patient selection for surgical procedures is a very difficult task and should be centralized to academic highly specialized centers. The physician should have extensive knowledge and experience of chronic cluster headache, a close professional relationship with the patient, and be prepared to dedicate time to test all possible medications and ascertain they are ineffective. The following criteria provide a basis for selecting patients for surgery[48]:

- Complete inefficacy of, or major contraindications to, all appropriate prophylactic medications for cluster headache
- Chronic headache for some time (about 2 years)
- Frequent attacks (daily or almost daily)
- Strictly unilateral headache
- Normal psychological profile
- No medical conditions contraindicating deep brain stimulation

The discovery that hypothalamic function is altered in cluster headache, documented by positron emission tomography and later by voxel-based morphometric analysis of magnetic resonance images, provided crucial support for the findings of numerous neuroendocrinological studies. Thus, for the first time, a lesion associated with a primary headache had been identified, and the lesion site suggested itself as a possible target for therapeutic intervention. The Italian group of Manzoni et al. proposed the use of electrode implant and stimulation to the inferior posterior hypothalamus in patients with severe intractable chronic cluster headache. The rationale was that stimulation to this area might inhibit the activation that PET had revealed. The technique of deep brain stimulation is already widely employed to control intractable movement disorders, and experience accumulated over a decade and more has shown it to be safe and associated with few side effects, although a case of fatal outcome has been reported. Eighteen hypothalamic implants have now been performed and reported by the Italian group with extremely encouraging results, whereas reports from other groups are quite scarce and with limited success.[49]

Although pain is reduced or disappears in about 50% of cases, a certain proportion experience a recurrence of pain attacks within the years after operation.[49] Promising results are accumulating for the less invasive greater occipital nerve blockade as well as bilateral nerve stimulation of the greater occipital nerve. We believe that these less invasive procedures should always be considered before deep brain stimulation.[50]

Occipital Nerve Stimulation (ONS) for CCH

Peripheral nerve stimulation in the occipital region for intractable headache patients was first tried in the 1990s for other chronic headaches or neuralgias, and the positive outcome led to ONS trials involving drCCH patients. Distal branches of the C2–C3 roots corresponding to the lesser and especially greater occipital nerve are the main targets of stimulation. The rationale for the ONS stimulation is thought to be related to a low-intensity and continuous activation of afferent nociceptive fibers corresponding to the respective dermatomes of the pain, and a secondary activation of brain plasticity leading to pain control. A common clinical fact is that pain originating in the

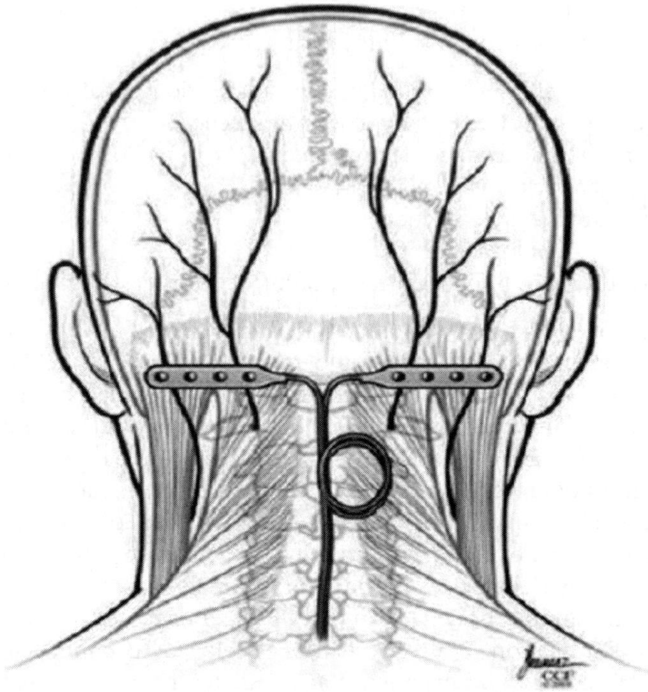

Figure 21-1 Illustration picturing bilateral occipital nerve stimulation

cervical region may spread to regions innervated by the trigeminal nerve, as well as the opposite, thereby suggesting a functional connection between these areas.

Clinical studies further support the convergence theory. A recent randomized controlled trial examining the effect of GON block in CH patients has shown positive results regarding duration, frequency and intensity of cluster attacks.[51] Currently a number of studies regarding ONS in altogether 27 drCCH patients are running and continually evaluated.[50,52] To date, the presented results are positive and promising, although only very few patients are attack free. Overall the frequency and intensity of attacks are reduced by around 50%, with a large inter-individual variation.[50,52]

The largest series by Burns et al. included 14 drCCH patients,[50] evaluated at a median follow up of 17.5 (range 4–35) months. All patients received bilateral ONS implantation. The first patient had a unilateral implant with good effect, but side-shift in pain lead to bilateral implantation in the patient and all subsequent patients. Ten (10) of 14 patients (71%) reported improvements between 20% and 90% primarily in frequency but also in severity or duration of attacks. Among them 5 had an improvement of 50% or better, usually considered the target for preventive treatments in headache.[50] Outcome measures were the patients' own estimate of effect compared to before implantation.

Eleven (11) of 14 patients were willing to recommend the procedure to others. None have become completely pain free.[50]

Another study by Magis et al involved eight drCCH patients receiving unilateral ONS.[52] At a mean follow up of 15.1 months (range 3–22), the mean attack frequency was reduced by 79.9% with a mean intensity reduction of 50%. Outcome was based on headache diaries. An update on this study includes a new patient and altogether nine patients with maximal follow-up of 32 months.[53] Results show a mean attack frequency reduction of 54% and intensity decrease of 47%.

In conclusion, over time, ONS probably induces neuromodulatory changes in central pain processing structures suggesting brain plasticity. However, the effect is reversible as the pain may return to normal shortly after interruption of the stimulation. Thus, the precise mechanism and the long term effect are yet to be determined.

Treatment of Other Trigeminal Autonomic Cephalalgias

Chronic Paroxysmal Hemicranias

Although there is no acute treatment, elective treatment with indomethacin is highly effective. Doses of 150 mg/day are recommended, although lower doses may sometime be effective. Moderate efficacy has been shown with verapamil. Hemicrania continua is a similar condition to paroxysmal hemicrania but is not considered as a trigeminal autonomic cephalgia; it too is highly sensitive to indomethacin.[54]

Short-Lasting Unilateral Neuralgiform Headache Attacks with Conjunctival Injection and Tearing

Short-lasting unilateral neuralgiform headache attacks with conjunctival injection and tearing (SUNCT) is a trigeminal autonomic cephalgia that at one time was considered totally resistant to pharmacological treatment. However, recent studies have shown that lamotrigine is effective in some SUNCT patients.[54,55]

Functional MRI studies have revealed that the posterior hypothalamus is activated during SUNCT attacks as also occurs in cluster headache. This finding, together with the close clinical similarities between SUNCT and cluster headache, suggested that hypothalamic stimulation might be useful in SUNCT.[56,57]

Cluster-Tic Syndrome

In this syndrome, attacks of cluster headache and of trigeminal neuralgia occur in the same patient. Usually the attacks occur at different times but sometimes they occur simultaneously. Treatment needs to be individualized combinations of verapamil and antiepileptics, specific for each condition (cluster headache and trigeminal neuralgia) even when both occur together.

New Daily Persistent Headache

New daily persistent headache (NDPH) has been recognized by the second edition of the IHS classification as a separate entity from chronic tension-type headache.[3] The current diagnostic criteria for NDPH appear in Table 21.3. As indicated by the name, NDPH is a daily, persistent headache which is unremitting from the moment of onset, typically in individuals who do not have a prior history of headache, and is usually refractory and resistant to treatment. The prevalence of NDPH is approximately 0.1% of the general population, and occurs in 2% to 10% of patients from headache clinics.[58,59] NDPH has a female predominance (2.5:1).[58] Diagnosed at all ages, NDPH usually begins in the second and third decade in women and in the fifth decade in men.

Typically, patients are able to pinpoint the exact date their headache started and in at least half the cases, headache begins in relation to an infection or flulike illness or a stressful life event. Unfortunately, the etiology of NDPH usually remains unknown.[60,61] Because NDPH begins simultaneously with a viral-like syndrome in some patients, an infectious cause has been proposed in relation to a postviral syndrome or to an unknown chronic infection.[60] In our personal experience, even when some patients reported an infection previous to the development of the headache, we could not serologically demonstrate it. Reactivation of Epstein-Barr virus or other infectious agents has been hypothesized as the trigger for the development of NDPH due to an activated immune response, setting up a state of continuous neurogenic inflammation. This hypothesis is far from being proved, and in about half of NDPH cases, there is no recognized trigger. Clinically the headache is similar to TTH, but there is no progressive evolution from a previous headache.

Table 21-3 Diagnostic Criteria for Primary New Daily Persistent Headache (ICHD-II)[3]

A. Headache for longer than 3 months fulfilling criteria B–D
B. Headache is daily and unremitting from onset or from less than 3 days from onset
C. At least two of the following pain characteristics:
  Bilateral location
  Pressing/tightening (nonpulsating) quality
  Mild or moderate intensity
  Not aggravated by routine physical activity such as walking or climbing stairs
D. Both of the following:
  No more than one: photophobia, phonophobia, or mild nausea
  Neither moderate or severe nausea nor vomiting
E. Not attributed to another disorder

Table 21-4 Secondary Causes of New Daily Persistent Headache

Cerebral vein thrombosis
Low–cerebrospinal fluid pressure headache
High–cerebrospinal fluid pressure headache
Medication overuse headache
Carotid or vertebral artery dissection

Pain is described as fairly constant and moderate to severe. Location is heterogeneous and not characteristic, and more than half of patients complain of migrainous-associated symptoms (in this order: nausea, phono/photophophia, vomiting).

Diagnosis of NDPH is one of exclusion. Secondary causes of NDPH and other chronic refractory headache appear in Table 21.4. Low–cerebrospinal fluid pressure headache due to spontaneous cerebrospinal fluid pressure leak, cerebral vein thrombosis, headache attributed to infection (particularly viral), and medication overuse headache can mimic NDPH presentation and should always be carefully ruled out with appropriate investigations.

NDPH is difficult to manage. These patients commonly receive preventive medications used to treat migraine, such as beta-blockers, topiramate, valproic acid, or chronic tension-type headache, such as amitriptyline, mirtazapine or combinations of those prophylactics.[60,62] It is also of utmost importance to inform the patients very carefully, that this type of headache is difficult and to provide them with realistic expectations.

Headache Attributed to Head and Neck Trauma

Acute posttraumatic headache following head trauma is the major complaint in the early phase, followed by nausea, photophobia, vertigo and impaired concentration. In most cases the symptoms resolve spontaneously within a few weeks. For a smaller proportion of patients the headache becomes chronic, refractory to treatment and often severely disabling.[63–66] Because of the high incidence of head trauma (350 per 100,000 in Europe, 180–220 per 100,000 in North America; 75% of these being mild head injury), and the consistency of symptoms, posttraumatic headache is a frequently occurring type of secondary headache. The prevalence of posttraumatic headache is approximately 0.5% to 1% in the general population, and occurs in 2% to 10% of patients from headache clinics.[66] The continuing presence of posttraumatic headache after injury varies between different studies. Recent studies have shown that 44% had headache after 1- to 3 months and up to 20% 3 years after head trauma.[63,64,66–68]

Despite these high numbers of posttraumatic headaches from prospective studies, there are no detailed reports with analysis of the exact headache frequency, duration, and impact in these individuals. Two percent to 10% of patients from headache clinics present with posttraumatic headache, representing probably the most severely affected individuals.[66,69] Chronic posttraumatic headache (CPTH) has a female predominance, with low education and a history of primary headaches as the major risk factors for CPTH in the female gender after a mild head trauma.[66]

CPTH has been a source of controversy for many years and opinions still differ in regard to its pathogenesis, natural course, the role of litigation and to what extent it could be explained as medication overuse headache. The debate of an organic versus psychogenic basis continues, but the evidence to support an organic basis is increasing.[68,70,71] The pathophysiology of traumatic acute headache results from damage to the skull, the dura, and increase in intracranial pressure but there is no clear causality to the chronic, refractory headache. Interestingly the persistence of headache is inversely correlated with the severity of the head trauma. Whiplash injuries may also lead to neck pain and headache, although the relation is less clear than in PTH. Most patients have normal findings in radiographs, CT or MRI of the cervical spine.

Posttraumatic headache has been recognized with detailed diagnostic criteria in the ICHD-II,[3] and has been subdivided in relation to the acute or the chronic phase and in relation to severity of the head trauma (Table 21.5). Clinically, CPTH presents as a dull, holocranial constant headache which may be aggravated by light, noise, physical and mental activity.[72] In a clinical series of 53 patients from a tertiary headache center, 50% patients also fulfilled the criteria for chronic tension-type headache, and 24% presented with a combination of CTTH and migraine without aura. In addition, 22 of 53 patients had additional MOH, and were detoxified with similar positive results as other patient populations with primary headaches.[72]

Table 21-5 The International Headache Classification, 2nd edition Diagnostic Criteria of Chronic Posttraumatic Headache[3]

5.2	New headache occurring <7 days after and lasting >3 months after head trauma or after regaining consciousness or memory
5.2.1	CPTH with moderate or severe head injury meaning at least one of the following: 1. Loss of consciousness >30 min 2. Glasgow Coma Scale <13 3. Posttraumatic amnesia >48 h 4. Imaging demonstration of a traumatic brain lesion (cerebral haematoma, brain contusion or skull fracture)
5.2.2	CPTH with mild head injury meaning all of the following: 1. No loss of consciousness, or loss of consciousness <30 min 2. Glasgow Coma Scale >13 3. Symptoms or signs diagnostic of concussion

Treatment of CPTH is often difficult and widely unspecific since treatment guidelines mostly copy the recommendations for treatment of the primary headache counterparts. Although less documented, multidisciplinary treatment strategies are usually recommended.[66,73] A pharmacological approach with tricyclics and antiepileptics is recommended similar to the treatment of tension-type headache and migraine but proper randomized controlled trials are lacking. Non-pharmacological treatment such as cognitive behavioral education and stress-pain management are widely used but in contrast to other chronic headache patients, CPTH patients also may suffer from other posttraumatic cognitive problems such as lack of concentration, fatigue, photophobia and phonophobia in addition to their debilitating chronic headache. These cognitive problems may complicate an intensive treatment program and in most short-term studies only minimal effect can be documented. In addition to pathophysiological studies in the acute posttraumatic phase, long lasting controlled interventional and regular follow-up studies are highly needed to optimize the extremely costly rehabilitation after head and neck traumas. The treatment of whiplash lesions are also unspecific and in most cases fairly disappointing.

Concluding Comments

In conclusion, diagnosis and management of refractory headaches other than migraine may be difficult and complex. Recently suggested guidelines have been published addressing when a treatment resistant migraine should be regarded as refractory, which will hopefully lead to further discussion and ultimately consensus for further clinical management and research.[74] Unless "refractory" is clearly defined (e.g., difficult to treat, but not untreatable), we express concern that patients, their relatives and the entire medical society may experience a certain degree of stigmatization by the term, which actually may or may not be correctly applied until patients are properly evaluated in an optimal tertiary headache center.

Searching the literature and in our clinical experience, the multidisciplinary, well organized management of these headache disorders may also be highly rewarding in clinical specialized practice. By means of a very systematic diagnostic approach and a multidisciplinary management strategy, it is actually possible to reduce the headache and the associated disability to an acceptable level leading to a major improvement in these patients' quality of life and function. Detailed patient information, realistic expectations and a continued scientific approach to these chronic headache disorders, primary or secondary, are the essential cornerstones in academic headache clinics. However, such a systematic treatment approach needs continuing evaluation studies. If proven to be successful and reliable, the multidisciplinary approach should be recommended to be implemented in future organizational and treatment guidelines.

References

1. Stovner LJ, Hagen K, Jensen R, Katsarava Z, Lipton RB, Scher AI et al. The global burden of headache: a documentation of headache prevalence and disability worldwide. *Cephalalgia.* 2007;27(3):193–210.
2. Bendtsen L, Jensen R. Tension-type headache: the most common, but also the most neglected, headache disorder. *Curr Opin Neurol.* 2006;19(3):305–309.
3. Headache classification subcommitee of IHS. The International Classification of Headache Disorders, 2nd ed. *Cephalalgia.* 2004;24(Supp 1):1–160.
4. Bendtsen L. Sensitisation: its role in primary headaches. *Curr Opin Invest Drugs.* 2002;3(3):449–453.
5. Bendtsen L, Ashina M. Sensitization of myofascial pain pathways in tension-type headache. In: Olesen J, Tfelt-Hansen P, Welch KM, eds. *The Headaches.* Lippincott-Raven;1999.
6. Bendtsen L. Central sensitization in tension-type headache—possible pathophysiological mechanisms. *Cephalalgia.* 2000;20(5):486–508.
7. Russell MB, Rasmussen BK, Brennum J, Iversen HK, Jensen RA, Olesen J. Presentation of a new instrument: the diagnostic headache diary. *Cephalalgia.* 1992;12:369–374.
8. Katsarava Z, Jensen R. Medication-overuse headache: where are we now? *Curr Opin Neurol.* 2007;20(3):326–330.
9. Ulrich V, Russell MB, Jensen R, Olesen J. A comparison of tension-type headache in migraineurs and in non-migraineurs: a population-based study. *Pain.* 1996;67:501–506.
10. Rasmussen BK, Jensen R, Schroll M, Olesen J. Interrelations between migraine and tension-type headache in the general population. *Arch Neurol.* [0003–9942] 1992;49:914–918.
11. Buchgreitz L, Lyngberg A, Bendtsen L, Jensen R. Increased prevalence of tension-type headache over a 12–year period is related to increased pain sensitivity. A population study. *Cephalalgia.* 2007;27(2):145–152.
12. Lyngberg AC, Rasmussen BK, Jorgensen T, Jensen R. Prognosis of migraine and tension-type headache: a population-based follow-up study. *Neurology.* 2005;65(4):580–585.
13. Holroyd KA, Martin PR, Nash JM. Psychological treatments of tension-type headache. In: Olesen J, Goadsby PJ, Ramadan N, Tfelt-Hansen P, Welch KM, eds. *The Headaches.* Philadelphia: Lippincott Williams & Wilkins;2005:711–719.
14. Holroyd KA. Assessment and psychological management of recurrent headache disorders. *J Consult Clin Psychol.* 2002;70(3):656–677.
15. Penzien DB, Rains JC, Lipchik GL, Creer TL. Behavioral interventions for tension-type headache: overview of current therapies and recommendation for a self-management model for chronic headache. *Curr Pain Headache Rep.* 2004;8(6):489–499.
16. Holroyd KA, O'Donnell FJ, Stensland M, Lipchik GL, Cordingley GE, Carlson BW. Management of chronic tension-type headache with tricyclic antidepressant medication, stress management therapy, and their combination: a randomized controlled trial. *JAMA.* 2001;285(17):2208–2215.
17. Jensen R, Roth JM. Physiotherapy of tension-type headaches. In: Olesen J, Goadsby PJ, Ramadan N, Tfelt-Hansen P, Welch KM, eds. *The Headaches.* Philadelphia: Lippincott Williams Wilkins;2005:721–726.

18. Torelli P, Jensen R, Olesen J. Physiotherapy for tension-type headache: a controlled study. *Cephalalgia.* 2004;24(1):29–36.
19. van Ettekoven H, Lucas C. Efficacy of physiotherapy including a craniocervical training programme for tension-type headache; a randomized clinical trial. *Cephalalgia.* 2006;26(8):983–991.
20. Soderberg E, Carlsson J, Stener-Victorin E. Chronic tension-type headache treated with acupuncture, physical training and relaxation training. Between-group differences. *Cephalalgia.* 2006;26(11):1320–1329.
21. Bove G, Nilsson N. Spinal manipulation in the treatment of episodic tension-type headache: a randomized controlled trial. *JAMA.* 1998;280(18): 1576–1579.
22. Graff-Radford SB, Canavan DW. Headache attributed to orofacial/ temporomandibular pathology. In: Olesen J, Goadsby PJ, Ramadan N, Tfelt-Hansen P, Welch KM, eds. *The Headaches.* Philadelphia: Lippincott Williams Wilkins;2005:1029–1035.
23. Biondi DM. Physical treatments for headache: a structured review. *Headache.* 2005;45(6):738–746.
24. Lenssinck ML, Damen L, Verhagen AP, Berger MY, Passchier J, Koes BW. The effectiveness of physiotherapy and manipulation in patients with tension-type headache: a systematic review. *Pain.* 2004;112(3):381–388.
25. Melchart D, Streng A, Hoppe A, Brinkhaus B, Witt C, Wagenpfeil S et al. Acupuncture in patients with tension-type headache: randomised controlled trial. *BMJ.* 2005;331(7513):376–382.
26. Endres HG, Bowing G, Diener HC, Lange S, Maier C, Molsberger A et al. Acupuncture for tension-type headache: a multicentre, sham-controlled, patient-and observer-blinded, randomised trial. *J Headache Pain.* 2007;8(5):306–314.
27. Ebneshahidi NS, Heshmatipour M, Moghaddami A, Eghtesadi-Araghi P. The effects of laser acupuncture on chronic tension headache–a randomised controlled trial. *Acupunct Med.* 2005;23(1):13–18.
28. Wang K, Svensson P, Arendt-Nielsen L. Effect of acupuncture-like electrical stimulation on chronic tension-type headache: a randomized, double-blinded, placebo-controlled trial. *Clin J Pain.* 2007;23(4):316–322.
29. Leinisch-Dahlke E, Jurgens T, Bogdahn U, Jakob W, May A. Greater occipital nerve block is ineffective in chronic tension type headache. *Cephalalgia.* 2005; 25(9):704–708.
30. Bendtsen L, Mathew NT. Prophylactic pharmacotherapy of tension-type headache. In: Olesen J, Goadsby PJ, Ramadan N, Tfelt-Hansen P, Welch KM, eds. *The Headaches.* Philadelphia: Lippincott Williams & Wilkins;2005:735–741.
31. Bendtsen L, Jensen R, Olesen J. Amitriptyline, a combined serotonin and noradrenaline re-uptake inhibitor, reduces exteroceptive suppression of temporal muscle activity in patients with chronic tension-type headache. *Electroencephalogr Clin Neurophysiol.* 1996;101:418–422.
32. Bendtsen L, Jensen R, Olesen J. A non-selective (amitriptyline), but not a selective (citalopram), serotonin reuptake inhibitor is effective in the prophylactic treatment of chronic tension-type headache. *J Neurol Neurosurg Psychiatry.* 1996;61:285–290.
33. Bendtsen L, Jensen R. Mirtazapine is effective in the prophylactic treatment of chronic tension-type headache. *Neurology.* 2004;62(10):1706–1711.

34. Zissis N, Harmoussi S, Vlaikidis N, et al. A randomized, double-blind, placebo-controlled study of venlafaxine XR in out-patients with tension-type headache. *Cephalalgia.* 2007;27(4):315–324.
35. Bendtsen L, Buchgreitz L, Ashina S, Jensen R. Combination of low-dose mirtazapine and ibuprofen for prophylaxis of chronic tension-type headache. *Eur J Neurol.* 2007;14(2):187–193.
36. Lampl C, Marecek S, May A, Bendtsen L. A prospective, open-label, long-term study of the efficacy and tolerability of topiramate in the prophylaxis of chronic tension-type headache. *Cephalalgia.* 2006;26(10):1203–1208.
37. Zeeberg P, Olesen J, Jensen R. Efficacy of multidisciplinary treatment in a tertiary referral headache centre. *Cephalalgia.* 2005;25(12):1159–1167.
38. Jensen R, Lyngberg A, Jensen R. Burden of cluster headache. *Cephalalgia.* 2007;27(6):535–541.
39. Ekbom K. Treatment of cluster headache: clinical trials, design and results. *Cephalalgia.* 1995;15:33–36.
40. Bussone G, Leone M, Peccarisi C, et al. Double-blind comparison of lithium and verapamil in cluster headache prophylaxis. *Headache.* 1990;30(7): 411–417.
41. Kudrow L. Lithium prophylaxis for chronic cluster headache. *Headache.* 1977;17(1):15–18.
42. Bussone G, Leone M, Peccarisi C, et al. Double-blind comparison of lithium and verapamil in cluster headache prophylaxis. *Headache.* 1990;30(7): 411–417.
43. Abdel-Maksoud MB, Nasr A, Abdul-Aziz A. Lithium treatment in cluster headache, review of literature. *Eur. J. Psychiatry.* 2009;23(1):53–60.
44. May A, Leone M, Afra J, et al. EFNS guidelines on the treatment of cluster headache and other trigeminal-autonomic cephalalgias. *Eur. J. Neurol.* 2006;13(10):1066–1077.
45. Leone M, D'Amico D, Moschiano F, Fraschini F, Bussone G. Melatonin versus placebo in the prophylaxis of cluster headache: a double-blind pilot study with parallel groups. *Cephalalgia.* 1996;16(7):494–496.
46. El Amrani M, Massiou H, Bousser MG. A negative trial of sodium valproate in cluster headache: methodological issues. *Cephalalgia.* 2002;22(3):205–208.
47. McGeeney BE. Topiramate in the treatment of cluster headache. *Curr Pain Headache Rep.* 2003;7(2):135–138.
48. Leone M, May A, Franzini A, et al. Deep brain stimulation for intractable chronic cluster headache: proposals for patient selection. *Cephalalgia.* 2004; 24(11):934–937.
49. Leone M. Deep brain stimulation in headache. *Lancet Neurol.* 2006;5(10): 873–877.
50. Burns B, Watkins L, Goadsby PJ. Treatment of medically intractable cluster headache by occipital nerve stimulation: long-term follow-up of eight patients. *Lancet.* 2007;369(9567):1099–1106.
51. Ambrosini A, Vandenheede M, Rossi P, et al. Suboccipital (GON) injection with long-acting steroids in cluster headache: a double-blind placebo-controlled study. *Cephalalgia.* 2003;23(7):734.
52. Magis D, Schoenen J. Neuro stimulation in chronic cluster headache. *Curr Pain Headache Rep.* 2008;12(2):145–153.

53. Magis D, Remacle JM, Schoenen J. Long term follow-up study of occipital nerve stimulation (ONS) for refractory chronic cluster headache: drastic change from short term outcome. *Cephalalgia.* 2006;26(11):1398.
54. May A. Update on the diagnosis and management of trigemino-autonomic headaches. *J Neurol.* 2006;253(12):1525–1532.
55. Lenaerts ME. Update on the therapy of the trigeminal autonomic cephalalgias. *Curr Treat Options Neurol.* 2008;10(1):30–35.
56. Leone M, Cecchini AP, Mea E, et al. Functional neuroimaging and headache pathophysiology: new findings and new prospects. *Neurol Sci.* 2007;28:S108–S113.
57. Wilbrink LA, Ferrari MD, Kruit MC, Haan J. Neuroimaging in trigeminal autonomic cephalgias: when, how, and of what? *Curr Opin Neurol.* 2009; 22(3):247–253.
58. Evans RW. New daily persistent headache. *Curr Pain Headache Rep.* 2003; 7(4):303–307.
59. Goadsby PJ, Boes C. New daily persistent headache. *J Neurol Neurosurg Psychiatry.* 2002;72 (Suppl 2):ii6–ii9.:ii6–ii9.
60. Evans RW, Rozen TD. Etiology and treatment of new daily persistent headache. *Headache.* 2001;41(8):830–832.
61. Couch J, Friedman JK, Williams BM. Characterization of new daily persistent headache (NDPH) and comparison with idiopathic chronic daily headache (ICDH). *Neurology.* 2006;66(5):A177.
62. Mack KJ. New daily persistent headache in children and adults. *Curr Pain Headache Rep.* 2009;13(1):47–51.
63. Bekkelund SI, Salvesen R. Prevalence of head trauma in patients with difficult headache: The North Norway Headache Study. *Headache.* 2003;43(1):59–62.
64. Evans RW. Posttraumatic headaches among United States soldiers injured in Afghanistan and Iraq. *Headache.* 2008;48(8):1216–1225.
65. Haas DC. Characteristics of chronic posttraumatic headache. *Headache.* 2002;42(2):162–163.
66. Keidel M. Posttraumatic headache. *Nervenheilkunde.* 2007;26(3):156–164.
67. Callaghan M, Abu-Arafeh I. Chronic posttraumatic headache in children and adolescents. *Dev Med Child Neurol.* 2001;43(12):819–822.
68. Faux S, Sheedy J. A prospective controlled study in the prevalence of posttraumatic headache following mild traumatic brain injury. *Pain Med.* 2008;9(8):1001–1011.
69. Pascual-Lozano AM, Salvador-Aliaga A, Lainez-Andres JM. Posttraumatic headache. Pathophysiology, clinical, diagnostic and therapeutic aspects. *Neurologia.* 2005;20(3):133–142.
70. Goryunova AV, Bazarnaya NA, Sorokina EG, et al. Autoantibodies to glutamate receptors in children with chronic posttraumatic headache. *Zhurnal Nevrologii I Psikhiatrii Imeni S S Korsakova.* 2006;106(8):50–53.
71. Obermann M, Nebel K, Gizewski ER, et al. Gray matter decrease in patients with posttraumatic headache following whiplash injury secondary to chronic pain. *Neurology.* 2008;70(11):A7.
72. Baandrup L, Jensen R. Chronic post-traumatic headache—a clinical analysis in relation to the International Headache Classification, 2nd ed. *Cephalalgia.* 2005;25(2):132–138.

73. Griffith JL. Posttraumatic stress disorder in headache patients: implications for treatment. *Headache.* 2009;49(4):552–554.
74. Schulman EA, Lake AE, Goadsby PJ, et al. Defining refractory migraine and refractory chronic migraine: proposed criteria from the refractory headache special interest section of the American Headache Society. *Headache.* 2008;48(6):778–782.

22

Caring for Patients with Refractory Migraine

Perils and Pearls

John F. Rothrock, MD

Introduction

To return to the office from a long, wearisome clinic replete with treatment-refractory chronic migraine patients and be welcomed by a thick stack of telephone messages from treatment-refractory chronic migraine patients may deflate even the most cheerfully optimistic clinician. The reality that one's colleagues generally may regard such patients as hypochondriacal nuisances, that a certain percentage *are*, in fact, hypochondriacal nuisances, the other psychiatric co-morbidities that are so common in this population, the relentless need to monitor patients' use of symptomatic medication and—last but not least—the current paucity of therapies for suppression of chronic migraine which can claim even a modest scientific basis for such use . . . all can combine to produce varying measures of frustration, hostility, ennui and a pervasive sense of helplessness. For those in an academic-based practice wherein career advancement is in no small part dependent upon research productivity and associated publications, the struggle simultaneously to fulfill those obligations while coping with a veritable tsunami of chronic migraine patients and their seemingly infinite needs poses a particular challenge.

While the potential perils and pitfalls that await the clinician who dares grapple with this disorder are seemingly infinite, and while those described here clearly overlap, they largely account for the high rate of treatment failure and disaffected clinicians associated with the attempted management of treatment-refractory chronic migraine. The advice offered for avoiding these pitfalls comes from one who has himself fallen into each on numerous occasions, and it is the author's sincere hope that the sharing of this experience will ease the journey of others who choose to follow a similar professional path.

While there may be a certain exhilaration that accompanies the effort to illuminate the *terra incognita* of chronic migraine, that effort also exacts an emotional toll from the clinician or clinical scientist who undertakes the mission. This chapter is dedicated to those individuals, and the pages that follow list some of the more common problems inherent in attempting to manage patients with chronic migraine, along with suggestions intended to assist the clinician in avoiding those pitfalls . . . or, at least, climbing out after he or she has tumbled within.

Perils and Pearls

If you are a clinician who devotes all or a large portion of your practice to the diagnosis and treatment of headache, many of the perils that may threaten your personal and professional sense of wellbeing stem from this simple fact: there are so many of them and so few of us. On the one hand, the headache subspecialist seldom need worry about patient volume (an old adage runs: "a physician willing to see headache patients will never be lonely"); instead you become part of a tremendous public health problem: how can the existing handful of experts in headache medicine hope to provide effective management to even a small minority of the millions of individuals who suffer from difficult-to-treat headache disorders?

More than 4% of the American population suffers from daily or near-daily headache, and roughly 1 in 50 of our citizens has chronic migraine, specifically.[1] In other words, as many as 6 million Americans actively are afflicted by a headache disorder for which—at this writing—there exists *no* therapy that possesses a U.S. Food and Drug Administration (FDA) indication for its treatment. Not surprisingly, it is this subpopulation with the chronic form of the disorder who account for a disproportionate share of the economic burden migraine imposes, and also not surprising is the fact that the waiting rooms of headache subspecialists are populated not by patients with episodic migraine who require the occasional nonsteroidal anti-inflammatory drug (NSAID) or triptan, but rather by patients afflicted with chronic migraine . . . and treatment-refractory chronic migraine at that.[2] Published studies from headache clinics consistently have reported that the majority of patients evaluated therein present with chronic daily headache, and the vast majority of *those* patients have chronic migraine.[3,4]

The old adage alluded to previously could be expanded to read: "the physician willing to see headache patients will never by lonely . . . *or rich*." To evaluate a treatment-refractory chronic migraine patient thoroughly—to take a meticulous headache history, identify and address comorbid conditions, construct an appropriate strategy for management and educate the patient in the hows and whys of the disorder and its treatment—is time consuming and hardly lucrative. Even with the aid of instruments intended to speed the process (e.g., a headache questionnaire completed by the patient prior to seeing the clinician), the 1:1 (one physician: one patient) paradigm is insufficient to the enormous task of managing the chronic migraine patient population adequately; once again, there are too many of them and too few of us.[5] Feeling over burdened and under-compensated, it's small wonder that the headache subspecialist may succumb to the bleak comfort of abject self-pity. Thus . . .

Pitfall 1: Frustration

The disorder of treatment-refractory chronic migraine is rife with codependence, and in many instances—regardless of whether the presentation is complicated by preexisting or acquired psychiatric comorbidity—the patient has abdicated his/her "locus of control." Such patients often are notable for the effusive and fulsome praise they offer up to you at the time of the initial evaluation ("I've heard so many wonderful things about you . . . I've been waiting *forever* to see . . . I know you're *so* popular . . . I just know *you're* the one who can help me . . . these headaches have taken over my life, etc"); in the next breath you're also likely to hear, "I've tried everything. Nothing works."

Don't be taken in. It's unlikely that you're the first physician to bask in this same warm praise and hear expressed this odd mélange of enthusiasm, desperation, and pessimism. One need not have borderline personality disorder (BPD), per se, to exhibit "borderline" behavior. As with BPD patients, it is useful to remember how rapidly one devolves from knight on white charger to being merely "like all the rest."

Quite literally, the patient may wish you to assume responsibility for his or her headaches, and the attempt to place the locus of control back where it belongs—that is, *internal*/with the patient—will be made more difficult if that patient already has an enabler—most often spouse or parent—who has served as a catalyst in the patient's abdication of control. It must be made clear from the start: the patient is the captain of this particular ship, and you are simply the navigator. Your role is to use your training and experience to clarify and to outline those management strategies which you consider to be most appropriate for this particular patient; it is the patient's responsibility to choose from the various courses available and wholeheartedly follow the course selected.

Remember, too, that there exist patients with treatment-refractory chronic migraine who at some level—conscious, subconscious, or unconscious—have embraced their headache disorder and will not (or cannot) give it up. In some patients it's as simple as secondary financial gain derived from obtaining formal medical disability consequent to chronic migraine. In others the origins of the symbiosis are less evident; especially in those with an Axis II personality disorderit's as if the patient is using the term "headache" as a metaphor for something far more complex and perhaps ultimately unfathomable. Whatever the source, it's fruitless to expect such patients to shed their headache disorder consequent simply to prescription of an oral prophylactic agent and a triptan or two.

Pitfall 2: *Tedium*

As previously stated, to evaluate thoroughly a patient with treatment-refractory chronic migraine can be a lengthy endeavor, and to provide follow-up care to these patients imposes additional layers of time, effort and responsibility. The histories initially provided can begin to sound depressingly familiar, and while it's true that no two patients are alike, in the case of chronic migraine—with the frequently associated psychiatric comorbidities, issues of symptomatic medication overuse, concomitant sleep disorders, hormonal dysfunction, other endocrine dysfunction, etc.—that's not necessarily an attractive proposition.

Telephone messages can be the bane of the headache subspecialist's existence. In their study of patient calls to a headache subspecialty practice, Loder and Geweke reported that the headache clinic under study received 3.17 calls per every hour of headache clinic scheduled and found that patients with chronic daily headache and personality disorders accounted for a disproportionately high number of these calls.[6] In another study that included the number of calls made by migraine patients to the physician as a secondary outcome variable, the investigators found that intensive patient education administered immediately after the initial clinic visit was associated with significantly fewer calls.[7] "The medicine's not working", "the medicine's making me sick", " I need more [opioid, butalbital containing compound, benzodiazepine, Stadol]" and—the author's personal favorite—the ubiquitous "I have a headache" . . . these and other messages can accumulate like the fallen leaves after an autumn wind storm, and responding to these messages inevitably drains one's time and psyche.

While it's impossible to eliminate totally the tedium of receiving and returning telephone messages from headache patients, this is one of the places where boundaries can and should be drawn. To extend the analogy, dealing effectively with a treatment-refractory chronic migraine patient in many ways resembles management of a patient with BPD. Prospectively establish with the patient what the goals of therapy are and indicate clearly the limits and extent of your own commitment. As regards telephone calls in particular, you may wish to specify those conditions under which a call may be considered appropriate and will be returned; the appendix provides an example of a written instrument for establishing those guidelines. If you are prescribing a medication with abuse potential or the potential for inducing medication overuse headache, then consider including on your prescription instructions as to the minimum period that medication is intended to last, and document this in the patient's chart. Emphasize to the patient that it is *his/her* responsibility to make that quantity last for the specified period and that requests for early refills (consequent to frequent headaches, the medication being lost, stolen or flushed down the toilet, etc.) will not be honored. If you are accepting responsibility for writing a controlled substance or any medication with the potential for abuse or inducing medication overuse headache, you may wish to indicate to the patient that he/she is not to seek or receive that medication from another source until or unless you have abdicated the responsibility for prescription writing. You may wish to confirm this understanding objectively with a controlled substance agreement signed by both parties and with copies to the chart and patient; one example of such an agreement has been published in the journal, *Headache*.[8]

What can you do to make yourself more efficient in clinic? Intake questionnaires meant to be completed by the patient prior to the physician's initial evaluation may prove quite helpful in expediting that process. While there exist well-validated, brief questionnaires effective in establishing the diagnosis of migraine, the Landmark Study results indicated that the vast majority of patients who present to a physician for evaluation of headache have migraine or probable migraine, and the added value of such brief, highly directed questionnaires in the clinic setting may be limited . . . especially for the headache subspecialist.[9] These questionnaires are perhaps of greatest utility when used in epidemiological studies involving large population samples. Other questionnaires completed by the patient may be helpful in assessing migraine—related functional disability, but these obviously do not constitute a headache history, per se.[10] Many physicians working at headache clinics devoted to evaluating large numbers of patients have developed their own intake questionnaires. While none admittedly is perfect or suited to the needs of all clinicians who frequently see headache patients, an example that the author has used and gradually modified over the years is available at www.uab.edu/neurology (link to Headache Program).

The importance of patient empowerment through education cannot be overemphasized. Patient education is key to maximizing compliance with therapy, in assisting the dysautonomous patient in recovering his or her locus of control and in engaging all chronic migraine patients in the management of their headache disorder. Like diabetes, migraine is often a lifelong or near lifelong disorder, and—as has been demonstrated with diabetes—therapeutic success is in large part dependent on patient autonomy and commitment.

A busy headache clinic is typically not an environment ideal for effective patient education; there is simply not enough time available to instruct a new patient with chronic migraine in the origins of his/her disorder, the basic guidelines for prophylactic therapy, the intricacies involved with taking, say, topiramate specifically, the general guidelines of acute therapy, detailed instructions regarding the use of, say, an oral triptan and injectable sumatriptan, the issue of medication overuse headache, etc., and even if there were, many patients understandably find it difficult in that setting to assimilate and retain the information imparted. Supplementary written materials can help to some extent, and many such materials have been published in *Headache*.[11–13]

To take this a long step further, multiple investigative groups have demonstrated that comprehensive migraine management programs that emphasize patient education may yield a more positive clinical outcome and other important benefits.[7,14,15] At this point such programs are few and far between, and new programs of this type are not simple to initiate. Regardless, the time for applying the disease management paradigm to chronic migraine is clearly past due, and in the future our present scatter-shot approach to management may evolve to take a more centralized, interdisciplinary, and effective form.[5,16]

Pitfall 3: Unrealistic Expectations

No matter how intelligent, articulate, clinically competent, and well-versed in the relevant medical literature another clinician may appear to be, *no one* achieves a spectacularly high rate of success in managing patients with treatment-refractory chronic migraine. I've long respected Dr. Neil Raskin for possessing those attributes just listed, and I can recall one occasion years ago—when I was a young assistant professor and before I came to know him better—when I called Dr. Raskin at his office in San Francisco to ask for his assistance with a challenging headache patient who was failing to respond to the "Raskin protocol" involving administration of dihydroergotamine. He politely waited until I'd completed my lengthy presentation and then replied in his dry manner, "John, I don't think much of *anything* works for migraine." Even the great ones have their moments of doubt.

If you set the goal of treatment in this population to render the patient headache-free or nearly so, expect frequent failure. In one study involving a consecutive series of previously refractory chronic migraine patients managed according to a uniform pharmacological treatment regimen, less than two-thirds experienced a 50% or greater reduction in headache days per month.[17] In that study, almost half of the responders required treatment with chronic methadone before reporting improvement, and subsequent studies have indicated that when the treatment response in such patients is scrutinized more closely and follow-up is extended, the success rate associated with chronic opioid therapy falls significantly.[18,19] Published reports from inpatient headache centers offering interdisciplinary therapies indicate a higher and more enduring success rate, but such centers are limited in number and may be inaccessible to many patients who require such intensive therapy.[20–22]

So what can you do? Or, more specifically, what can you reasonably expect to accomplish when you seek to grapple with treatment-refractory chronic migraine? First, use what information exists in the published literature in conjunction with what you derive from your evaluation to determine a realistic treatment goal for the individual patient. For example, patients with chronic migraine who have experienced daily headache for more than 6 months appear to be particularly resistant to treatment with the pharmacological therapies we typically prescribe or administer; only a small minority of such patients experience remission to episodic migraine.[23,24]

At the inpatient unit of the Michigan Neurologic and Head Pain Institute, staff members attempt to treat what may represent the most difficult and challenging patients within the treatment-refractory migraine population. Lake et al have emphasized that despite the time and interdisciplinary effort expended upon their patients, what constitutes treatment "success" must be calculated in the context of each patient's status at baseline, and they emphasize that whatever short-term gains result from the hospitalization will not be sustained if (1) the patient lacks sufficient motivation, or (2) after discharge there is not available to the physician a healthcare provider willing and able to work closely with that patient in continuing to implement the management plan initiated during hospitalization.[22]

Certain patients will fail to improve no matter how modest the treatment goal you've set. Psychiatric comorbidity is exceedingly common in patients with migraine, and such comorbidity may further diminish an already modest chance of treatment success.[25,26] In one study from a university-based outpatient headache clinic, patients with chronic migraine and BPD were far less likely to report any benefit from treatment relative to age- and gender-matched chronic migraine patients lacking BPD and receiving the same therapeutic interventions for their headache disorder.[27] Saper and Lake have written that in patients with BPD ". . . opioids may result in an escalation . . . of harmful behaviors," and other investigators have reported that opioid therapy may provoke psychiatric destabilization in patients with BPD.[27,28]

In summary, it's often necessary to set the bar low in determining what you or your patients reasonably can expect from even the most expert application of the therapies currently available.

Pitfall 4: Alienation

Although at times it may seem so, *you're not alone.* There is a small but expanding community of clinicians, clinical scientists, and basic scientists currently working in the field of headache medicine, and there exist numerous opportunities for interacting with your brethren. Join at least one of the national or international professional societies devoted to headache medicine. Subscribe to and read their journals. Submit your own work for publication, be it a letter to-the-editor that expresses your opinion of a published article, a report of a particularly unusual or challenging case or the results of your own original research. Visit their Web sites. Attend their meetings; those individuals considered to be experts in the field are generally a congenial lot, approachable and quite willing to share with you their own opinions and suggestions. If you have the opportunity to engage in collaborative clinical research involving headache, do so; the knowledge that you are assisting in a group effort to raise the existing standard of care can be refreshing and provide a much-needed jolt of enthusiasm.

To attempt to manage a large volume of patients with treatment-refractory chronic migraine is not for the faint of heart, and even those who initially

Pearls to Remember in Caring for Patients with Refractory Migraine

- Establish clear limits about your availability and appropriate patient requests.
- Encourage patients to take responsibility for their disorder: "The patient is the captain of this particular ship, and you are simply the navigator."
- Make use of written or online patient education materials and educational programs.
- Set realistic treatment goals for individual patients.
- Encourage appropriate, modest expectations of treatment benefit: "Remember that no one achieves a spectacularly high rate of success in managing patients with treatment-refractory chronic migraine."
- You are not alone: Seek support and advice from colleagues.

embrace the challenge will experience their low moments. Don't add to the demands of your job by alienating yourself from your peers.

Summary

To attempt to manage large numbers of patients with treatment-refractory chronic migraine requires energy, perspective, humor, and the oft-difficult task of attempting to maintain compassion while at the same time refusing to compromise one's personal and professional boundaries. The pitfalls outlined and summarized here are all too real, and few who accept the challenge of dealing with this patient population will remain unscathed by the experience.

That said, the author wishes to acknowledge the contributions of that small band of brothers (and sisters) who initially undertook the challenge of treating what we now term chronic migraine. To them belongs the greatest share of the credit for bringing out of the shadows and into the lights this headache disorder that afflicts so many millions. May we be successful in carrying on the work they began.

References

1. Bigal M, Lipton R, Tepper S, Rapoport A, Sheftell F. Primary chronic daily headache, its subtypes in adolescents and adults. *Neurology.* 2004;63:843–847.
2. Munakata J, Hazard E, Serrano D, Klingman D, et al. Economic burden of transformed migraine. Results from the American Migraine Prevalence and Prevention (AMPP) Study. *Headache.* 2009;49:498–508.
3. Mendizabal J, Rothrock J. An inter-regional comparative study of headache clinic populations. *Cephalalgia.* 1998;18:57–59.
4. Dowson A. Analysis of the patients attending a specialist UK headache clinic over a 3–year period. *Headache.* 2003;43:14–18.
5. Rothrock J. La sistema decompuesto. *Headache* 2008; 48:328–329.
6. Loder E, Geweke L. Volume and nature of telephone calls in a specialty headache practice. *Headache.* 2002;42:883–887.

7. Rothrock J, Parada V, Sims C, Key K, Walters N. The impact of intensive patient educations on clinical outcome and patient behavior. The USA Headache School. *Headache.* 2006;46:726–731.
8. Rothrock J. Controlled medication agreement. *Headache.* 2006;46:549.
9. Tepper S, Dahlof C, Dowson A, et al. Prevalence and diagnosis of migraine in patients consulting their physician with a complaint of headache. Data from the Landmark Study. *Headache.* 2004;44:856–864.
10. Stewart W, Lipton R, Kolodner K. Migraine disability assessment (MIDAS) score: relation to headache frequency, pain intensity and headache symptoms. *Headache.* 2003;43:258–265.
11. Rothrock J. Chronic migraine: medication overuse headache. *Headache.* 2007; 47:467–468.
12. Rothrock J. Migraine “chronification”. *Headache.* 2008;48:181–182.
13. Rothrock J. Acute migraine: treating early. *Headache.* 2009;49:635–636.
14. Blumenfeld A, Tischio M. Center for excellence for headache care: group model at Kaiser Permanente. *Headache.* 2003;43:431–440.
15. Maizels M, Saenz V, Wirjo J. Impact of a group-based model of disease management for headache. *Headache.* 2003;43:621–627.
16. Loder L, Biondi D. Disease modification in migraine: a concept that has come of age? *Headache.* 2003;43:135–143.
17. Rothrock J, Management of chronic daily headache utilizing a uniform treatment pathway. *Headache.* 1999;39:650–653.
18. Saper J, Lake A, Hamel R, et al. Daily scheduled opioids for intractable head pain: Long-term observations of a treatment program. *Neurology.* 2004; 62:1687–1694.
19. Saper J, Lake A. Continuous opioid therapy (COT) is rarely advisable for refractory chronic daily headache: limited efficacy, risks, and proposed guidelines. *Headache.* 2008;48:838–849.
20. Saper J. Pearls from an inpatient headache unit. *Headache.* 2008;48:820–827.
21. Freitag F, Lake A, Lipton R, Cady R on behalf of the U.S. Headache Guidelines Consortium. Inpatient treatment of headache: an evidence-based assessment. *Headache.* 2004;44:342–360.
22. Lake A, Saper J, Hamel R. Comprehensive inpatient treatment of refractory chronic daily headache. *Headache.* 2009;49:555–562.
23. Rothrock J, Parada V, Sims C, key K Walters N, Zweifler R. Predictors of a negative response to topiramate therapy in patients with chronic migraine. *Headache.* 2005;45:932–935.
24. Conway S, Delplanche C, Crowder J, Rothrock J. Botox J. Botox therapy for refractory chronic migraine. *Headache.* 2005;45:355–357.
25. Hamelsky S, Lipton R. Psychiatric co-morbidity of migraine. *Headache.* 2006;46:1327–1333.
26. Jette N, Patten S, Williams J, Becker W, Wiebe S. Comorbidity of migraine and psychiatric disorders-a national population-based study. *Headache.* 2008;48:501–516.
27. Rothrock J, Lopez I, Zweifler R, Andress-Rothrock D, Walters N. Borderline personality disorder and migraine: detection, epidemiology and therapeutic response. *Headache.* 2007;47:22–26.
28. Saper J, Lake A. Borderline personality disorder and the chronic headache patient. Review and management recommendations. *Headache.* 2002;42:663–674.

Appendix 22-1

To Our Headache Patients: When to Call

The volume of telephone calls generated by our headache patient population is quite high, and while we can understand a patient's desire to discuss his or her headache management via phone or email, we simply do not have the resources available to offer that service. It's consequently important that you understand when and for what purpose to call our office or clinic.

Reasons to call our office:

1. If you have an *urgent* problem related to the care you've received from us (for example, a possible allergic reaction or serious side effect from a medication prescribed for you). For what you consider to be a true *emergency*, either call 911 or present immediately to an emergency medical facility.
2. If you have an acute, severe headache that has persisted despite self-administered therapy, and you wish to come in that same day for in-clinic treatment of your headache. This treatment option will be open to you only at those times that our staff is in clinic and available. Call early in the day to arrange treatment; we cannot offer this service if your call is received as the clinic is about to close.
3. For prescription refills. Again, due to the high volume of calls we receive, we cannot guarantee your prescription will be refilled the same day you call; for that reason, we urge you to anticipate when you will be running out of a given medication and call at least 3 days in advance. If you call on a Friday, your prescription may not be refilled until the Monday following.

Reason to call our clinic:

1. If you are not doing well generally in regard to your headache control and would like to schedule an earlier appointment

23

Assessing and Preventing Disability in Refractory Migraine

Jonathan M. Borkum, PhD

Introduction

And so, 6 years of advanced training, specialty boards, two decades of clinical experience, and one year of treating this particular patient have come down to this: Is the claimant totally disabled? On what date will they be able to return to work? *Please give objective supporting evidence.*

Arguably, these are administrative and not clinical questions. To give shape to them, and to provide rational answers, will seemingly take us far afield of medicine. Let us begin, though, by refreshing our memories about the extent of disability in migraine.

Disability Prevalence

Population-based studies demonstrate that migraine can indeed be disabling. The average migraineur loses 4.6 workdays per year,[1] but the distribution of lost work time is highly skewed: 10% of male migraineurs and 18% of women report losing 11 or more days.[2] Chronic headaches in general (present on at least 90 of the preceding 180 days) have been associated with an unemployment rate of 18.7% versus 7.5% for those with 30 or fewer headache days.[3] Studies on migraine in particular suggest a doubling in the unemployment rate for people with the chronic form of the disorder (see Table 23.1). In other

Table 23-1 Headache Clinic-Based Studies of the Migraine Disability Assessment (MIDAS) Questionnaire in Chronic Migraine

Source	Country	Migraine Type	*N*	Age	% Female	Duration	Severity[a]	% Employed	MIDAS	Missed Workdays[b]	% MIDAS >11
Bigal[76]	USA	Episodic	86	36.1	68.6		7.4		19.3	2.3	72.2
		Chronic	182	38.3	72.5		6.3		34.9	5.3	86.3
Canuet[33]	Cuba	Episodic	82				8.3		24.7		
		Chronic`	34				8.8		79.4		
Cassidy[77]	Ireland	Episodic	107	39.1		12.6	7.4	65.2	16.5	2.2	
		Chronic	33	36.7		9.6	7.1	64.5	60.1	16.4	
D'Amico[37]	Italy	Chronic	150	45.5	83.3	25.6			79.2	58	87.3
D'Amico[78]	Italy	Episodic	264	37.6	74.6	18.8	7.7	83.3	23.4	2.2	73.1
		Chronic	247	44.7	84.6	24.6	7.0	69.6	84.1	7.1	89.1
Meletiche[79]	USA	Episodic	44	39.3	81.8		7.1		27.3		
		Chronic	46	41.3	80.4		6.6		70.7		
Rossi[53]	Italy	Episodic	121	36.6	68.6	17.5	8.0	81.8	23.7		66.1
		Chronic	79	41.2	79.7	18.5	7.7	40.5	57.7		77.2

[a]Average pain intensity on a scale of 0–10 over preceding 3 months (by recall).

[b]In the last 3 months (by recall).

large population based studies in Norway[4] and the United States,[5] people with chronic migraine report losing 15 to 20 workdays per year.

Not surprisingly, then, in the World Health Organization's consensus-based metric, severe migraine is classified alongside quadriplegia, active psychosis, and dementia as an important cause of disability.[6]

No studies have yet quantified the disability attributable to refractory migraine. However, since triptans have been shown to reduce the considerable absenteeism experienced by patients with episodic migraine, it stands to reason that those with refractory migraine have an even higher disability burden.[7,8] And with treatment at an endpoint, there often seems little for these patients to do other than file a disability claim. But on what grounds might refractory migraine become a cause for disability?

Disability Determination

To begin framing the problem, consider the American Medical Association's *Guides to the Evaluation of Permanent Impairment.* Here, a distinction is drawn between impairment, which is "a loss, loss of use, or derangement of any body part, organ system, or organ function" and disability, "an alteration of an individual's capacity to meet personal, social, or occupational demands or statutory or regulatory requirements because of an impairment" (ref. 9, pp. 2 and 8). In essence, impairment is an alteration in the structure or function of an organ or body part, while disability is a limitation in the behavior of the whole person.[10] Intermediate between these two is "functional limitation"—difficulty in the performance of a specific activity such as walking or driving. Disability is reduced participation in a social role caused by functional limitations from impairment.

Thus, disability is not, strictly speaking, a medical term. For unlike a disease, it pertains not to a person, but to the interaction of the person with their environment.[11] Disability is strongly influenced by such contextual factors as the physical setting (e.g., lighting, sound level, and exposure to fumes); the availability of health care, assistive technology, and social support; and attitudes such as stigmatization.[12] Personal factors such as emotional resilience, self-efficacy, and economic resources surely contribute as well.

The problem becomes more complicated still for purely subjective experiences such as migraine, in which the disability experienced is not clearly associated with an observable impairment of body structure or function.

Legally, disability is not even a single construct, because different compensation systems use different conceptual and operational definitions. We examine six of these systems in particular: Social Security Disability, the Railroad Retirement System, workers' compensation, private disability insurance, the Family and Medical Leave Act, and Veterans' disability ratings.

> Challenges in Determining Disability in Refractory Migraine
>
> - Disability is not a medical term and not a single construct.
> - Disability is greatly influenced by contextual and personal factors.
> - Most systems of disability determination are heavily focused on the presence of objective signs of impairment.

Social Security Disability

Under the United States Social Security Act, disability is "the inability to engage in any substantial, gainful activity by reason of a medically determinable physical or mental impairment(s), which can be expected to result in death or which has lasted or can be expected to last for a continuous period of not less than 12 months" (Code of Federal Regulations, 20 CFR 404.1505). Thus, disability requires (1) an underlying condition, i.e., "anatomical, physiological, or psychological abnormalities which can be shown by medically acceptable clinical and laboratory diagnostic techniques" (20 CFR 404.1508); (2) an impairment, or limitation in functioning, that can be attributed to the condition; and (3) occupational disability as a result of the impairment.

Diagnosis is required based on "medical evidence consisting of signs, symptoms, and laboratory findings—not only by the individual's statements of symptoms" (e.g., 20 CFR 404.1529). This requirement is difficult to meet for subjective disorders such as migraine, so it is not surprising that half of all Social Security Disability disputes to reach federal court involve some type of chronic pain.[13]

At present, the diagnostic criteria for migraine, as with other primary headache disorders, are based on subjective patient report, making it difficult to establish legally that the condition exists.[14] Migraines are not included among the roster of impairments listed as qualifying for Social Security Disability; in fact, headache is included only as a symptom of toxoplasmosis or as a side effect of antiretroviral treatment (20 CFR 404, Appendix 1). Thus, legal case discussions of migraines may include such statements as "Defendant admitted that [her neurologist] found no physical abnormalities accounting for her migraines."[15]

Paradoxically, psychological disorders, which like migraine lack objective clinical signs, are considered forms of impairment in Social Security Disability. And among these accepted disorders is somatoform pain disorder, a diagnosis in which the etiology of the pain is attributed principally to psychological factors (20 CFR 220 Appendix 1).

In part, the Social Security Administration has dealt with the problem of subjectivity by establishing liberal criteria for what constitutes an objective clinical sign, allowing, for example, the tender point examination for fibromyalgia.[16] More commonly, however, in the absence of laboratory data, the focus shifts to the credibility of the patient's claims.[16] Thus, commissioners may rely on the length of time the physician has known the patient, the number of healthcare providers who arrived at the same diagnosis, whether the patient was taking medication for the condition, and the level of functioning during the period of alleged disability.[15,17]

For physicians trained in the scientific method, such disability determination may seem like an exercise in arbitrary inference. Yet subjective variables such as pain, fatigue, nausea, and vertigo are often the true core of a disability claim. For "most diseases and injuries do not prevent people from working by mechanical failure. Rather, people are incapacitated by a variety of unbearable sensations when they try to work" (ref. 18, p. 28). And adjudication is as much about dispute resolution as it is about fact finding. For if the main goal in court were scientific certainty, evidence would never be excluded merely because it was improperly obtained, for example, through a breech of confidentiality or through unreasonable search and seizure.[19]

Role of the Physician

The physician plays a key role in the Social Security system of disability determination. In part, this is by identifying any objective clinical signs, no matter how faint, to substantiate the diagnosis. Mechanical allodynia in the region of pain, a distended superficial temporal artery, and local autonomic symptoms such as lacrimation, ptosis, or conjunctival injection would carry significant weight, for example, in the determination of a disability claim for particular kinds of headaches. Once the existence of the disorder has been in some sense verified, subjective reports of pain, nausea, and photosensitivity become more credible.

Absent such signs, the physician is likely the best person in the process to judge the severity of the disorder, the degree to which the patient's reports are consistent with each other and with the diagnosis, and the likelihood that such a condition would produce impairments and functional limitation lasting for at least another 12 months.

Note that the Social Security Administration considers the claimant's "impairment or combination of impairments" in determining disability.[17] Thus, documenting comorbidities such as depression or panic disorder may be as important as the primary diagnosis.

Disability itself is not decided by the physician, who is usually not especially knowledgeable about the characteristics of the claimant's workplace or their capacity for modification. Rather, it is determined by the administrative law judge based on information from a wide variety of sources.

Railroad Retirement System

In the United States, disabled employees with at least 10 years (120 months) of service to a railroad are covered under the Railroad Retirement System rather than the Social Security system.[20] The disability criteria, however, are the same as for Social Security (20 CFR 220.114).

Workers' Compensation

Workers' compensation is a form of insurance carried by employers in the United States and other developed countries. It provides compensation to workers who are injured on the job. In most cases, employees who accept workers' compensation forgo their right to sue the employer for negligence. Workers' compensation insurance carriers in the United States often use the AMA's *Guides to the Evaluation of Permanent Impairment*[9] in determining loss of function. In doing so, they are confronted by the same dilemma as in Social Security: "to incorporate the subjectivity associated with pain into an impairment rating system whose fundamental premise is that impairment assessment should be based on objective findings" (ref. 21, p. 569). The *Guides*, in fact, embody this tension.[10] For most disorders, the ratings are based on objective criteria such as electromyographic evidence of a lumbar radiculopathy. That the radiculopathy involves pain is simply assumed and receives no special rating.

In a separate chapter, however, the AMA *Guides* allow impairment ratings based on subjective data, provided that the disorder and the patient meet certain criteria. The disorder must be a known medical condition felt to have a biological underpinning—migraines qualify. The patient's reports must be complete enough to allow a rating, credible and internally consistent to allow confidence in that rating, and consistent with the disorder. Provided these requirements are fulfilled, impairment is based on data (especially psychometric data) on pain, mood, and pain-interference in daily activities, and behavioral observations of pain behavior. The impairment is scored qualitatively as none, mild, moderate, moderate-severe, or severe.[21]

Thus, the pain chapter in the *Guides* is a systematic version of the approach taken in practice by Social Security Disability. This does not seem unreasonable. That sensation can be measured accurately is shown by the reproducible, indeed mathematical, relationship between the magnitude of pain and the intensity of the eliciting stimulus, and the dose-response curves for analgesic medication (e.g., ref. 22). The problems, rather, are the credibility of the patient when compensation issues are involved, and the plethora of factors that can influence how pain is perceived. The former problem is dealt with in the *Guides* through physician judgment. We touch on the latter problem in the text that follows, in discussing how to prevent disability.

In workers' compensation cases, a further level of dispute can arise: whether the migraines arose out of the individual's employment. For example, the claims may focus on occupational exposure to odors (e.g., from work near diesel fumes or at a perfume counter). In other cases, the migraines are one component of more general pain arising from occupationally related neck, head, or upper back trauma. In these cases the physician will generally be asked to verify that the disorder was caused or significantly exacerbated by the occupational injury or exposure. Also, particular emphasis may be placed on functional limitations (for example, in lifting or climbing ladders) and environmental intolerances (e.g., to noise or fumes) relevant to job placement.

Private Disability Plans or Policies

In private disability plans, disability is generally defined by the policy and "some plans have been interpreted by plan administrators or insurers such that one would have to be virtually on a deathbed or in a coma before one would meet the definition of disability" (ref. 23, p. 285). Note in particular that in an "any occupation" policy, in which one is not considered disabled if capable of performing *any* type of work, the availability of such jobs within one's geographic area usually is not germane in deciding the claim. "From the insurance company's perspective, they are not going to get in the business of finding a job for the claimant" (ref. 23, p. 285). In some plans subjective data is discounted altogether and positive imaging studies are required to accept the claim. Other policies may accept "self-reported conditions" such as migraine but limit benefits to a set period, such as 12 or 24 months.[23] Similarly, private disability plans will sometimes classify chronic pain as a mental disorder. Depending on the policy, this may reduce benefits or disallow them altogether.[16]

Role of the Physician

In theory, the physician's role is much the same as in Social Security Disability and workers' compensation—to identify the diagnosis, prognosis, impairments, and perhaps functional limitations. Depending on the plan, however, particular emphasis may be placed on distinguishing subjective from objective data. Moreover, while disability is technically determined by the plan administrator, in practice the physician's judgment may be the determining factor.

Family and Medical Leave Act (FMLA)

In the United States, the Family and Medical Leave Act (FMLA) provides for up to 12 weeks of unpaid leave for employees following the adoption or birth of a child, or for a "serious health condition" that leaves the employee unable to perform their job responsibilities or functions, or to care for a parent or child with such a health condition. It applies to U.S. and state government employees, and to workers for companies with 50 or more employees in a 75-mile radius. To be covered by FMLA, the employee must have been with the employer for at least one year, including 1250 hours of employment in the preceding 12 months, and must give the employer notice as soon as is practicable that the leave will be needed (29 USCS 2611-2614).

FMLA defines a "serious health condition" as one that involves a period of incapacity of more than three consecutive calendar days, and at least two treatments by a health care provider, or an ongoing course of treatment (such as prescription medication). Specifically excluded are minor illnesses such as "headache other than migraine."

Migraines, on the other hand, are accepted as a serious health condition under FMLA.[24] Particularly relevant is that the time off can be implemented as an "intermittent or reduced [work] schedule basis," which allows for repeated, brief periods of incapacity (29 CFR 825.306).

Role of the Physician

In FMLA, disability is determined largely by the physician. To qualify for the leave, the worker submits a disability form—Form WH-380-E, "Certification of Health Care Provider for Employee's Serious Health Condition," completed in part by the health care provider. This form removes some of the ambiguities in disability determination. The "medical facts" supporting the claim are simply diagnosis, symptoms, doctor visits, and ongoing treatment (29 CFR 825.306). And while the health care provider is asked to certify that the employee is unable to perform at least one of his or her job functions, a list of these functions must be provided to the physician by the employer or, failing that, the employee.[25]

Department of Veterans' Affairs

Simplest of all are the disability ratings applied to veterans, which, for migraines, are based simply on the frequency of attacks, as shown in Table 23.2 (38 CFR 4.124a). These ratings are made by physicians within the VA system.

Table 23-2 Disability Ratings for Migraines in the Department of Veterans Affairs

Average Frequency of "Characteristic Prostrating Attacks"	Disability Rating
Less than once every 2 months	0
One in 2 months over last several months	10
Once a month over last several months	30
Very frequent completely prostrating and prolonged attacks productive of severe economic inadaptability	50

From Code of Federal Regulations, 38 CFR 4.124a.

Some Common Systems of Disability Determination and Compensation

- Social Security Disability
- Railroad Retirement System
- Workers' Compensation
- Private Disability Insurance
- Family and Medical Leave Act
- Veterans' Administration

Clinical Assessment of Disability

In all of the systems we have reviewed, disability determination in migraine is dependent on an assessment of severity of the disease. At this point, of course, there are no objective measures of disease severity for migraine. In the future, plasma levels of calcitonin gene-related peptide or substance P,[26] functional imaging of pain modulatory circuits,[27] glutamate concentration in cerebrospinal fluid,[28] or determination of the grey matter volume of somatosensory cortex[29] may fulfill this role (although brain imaging studies may also give rise to legal controversies over the invasion of privacy[30]).

In the meantime, disability is best assessed by asking about the extent of interference in daily activities. This can be placed on a more quantitative basis, and coordinated with the research literature, by using a validated psychometric measure of some kind. Two are in common use for disability assessment in headache sufferers: the Migraine Disability Assessment (MIDAS) questionnaire,[31] and the Headache Impact Test (HIT[32]).

It should be noted that interference in functioning is one component, along with emotional state and sense of physical well-being, in quality of life.[33] Thus, quality of life measures such as the Headache Disability Inventory,[34] the Migraine Specific Quality of Life scale,[35] or the life interference scale of the West Haven-Yale Multidimensional Pain Inventory[36] are sometimes used instead of MIDAS or HIT. The MIDAS questionnaire quantifies the impact of headaches on occupational and social functioning. Its five items cover the number of days in the last ninety on which, because of a headache, the respondent (1) missed work or school; (2) was unable to do household work; (3) missed family, social, or leisure activities; or (4) had a 50% or greater reduction in productivity at work or (5) in household work.

The MIDAS has the advantages of internal consistency, stability over time,[31] some sensitivity to treatment effects[37,38] and validation against physician judgments[39] and diary measures of disability ($r = 0.59$, in 40; $r = 0.63$).[41] Further, it has been used to increase the efficiency of treatment by stratifying patients according to the severity of their disorder.[42] Results are consistent across studies. As show in Table 23.1, the functional impact of chronic migraine is very high as indexed by both the total MIDAS score and the number of lost workdays due to headache.

For disability determination in the legal sense, however, the MIDAS seems best regarded as an example of the self-report scales discussed in the AMA *Guides*. That is, scores would inform decision-making only in the context of the diagnosis, credibility, and consistency of the patient. As a retrospective measure, it is presumably subject to errors and bias in recall. Question 1, the number of lost workdays, has a modest correlation coefficient of only 0.41 with a prospective diary measure of the same variable.[41] There appears to be a systematic bias as well, as the score on Question 1 appears to be about 77% higher than the corresponding diary measure.[41] Moreover, MIDAS scores are surprisingly independent of work status; they remain valid in people who are unemployed, retired, or disability-retired.[43] Thus, the MIDAS score is not clearly measuring the sort of disability that is important for legal purposes.

> Instruments for the Clinical Assessment of Disability in Refractory Migraine
>
> - Migraine Disability Scale (MIDAS)
> - Headache Impact Test (HIT)
> - The Headache Disability Inventory (HDI)
> - The life interference scale of the West Haven-Yale Multidimensional
> - Pain Inventory

Preventing Disability

High mean disability scores on the MIDAS may mask an equally high variability. Thus, while in one clinic-based study of chronic migraine the average respondent reported losing 19 days of work a month, 61% of respondents lost no work time at all.[37] Similarly, while another study found that chronic migraine caused a high disability burden in the population, 76% of respondents reported no absenteeism due to headache in the preceding 90 days.[5]

Thus, for hints about how to prevent disability, it will be helpful to understand more precisely who becomes disabled. In Table 23.3 the main variables that have been studied in migraine-related disability are summarized, along with the strength of association given as the Pearson correlation, *r*. (When correlations were not reported in the source article they could often be derived. For frequency counts, this was accomplished by collapsing the data into 2 × 2 tables and calculating *r* as the phi coefficient. For continuous data, the standardized mean difference was first computed and then converted into *r* using the point-biserial formula [see ref. 44, pp. 47, 48, and 62].)

The variable most consistently associated with disability is pain intensity, with all studies showing a correlation between 0.31 and 0.35, regardless of the exact disability measure used. The effect of headache frequency seems more variable, but the majority of studies show an effect. Nausea (at least in adults) and some combination of photophobia and phonophobia, although having seemingly less impact than pain intensity, add significantly to the burden as well.

Other less well-studied variables also seem predictive. Neck pain during migraines may be associated with greater disability,[45] perhaps as a marker for allodynia, which is disproportionately present in higher disability classes.[46] Premenstrual migraines may be more disabling than non-menstrual headaches.[47]

Table 23-3 Predictors of Disability in Migraine

Source (First Author)	Sample Type	*N*	Age	% Female	Diagnosis	Disability Measure	Effect Size (as Pearson *r*)
Headache Intensity							
Gesztelyi[80]	Clinic	231	37	84	EM + CM	MIDAS	0.34***
Magnusson[81]	Clinic	115	38	90	EM + CM	HDI	—*
Park[82]	Clinic	92	37	82	EM	Diary	0.31*
Stewart[43]	Population	794	38	78	EM + CM	MIDAS	0.35***
Tkachuk[83]	Community	37	14	51	EM	Diary	0.35*
Headache Frequency							
Brown [84]	Clinic + Prim Care	146	44	87	EM	MIDAS	0.47***,[b]
Ford[45]	Clinic	141	37	87	EM + CM	HIT-6	0.26**
Gesztelyi[80]	Clinic	231	37	84	EM + CM	MIDAS	0.55***
Holroyd[40]	Community	232	38	79	EM + CM	MIDAS	0.35***
Magnusson[81]	Clinic	115	38	90	EM + CM	HDI	*ns*
Stewart[43]	Population	794	38	78	EM + CM	MIDAS	0.25***
Tkachuk[83]	Community	37	14	51	EM	Diary	0.13 (*ns*)
Headache Is Accompanied by Nausea							
Ford[45]	Clinic	141	37	87	EM + CM	HIT-6	0.20*
Park[82]	Clinic	92	37	82	EM	Diary	0.34*
Tkachuk[83]	Community	37	14	51	EM	Diary	0.03 (*ns*)
Other Associated Symptoms							
Ford[45]	Clinic	141	37	87	EM + CM	HIT-6	0.20* (neck pain)
Holroyd[40]	Community	232	38	79	EM + CM	MIDAS	0.35*** (photo + phono + nausea)
Park[82]	Clinic	92	37	82	EM	Diary	0.24* (photophobia)

(continued)

Table 23-3 Predictors of Disability in Migraine (Continued)

Source (First Author)	Sample Type	*N*	Age	% Female	Diagnosis	Disability Measure	Effect Size (as Pearson *r*)
Park[82]	Clinic	92	37	82	EM	Diary	0.15 (*ns*; phonophobia)
Tkachuk[83]	Community	37	14	51	EM	Diary	0.39** (photo + phono)
Premenstrual vs. Nonmenstrual Migraine							
Granella[47]	Clinic	64	35	100	EM + CM	Diary	0.18*,[c]
Coping Response							
Ford[45]	Clinic	141	37	87	EM + CM	HIT-6	0.44**
Catastrophizing							
Holroyd[40]	Community	232	38	79	EM + CM	MIDAS	0.24***
Depression							
Gesztelyi[80]	Clinic	231	37	84	EM + CM	MIDAS	0.45***
Holroyd[40]	Community	232	38	79	EM + CM	MIDAS	0.14*
Rossi[53]	Clinic	79	41	80	CM	MIDAS	0.32**
Tietjen[85]	Clinic	142	39	84	Migraine	MIDAS	0.07[b, d] (*ns*)
Posttraumatic Stress Disorder							
Ifergane[86]	Clinic	92	43	77	EM	MIDAS	0.20[c] (*ns*)
Peterlin[87]	Clinic	390	43	91	EM	HIT-6	0.21***,[c]

[a]*$p < 0.05$; **$p < 0.01$; ***$p < 0.001$.

[a]Partial correlation.

[b]Derived as phi coefficient from contingency table.

[c]Derived as point-biserial coefficient from standardized mean difference.

[d]For comorbid depression, anxiety, and/or fibromyalgia.

Among psychological variables, disability seems to be associated with catastrophizing—that is, the tendency to feel overwhelmed by pain, to ruminate on it, and to overestimate its likely negative impact.[48] In prospective clinical studies, catastrophizing has emerged as a predictor of new-onset disabling low back pain,[49] of a deteriorating course of pain intensity, depression, and disability in rheumatoid arthritis,[50] and of pain intensity in postherpetic neuralgia.[51] In laboratory studies, individuals who catastrophize show a more pronounced windup of pain sensitivity with repeated stimulation (e.g., ref. 52). Thus, a malignant role for catastrophizing in migraine-disability seems plausible.

There is also evidence for the role of depression, when measured psychometrically, and possibly also for posttraumatic stress disorder, as important factors in migraine-associated disability. Insecure attachment[53] and borderline personality disorder[54] have similarly been associated with disability in migraine.

Logically, we might also expect the link between migraine and disability to be moderated by such variables as vocational resourcefulness (education level, amount of time in the workforce, urban dwelling/availability of a variety of jobs), personal resourcefulness (self-efficacy, strong health appraisal, limited perceived impact of the migraines) and the number of comorbid conditions (e.g., ref. 55).

Opioid use may deserve study, even apart from its role in medication-overuse headache. In chronic low back pain, having once been dependent on prescription opioids[56] or having taken high doses[57] is associated with a markedly greater disability status one year after tapering from the medications, even after controlling for pain and comorbid psychological disorders. However, whether this represents a causal effect of opioids or is simply a marker for some unmeasured personality or disease-related variable is uncertain. Moreover, an association with disability has not always been replicated across studies.[58]

Of note, the psychological variables seem to contribute independently of the characteristics of the headaches themselves. Thus, in refractory migraine, in which a reduction in headaches has by definition not occurred despite appropriate traditional treatment, reducing psychological comorbidity and improving pain coping may provide an alternate means of approach.

Moreover, psychological variables may be especially significant in refractory migraine. Patients are keenly aware, of course, of the accumulated treatment failures. Feeling overwhelmed by pain, afraid of its impact, or resigned to suffering would scarcely seem irrational. Reconstructing a sense of control over the migraines, or over one's emotional and cognitive response to the migraines, through cognitive–behavioral therapy can be important for restoring quality of life.[59] Indeed, it seems relevant to consider disability, along with comorbidity, medication overuse, and headache frequency, as an important criterion for staging patients to a more intensive and multidisciplinary level of care.[60]

Characteristics of the work environment are surely also relevant. There has been little study of this area so far. However, migraine itself has been found to correlate with exposure to fumes (in women[61]) and to the concentration of mold spores in workplace dust.[62] Migraines may also correlate with certain aspects of job stress. Among men, these aspects are lack of support from coworkers and a demanding work environment with little authority or decision latitude (high demand-low control). Among women, job insecurity seems to be especially important.[63] Reverse causality, however, (that migraines may be leading people to experience their jobs as more stressful) has not been ruled out. A stronger case can be made for the perception that one's job entails more effort than reward. This aspect of work stress correlates with later onset of migraines in those initially free of the disorder.[64]

Some Factors that Contribute to Migraine-Related Disability

- Pain intensity
- Headache frequency
- Nausea, photo and phonophobia
- Premenstrual attacks
- Neck pain
- Catastrophizing
- Depression

Encouraging Functioning

Patients may see disability as their only option for meeting their basic financial needs, a view perhaps exacerbated by the tendency of thought to become less subtle and complex—to "lose dimensionality"—under stress. Yet for a number of reasons, patients should be encouraged from the outset to consider alternative solutions.

Depending on the payer, the disability determination process can be agonizingly slow. For Social Security Disability, the time to initial decision is approximately 97 days; while for complex cases (of which refractory migraines are likely an example) final resolution can take up to 3 years.[65] Surely this is not the safety net most patients have in mind when they file.

The decision time for private disability insurance is regulated by law, at least if the policy is provided by the employer However, a claimant may not qualify for disability benefits until after, say, the first 180 days (the elimination period), after which the case decision and one or more appeals may need to take place.[23]

Moreover, disability status, once acquired, tends to persist. In one prospective population study, 92% of patients who initially had moderate or high disability from headache were still disabled 3 years later.[66] Although this does not prove a causal role for disability compensation, it fits with the idea that the transition to disability is life-altering.

And not necessarily for the better. Disability often entails diminished income, severing of the social identity provided by work, stigmatization, isolation and withdrawal, diminished self-esteem and sense of effectiveness, and chronic sorrow for the loss of functioning.[67] Reactions to the illness such as depression, anger (directed internally or at the pain), and substance abuse are not resolved by disability and may be intensified. In solving the problem of work demands that are incompatible with the illness, disability status brings into play the new problem of reconstructing a meaningful life, with its implications of restored psychosocial homeostasis, functioning, and person–environment fit.[67] Not surprisingly, then, disability is both a component and a correlate of impaired quality of life in migraine.[33]

The Americans with Disabilities Act

Some support for remaining at work despite disability is provided by the Americans with Disabilities Act (ADA; 42 USC 12101), which makes it unlawful for an employer to discriminate against an otherwise qualified individual with a disability. Moreover, the law requires reasonable accommodation when the accommodation would allow the otherwise qualified individual to perform the job. Reasonable accommodations may include physical access, providing equipment or devices, modifying the work schedule, or restructuring the job. The accommodation generally follows good faith discussions between employee and employer stemming from a specific request by the employee.[68]

For ADA purposes, migraines have been accepted as a disabling condition[69] and thus such changes as alterations of migraine-aggravating lighting or computer screens would likely be mandated. However, there are numerous limitations in the ADA that make it far from a panacea. For example, it applies only to firms with 15 or more workers. It does not require changes that would be a significant hardship to the operation of the business. And the employee must otherwise be able to perform the essential functions of the job.

Now, for most jobs, attendance is an essential function. Thus, while the ADA may support leaves of known duration, it does not require retaining an employee with unpredictable absences. The courts have been divided as to whether working from home is a reasonable accommodation.[68] Although a stressed and aggrieved patient may see the ADA mostly as grounds for a lawsuit, the courts have sided with the employer between 95% and 98% of the time.[68] Therefore the real power of the act is in the good faith discussions that it requires.

Much good can come from these discussions, including modification of occupational exposures to fumes, lighting, or noise; alterations in work schedule; and, although likely not mandated by the ADA, a restructuring of the job to reduce stress. The simple fact that the discussion takes place can help maintain the motivation and self-efficacy of the employee and prevent a spiral of mutual distrust. Not surprisingly, then, a recent Cochrane review found moderate-quality evidence that such discussions reduce disability in musculoskeletal disorders when compared with clinical care alone.[70] Of note, health care does not seem to reduce disability, and workplace intervention does not seem to improve health; rather, the two domains appear relatively independent.

The physician, as a headache specialist who likely has authority in the workplace, knowledge of the disorder, and the trust of the patient, is in a good position to facilitate and contribute to these discussions.

The Americans with Disabilities Act (ADA) and Refractory Migraine

- The ADA requires employers to make "reasonable accommodations" for people with disabilities—but employees must be able to perform the essential functions of their jobs.
- Migraine is considered a disabling condition under the ADA, but attendance is an essential function
- Thus, ADA is most useful as a way of opening discussions with an employer about improved work conditions.
- ADA may not provide protection for unpredictable work absences.

Vocational Rehabilitation

Once a person qualifies for Social Security Disability, access to vocational rehabilitation services increases. However, there can be long waiting lists for vocational rehabilitation services, which are most useful to people who have already begun thinking about alternative career directions. Thus, the application for long-term or permanent disability is not too soon for the patient to begin thinking about different types of work.

Classically, vocational counseling utilizes information on a person's aptitude, skills, personality, and mix of vocationally oriented traits to find a good person-environment fit.[71] Personality assessment generally uses the five factor model[72]—for example, matching extroverts to occupations involving human interaction. Vocationally oriented traits are most frequently those proposed by Holland: Realistic (e.g., a machinist), Investigative (e.g., a scientist), Artistic (or creative; e.g., an architect or clothes designer), Social (e.g., a coach or a caterer), Enterprising (e.g., a buyer, personnel manager, or small business owner), and Conventional (e.g., a bookkeeper or transcriptionist). People and their corresponding job matches have a hierarchy of traits—for example, physicians tend to be investigative first, but also social and artistic.[73] (It is thus not surprising that changes that make medicine less social and creative have had significant effects on job satisfaction of doctors[74]).

Even outside of formal theory, it may become clear from an individual's description of their previous jobs that they possess intangible, transferable skills. For example, a tractor mechanic's carefully reasoned troubleshooting may apply equally well, with training, to auditing a balance sheet in an office far removed from diesel fumes.

Also relevant is past training, including training that was never utilized—an art school graduate who ended up, because of circumstances long since resolved, selling men's clothing. And even when an individual is most convinced they will never work again, one may discern a surprising degree of industriousness in their crafts or hobbies. Even if these are impractical as a primary means of support, they may allow a small supplementary income after disability.

Across all conditions, vocational rehabilitation is successful approximately 62% of the time, ranging from 75% for people with sensory or communication deficits to 55% of people with mental impairments.[75] Vocational counseling is its own specialty, of course, and requires a luxury of time not usually available to the medical practitioner in the consulting room. But asking about the positive aspects of previous jobs, past accomplishments in the workplace, and reinforcing any spark of interest or pride, can help shift a person from dichotomizing between their former occupation and lifelong disability. Even if they are too worried about finances to think creatively now, remembering their potential will be important once they are receiving disability.

Seen in this light, disability determination is perhaps a clinical question after all, and not so far afield of medicine. For in the end, disability is not about a form, a policy, or a hearing, but about navigating a life transition with creativity, courage, and grace.

References

1. Steiner TJ, Scher AI, Stewart WF, Kolodner K, Liberman J, Lipton RB. The prevalence and disability burden of adult migraine in England and their relationships to age, gender and ethnicity. *Cephalalgia.* 2003;23:519–527.
2. Stewart WF, Lipton RB, Simon D. Work-related disability: results from the American Migraine Study. *Cephalalgia.* 1996;16:231–238.
3. Stang P, Von Korff M, Galer BS. Reduced labor force participation among primary care patients with headache. *J Gen Intern Med.* 1998;13:296–302.
4. Fiane I, Haugland ME, Stovner LJ, Zwart J-A, Bovim G, Hagen K. (2006). Sick leave is related to frequencies of migraine and non-migrainous headache—The HUNT study. *Cephalalgia.* 2006;26:960–967.
5. Bigal ME, Serrano D, Reed M, Lipton RB. Chronic migraine in the population: Burden, diagnosis, and satisfaction with treatment. *Neurology.* 2008;71:559–566.
6. Murray CJL, Lopez AD. Regional patterns of disability-free life expectancy and disability-adjusted life expectancy: Global Burden of Disease study. *Lancet.* 1997;349:1347–1352.
7. Davies GM, Santanello N, Gerth W, Lerner D, Block GA. Validation of a migraine work and productivity loss questionnaire for use in migraine studies. *Cephalalgia.* 1999;19:497–502.
8. Lofland JH, Kim SS, Batenhorst AS, et al. Cost-effectiveness and cost-benefit of sumatriptan in patients with migraine. *Mayo Clin Proc.* 2001;76:1093–1101.

9. Cocchiarella L, Andersson GBJ. *Guides to the Evaluation of Permanent Impairment*, 5th ed. Chicago: AMA Press, 2001.
10. Robinson JP, Turk DC, Loeser JD. Pain, impairment, and disability in the AMA Guides. *J Law Med Ethics.* 2004;32:315–326.
11. Brandt EN Jr, Pope AM. *Enabling America: Assessing the Role of Rehabilitation Science and Engineering.* Washington, DC: National Academy Press; 1997.
12. World Health Organization. *International Classification of Functioning, Disability and Health.* Geneva: World Health Organization, 2001.
13. Bierman AE. The medico-legal enigma of fibromyalgia: Social Security Disability determinations and subjective complaints of pain. *Wayne Law Rev.* 1998;44:259–273.
14. Loder E, Loder J. Medicolegal issues in cluster headache. *Curr Pain Headache Rep.* 2004;8:147–156.
15 *Olsowka v. Sugendrini, LEXIS 2339* (Michigan Court of Appeals, 2008).
16. Finch M. Law and the problem of pain. *University of Cincinnati Law Review* 2005;74:285–327.
17 *Flaherty v. Astrue, LEXIS 23269 Soc. Sec. Rep. Service 621* (U. S. Court of Appeals for the Tenth Circuit, 2007).
18. Osterweis M, Kleinman A, Mechanic D. (eds.), *Pain and Disability: Clinical, Behavioral, and Public Policy Perspectives.* Washington, DC: National Academy Press;1987.
19. Agatstein DJ. Beyond the threshold: wincing at Social Security's process of evaluating pain. *J Natl Assoc Admin Law Judges.* 1997;17:231–283.
20. U. S. Railroad Retirement Board. *Railroad retirement handbook 2006.* Chicago: U. S. Railroad Retirement Board, 2006.
21. Turk DC, Robinson JP, Loeser JD, Covington E, Lippe P. Pain. In: Cocchiarella L, Andersson GBJ (eds.), *Guides to the Evaluation of Permanent Impairment*, 5th ed. Chicago: AMA Press;2001:565–591.
22. Price DD. *Psychological Mechanisms of Pain and Analgesia.* Seattle: IASP Press;1999.
23. Martin DP. The subtle snake: long-term disability insurance under ERISA. *The Alabama Lawyer.* 2005;66:279–287.
24 *Rebecca Sills v. Bendix Commercial Vehicle Systems, LLC, LEXIS 25425* (U.S. District Court for the Northern District of Indiana, Fort Wayne Division, 2005).
25. Department of Labor. Form WH-380–E. OMB Control Number 1215–0181, January 2009.
26. Fusayasu E, Kowa H, Takeshima T, Nakaso K, Nakashima K. Increased plasma substance P and CGRP levels, and high ACE activity in migraineurs during headache-free periods. *Pain.* 2007;128:209–214.
27. Moulton EA, Burstein R, Tully S, Hargreaves R, Becerra L, Borsook D. Interictal dysfunction of a brainstem descending modulatory center in migraine patients. *PLoS ONE.* 2008;3(11): e3799.
28. Peres MFP, Zukerman E, Senne Soares CA, Alonso EO, Santos BFC, Faulhaber MHW. Cerebrospinal fluid glutamate levels in chronic migraine. *Cephalalgia.* 2004;24:735–739.
29. DaSilva AFM, Granziera C, Snyder J, Hadjikhani N. Thickening in the somatosensory cortex of patients with migraine. *Neurology.* 2007;69:1990–1995.

30. Kolber AJ. Pain detection and the privacy of subjective experience. *Am J Law Med.* 2007;33:433–456.
31. Stewart WF, Lipton RB, Whyte J, Dowson A, Kolodner K, Liberman JN, Sawyer J. An international study to assess reliability of the Migraine Disability Assessment (MIDAS) score. *Neurology.* 1999;53:988–994.
32. Ware JE Jr., Bjorner JB, Kosinski M. Practical implications of item response theory and computerized adaptive testing. *Med Care.* 2000;38 (Suppl. II): II-73—II- 82.
33. Canuet L, Ishii R, Fernandez-Concepcion O, Iwase M, Takeda M. Severity of depressive symptoms as predictor of impairment of quality of life in chronic migraine: Comparison with episodic migraine. *Psychiatr Clin Neurosci.* 2008;62:738–740.
34. Jacobson GP, Ramadan NM, Aggarwal SK, Newman CW. The Henry Ford Hospital Headache Disability Inventory (HDI). *Neurology.* 1994;44: 837–842.
35. Martin BC, Pathak DS, Sharfman MI, Adelman JU, Taylor F, Kwong J, Jhingran P. Validity and reliability of the Migraine-Specific Quality of Life Questionnaire (MSQ Version 2.1). *Headache.* 2000;40:204–215.
36. Kerns RD, Turk DC, Rudy TE. The West Haven-Yale Multidimensional Pain Inventory (WHYMPI). *Pain.* 1985;23:345–356.
37. D'Amico D, Usai S, Grazzi L, et al. Quality of life and disability in primary chronic headaches. *Neurol Sci.* 2003;24:s97–s100.
38. García ML, Baos V, Láinez M, Pascual J, López-Gil A. Responsiveness of Migraine-ACT and MIDAS questionnaires for assessing migraine therapy. *Headache.* 2008;48:1349–1355.
39. Lipton RB, Stewart WF, Sawyer MB, Edmeads JG. Clinical utility of an instrument assessing migraine disability: The Migraine Disability Assessment (MIDAS) questionnaire. *Headache.* 2001;41:854–861.
40. Holroyd KA, Drew JB, Cottrell CK, Romanek KM, Heh V. Impaired functioning and quality of life in severe migraine: the role of catastrophizing and associated symptoms. *Cephalalgia.* 2007;27:1156–1165.
41. Stewart WF, Lipton RB, Kolodner K, Sawyer J, Lee C, Liberman JN. Validity of the Migraine Disability Assessment (MIDAS) score in comparison to a diary-based measure in a population sample of migraine sufferers. *Pain.* 2000;88:41–52.
42. Lipton RB, Stewart WF, Stone AM, Lainez MJ, Sawyer JP. Stratified care vs. step care strategies for migraine. *JAMA.* 2000;294:2599–2605.
43. Stewart WF, Lipton RB, Kolodner K. Migraine Disability Assessment (MIDAS) score: relation to headache frequency, pain intensity, and headache symptoms. *Headache.* 2003;43:258–265.
44. Lipsey MW, Wilson DB. *Practical Meta-analysis.* Thousand Oaks, CA: Sage; 2001.
45. Ford S, Calhoun A, Kahn K, Mann J, Finkel A. Predictors of disability in migraineurs referred to a tertiary clinic: neck pain, headache characteristics, and coping behaviors. *Headache.* 2008;48:523–528.
46. Bigal ME, Ashina S, Burstein R, Reed ML, Buse D, Serrano D, Lipton RB. Prevalence and characteristics of allodynia in headache sufferers: a population study. *Neurology.* 2008;70:1525–1533.

47. Granella F, Sances G, Allais G, et al. Characteristics of menstrual and nonmenstrual attacks in women with menstrually related migraine referred to headache centres. *Cephalalgia.* 2004;24:707–716.
48. Sullivan MJL, Bishop SR, Pivik J. The Pain Catastrophizing Scale: development and validation. *Psychol Assess.* 1995;7:524–532.
49. Picavet HSJ, Vlaeyen JWS, Schouten JSAG. Pain catastrophizing and kinesiophobia: Predictors of chronic low back pain. *Am J Epidemiol.* 2002;156: 1028–1034.
50. Keefe FJ, Brown GK, Wallston KA, Caldwell DS. Coping with rheumatoid arthritis pain: catastrophizing as a maladaptive strategy. *Pain.* 1989;37:51–56.
51. Haythornthwaite JA, Clark MR, Pappagallo M, Raja SN. Pain coping strategies play a role in the persistence of pain in post-herpetic neuralgia. *Pain.* 2003;106:453–460.
52. Edwards RR, Smith MT, Stonerock G, Haythornthwaite JA. Pain-related catastrophizing in healthy women is associated with greater temporal summation of and reduced habituation to thermal pain. *Clin JPain.* 2006;22: 730–737.
53. Rossi P, Di Lorenzo G, Malpezzi MG, et al. Depressive symptoms and insecure attachment as predictors of disability in a clinical population of patients with episodic and chronic migraine. *Headache.* 2005;45:561–570.
54. Rothrock J, Lopez I, Zweilfer R, Andress-Rothrock D, Drinkard R, Walters N. Borderline personality disorder and migraine. *Headache.* 2007;47:22–26.
55. Bishop M. Determinants of employment status among a community-based sample of people with epilepsy: implications for rehabilitation interventions. *Rehabil Counsel Bull.* 2004;47(2):112–120, 122.
56. Dersh J, Mayer TG, Gatchel RJ, Polatin PB, Theodore BR, Mayer EA. Prescription opioid dependence is associated with poorer outcomes in disabling spinal disorders. *Spine.* 2008;33:2219–2227.
57. Kidner CL, Mayer TG, Gatchel RJ. Higher opioid doses predict poorer functional outcome in patients with chronic disabling occupational musculoskeletal disorders. *J Bone Joint Surg Am Vol.* 2009;91:919–927.
58. Soin A, Cheng J, Brown L, Moufawad S, Mekhail N. Functional outcomes in patients with chronic nonmalignant pain on long-term opioid therapy. *Pain Practice.* 2008;8:379–384.
59. Branca B. Pain and disability: Part 1. Assessing and determining disability in the complex migraine pain patient. *fDirect Psychiatry.* 2007;27(4):303–311.
60. Saper J, Lake A III, Lipton R. Staging headache cases: reconciling the complexity of a case with the required intensity of treatment. *Headache.* 2007;47:90–93.
61. Rasmussen BK. Migraine and tension-type headache in a general population: Psychosocial factors. *Int J Epidemiol.* 1992;21:1138–1143.
62. Vincent D, Annesi I, Festy B, Lambrozo J. Ventilation system, indoor air quality, and health outcomes in Parisian modern office workers. *Environ Res.* 1997;75:100–112.
63. Wilkins K, Beaudet MP. Work stress and health. *Health Rep.* 1998;10(3): 47–62.
64. Mäki K, Vahtera J, Virtanen M, Elovainio M, Keltikangas-Järvinen L, Kivimäki M. Work stress and new-onset migraine in a female employee population. *Cephalalgia.* 2008;28:18–25.

65. Tulu B, Horan TA. The electronic disability record: purpose, parameters, and model use case. *JAm Med Informat Assoc.* 2009;16:7–13.
66. Von Korff M, Ormel J, Keefe FJ, Dworkin SF. Grading the severity of chronic pain. *Pain.* 1992;50:133–149.
67. Livneh H, Antonak RF. Psychological adaptation to chronic illness and disability: a primer for counselors. *J Counsel Dev.* 2005;83:12–20.
68. Matejkovic JE, Matejkovic ME. What is reasonable accommodation under the ADA? Not an easy answer; rather a plethora of questions. *Mississippi Coll Law Rev.* 2008/2009;28:67–96.
69. *Hankins v. The Gap, LEXIS 12307* (U.S. Court of Appeals, 6th Circuit, 1996). Also LEXIS 21887 (U.S. District Court for the Eastern District of Kentucky, Covington Division).
70. Van Oostrom SH, Driessen MT, de Vet HCW, et al. Workplace interventions for preventing work disability. *Cochrane Database of Systematic Reviews* 2009;Issue 2. Art. No.: CD006955.
71. Phillips SD, Jome LM. Vocational choices: What do we know? What do we need to know? In: Walsh WB, Savickas, ML (eds.), *Handbook of Vocational Psychology: Theory, Research, and Practice,* 3rd ed. Mahwah, NJ: Lawrence Erlbaum;2005:127–153.
72. Walsh WB, Eggerth DE. Vocational psychology and personality: the relationship of the five-factor model to job performance and job satisfaction. In: Walsh WN, Savickas L (eds.), *Handbook of Vocational Psychology: Theory, Research, and Practice,* 3rd ed. Mahwah, NJ: Lawrence Erlbaum; 2005:267–295.
73. Holland JL. *Making Vocational Choices,* 2nd ed. Odessa, FL: Psychological Assessment Resources, 1992.
74. Hueston WJ. Rekindling the fire of family medicine. *Fam Pract Manage.* 2006;13:15–17.
75. Dutta A, Gervey R, Chan F, Chou C-C, Ditchman N. Vocational rehabilitation services and employment outcomes for people with disabilities: a United States study. *J Occup Rehabil.* 2008;18:326–334.
76. Bigal ME, Rapoport AM, Lipton RB, Tepper SJ, Sheftell FD. Assessment of migraine disability using the Migraine Disability Assessment (MIDAS) Questionnaire: a comparison of chronic migraine with episodic migraine. *Headache.* 2003;43:336–342.
77. Cassidy EM, Tomkins E, Hardiman O, O'Keane V. Factors associated with burden of primary headache in a specialty clinic. *Headache.* 2003;43: 638–644.
78. D'Amico D, Grazzi L, Usai S, Rigamonti A, Curone M, Bussone G. Disability pattern in chronic migraine with medication overuse: a comparison with migraine without aura. *Headache.* 2005;45:553–560.
79. Meletiche DM, Lofland JH, Young WB. Quality-of-life differences between patients with episodic and transformed migraine. *Headache.* 2001;41:573–578.
80. Gesztelyi G, Bereczki D. Determinants of disability in everyday activities differ in primary and cervicogenic headaches and in low back pain. *Psychiatr Clin Neurosci.* 2006;60:271–276.
81. Magnusson JE, Becker WJ. Migraine frequency and intensity: relationship with disability and psychological factors. *Headache.* 2003;43:1049–1059.

82. Park JW, Shin HE, Kim JS, Lee KS. Assessing migraine disability by diary-based measurement: relationship to the characteristics of individual attacks. *Eur J Neurol.* 2008;15:817–821.
83. Tkachuk GA, Cottrell CK, Gibson JS, O'Donnell FJ, Holroyd KA. Factors associated with migraine-related quality of life and disability in adolescents: a preliminary investigation. *Headache.* 2003;43:950–955.
84. Brown JS, Neumann PJ, Papadopoulos G, Ruoff G, Diamond M, Menzin J. Migraine frequency and health utilities: findings from a multisite survey. *Value Health.* 2008;11, 315–321.
85. Tietjen GE, Herial NA, Hardgrove J, Utley C, White L. Migraine comorbidity constellations. *Headache.* 2007;47:857–865.
86. Ifergane G, Buskila D, Simiseshvely N, Jotkowitz A, Kaplan Z, Cohen H. Post-traumatic stress disorder is not over-represented in a sample population of migraine patients. *Eur J Intern Med.* 2009;20:182–185.
87. Peterlin BL, Tietjen GE, Brandes JL, Rubin SM, Drexler E, Lidicker JR, Meng S. Posttraumatic stress disorder in migraine. *Headache.* 2009;49:541–551.

24

Coding and Reimbursement for Services to Patients with Refractory Migraine

Stuart Black, MD

Introduction

In the beginning, there was fee for service! In earlier years, medical practitioners were paid through trade, exchange, or by monetary reimbursements. Throughout the 19th century, most patients were treated in their homes. Even surgery was often performed in homes. At that time, the market for health insurance in the United States was not a priority. Medical technology was quite elemental, people had relatively low medical expenditures, and, comparatively speaking, there was not a significant reliance on doctors or hospitals for medical services. That was soon to change.

By the end of the 19th century and in the early 20th century, industrialization in America was associated with changes in the economy and family dynamics. There was a population shift from rural environments to urban centers. The household economy became dependent on the labor of the primary wage earner, and any illness or injury had a direct impact on the economic viability of the entire family. By the 1920s medicine began to play a larger role in people's lives. Hospitals became the centers for surgery and more advanced medical care. Because sickness now interrupted the family income and imposed additional unforeseen expenses, people began to visit physicians more regularly. As medical technology advanced, physician quality also improved. However, along with the advances in the medical delivery system, the cost of providing medical care escalated. By the end of the 1920s, as families began to demand greater access to medical services and the cost of care increased, there became a need for a different type of reimbursement system than the traditional methods of payment in preindustrial America.

By 1929, money in America was scarce. The Great Depression made hospitals economically unstable, and individuals suffered the hardships of lost jobs and lost income. Any illness brought even greater direct and indirect economic burden to families. However, with an increased urban migration, the demand for hospital care increased. As the increased need for hospital utilization escalated, an alternative payment system for medical services, which would ultimately revolutionize the health care industry, emerged. This new payment innovation, which many believe was the beginning of modern-day, prepaid health insurance, had its origin in Dallas, Texas. In 1929 a group of Dallas teachers contracted with Baylor University Hospital (now Baylor University Medical Center at Dallas) to provide 21 days of hospitalization for a fixed rate of 50 cents a month or $6.00 per year. The initial enrollment into this first model of a group health plan was 1250 Dallas area teachers. Within a short period of time, other groups of Dallas employees joined the program, which began to attract attention across the United States. Similar plans, following the Dallas prototype, began to emerge nationwide, some of which offered patients a choice of different hospitals within their community. This plan became the precursor or model for Blue Cross Insurance. The name of Blue Cross was adopted in 1934 by the St. Paul, Minnesota's group health plan, and by 1935 there were 15 Blue cross plans in 11 states. The concept of prepaid hospital insurance, which guaranteed hospital coverage and ensured the hospital charge would be paid, grew during the years of the Great Depression. The innovative Baylor plan had the support of the American Hospital Association, which encouraged networking with different hospital groups coordinating them into the Blue Cross network. This organization also reduced interhospital competition during a time when consumers suffered from reduced incomes and hospitals suffered from falling revenue. Blue Cross was given tax-exempt status by different states, allowing growth as a nonprofit organization. Tax exempt status also allowed this new insurance group to be free from the unusual insurance regulations.

Blue Shield, which covered the reimbursement of physician's services, emerged several years after Blue Cross. In 1939, the California Medical Association started the California Physician's Service (CPS), which was the first prepayment plan to cover physician fees. Individuals earning less than $3000 per year were eligible for enrollment. Employee groups were enrolled for a fee of $1.70 per employee per month. Different state and local medical societies began to form their own individual insurance plans. In 1946, the different physician-sponsored plans affiliated into what became Blue Shield. Like the Blue Cross plans, Blue Shield plans were to operate as nonprofits and were given tax exempt status. Both organizations were required to charge the different insured employee groups the same premium regardless of membership health status. This is known as community rating, which requires the company to charge the same premium for sicker people as for healthy people. By 1948, Blue Cross and Blue Shield planned to merge. The merger was not supported by the American Medical Association (AMA), which felt that the joint venture between hospitals and physicians could lead to issues regarding restraint in trade. Although remaining independent organizations, the Blues began working together on various policy issues. As the years passed, different corporate coordinating agencies were formed to direct the activities of their different member plans. The long-awaited merger of Blue Cross and Blue Shield was not completed until 1982.[1]

It was not long before the success of the Blues attracted competition from other for-profit insurance companies. During the ensuing years, there was a rise in the private health insurance industry. Because the new for-profit insurance companies were not tax exempt, they were also not under the same regulations as Blue Cross and Blue Shield. The commercial for-profit insurance companies were not required to community rate their policies and could undercut the Blues by offering lower premiums to healthier people while charging sicker individuals higher premiums. As competition intensified throughout the 1940s, the marketplace for private health insurance grew significantly from what had started out as the Baylor Plan in 1929. However, the explosive growth in health insurance coverage in the 1940s was not due just to competition. Other events including a series of government policies passed in the 1940s and 1950s changed the entire industry.

After America entered World War II in 1941, there was a labor shortage, yet companies needed to recruit employees. This could have lead to a wage war with employers forced to raise wages in order to compete for the scarce labor. The federal government reacted by imposing wage and price controls under the 1942 Stabilization Act.[2] But, while Congress imposed price and wage freezes, this act did allow employers to expand their benefit offers to attract employers. In addition to vacations and pensions, the new benefits included adoption of employee health insurance plans. These new health benefit packages turned out to be an important vehicle in securing workers, and provided private insurers a greater market for their products. The legislation eventually included provisions making employer-provided health coverage nontaxable, which was equivalent to receiving more salary without paying additional payroll tax. In 1945, the War Labor Board ruled that employers could not change or cancel the employee's insurance plan during the contracted period. The concept of employers providing and paying for the workers' medical insurance grew rapidly, and it became the primary mechanism for providing health insurance coverage in America.

By the 1950s, employment-based health insurance was firmly in place, and by the 1960s the private health insurance system was well established. However, healthcare expenses were also rising. This meant that the employer's cost of providing health insurance for employees was escalating. In addition, before 1965, private health insurance was the only widely available source of payment for health care. This meant it was available primarily to working people and their families. In a now prosperous economy, the political atmosphere became more favorable toward ensuring at least a minimum level of health care for its citizens, especially senior Americans who were no longer working and did not have employment-based coverage. Twenty years after the end of World War II, in 1965, Congress enacted Medicare as part of President Lyndon B Johnson's Great Society program. At the July 30, 1965 Medicare signing ceremony that took place in Independence, Missouri, President Johnson enrolled former President Harry Truman as the first Medicare beneficiary and presented him with the first Medicare card.[3]

Soon, as the expansion of medical technology and overall improvement in medical services occurred, along with increasing demand for medical care, overall medical costs began to rise dramatically. There were also increased requirements regarding the standards of quality for physicians and hospitals. With the introduction of Medicare and the evolution of a different physician evaluation and management documentation system, a new set of coding rules emerged that did not follow the traditional medical training and documentary skills taught in medical school.

The transformation of health care in our country from the rudimentary state of medical technology before 1920 to the sophisticated medical system that currently exists is associated with significant changes in how physicians practice and are reimbursed for services rendered. To have a successful practice and maintain compliance with the new coding principals, it is critical for physicians to understand the Medicare Evaluation and Management (E/M) coding system plus the rules published in the AMA Current Procedural Terminology (CPT) codebook and the CMS *Documentation Guidelines for Evaluation and Management Services.* Non-Medicare insurers also base reimbursements on the Medicare CPT definitions and interpretations for reporting documentation and coding.

Under the initial Medicare legislation, physicians were reimbursed according to the "usual, customary, and reasonable rate." Physicians were to bill patients directly for services rendered and the patient had to be reimbursed by Medicare. There were significant increases in medical costs, and Medicare expenditures also rose during the 1970s. To curb inflation, President Richard Nixon implemented the Economic Stabilization Program in 1971. This program included wage and price controls in an effort to contain escalating prices. In 1972, Professional Standards Review Organizations were created with the intent to limit the expansion of Medicare costs through oversight of physician practices. Despite additional congressional legislation, Medicare expenditures continued to rise sharply during the 1970s and 1980s. This escalation of health care expenditures precipitated more direct government intervention into how physicians were paid for services rendered.

In the 1980s, Congress passed different legislation involving Medicare and ultimately restructured the way physician services were reimbursed. In 1983, the Medicare reimbursement policy changed from reimbursing according to the "usual and customary" rates to a prospective payment system.

The Consolidated Omnibus Budget Reconciliation Act of 1985 (COBRA) mandated Medicare coverage for newly hired state and local government employees. In 1986, the Omnibus Budget Reconciliation Act (OBRA 1986) changed some of the payment procedures for different Medicare services in an effort to slow down Medicare spending. The Omnibus Budget Reconciliation Act of 1987 (OBMA 1987) dealt with quality standards for Medicare- and Medicaid-certified nursing homes. Because of continued rise in health care expenditures, the Balanced Budget and Emergency Deficit Control Reaffirmation Act of 1987 froze all Medicare payment rates. In 1988, Clinical Laboratory Improvement Amendments were enacted. This was intended to strengthen the quality requirements for clinical laboratories. In 1989, the Omnibus Budget Reconciliation Act (OBRA 1989) was signed into law by President George H. W. Bush. This Act, which went into effect in January 1992, significantly redefined the way Medicare paid for physician services. Instead of basing reimbursements on charges, the federal government established a Medicare fee schedule for physician services.

Coding and Billing for Physician Services in the United States

In place of paying physicians according to what they billed, the federal government established a standardized payment schedule based on a resource-based relative value scale (RBRVS). This is a system that originated in the late 1970s at the Harvard School of Public Health. A research team funded by what was then known as the Health Care Financing Administration (HCFA), and is now known as the Centers for Medicare and Medicaid Services (CMS), originally developed the methodology behind RBRVS. The principal investigators were William Hsiao, PhD, and Peter Braun, MD.[4] The research was done to identify and develop objective measures of physician work and a more cost-effective payment system for physicians across all specialties. The RBRVS system was designed to address the soaring cost of health care in the United States. In this system, payments for services rendered were quantified by determining the resource costs needed to provide them. After passage of the Omnibus Budges Reconciliation Act of 1989, legislation established the RBRVS for United States physicians, replacing prior charge-based payments. Under this new legislation, physicians were also prohibited from referring Medicare patients to clinical laboratories in which they had a financial interest. The RBRVS is used today by Medicare and most private insurers and remains the method for determining physician compensation for services provided. The new Evaluation and Management (E/M) model was part of the RBRVS system. Reimbursement policies for most cognitive medical specialties, including headache medicine, are based on compliant coding for E/M services. To receive appropriate compensation for the time and effort spent treating more complex patients, including the patient with refractory migraine, the headache physicians must understand better the complexities of RBRVS that produced the current CPT payment system and codes.

The RBRVS was developed to produce four main outcomes: (1) uniform policies nationwide, (2) a national fee schedule, (3) new CPT codes (particularly Evaluation and Management codes), and (4) establishment of relative values on the basis of the resources used by physicians to perform a particular service (physician work and practice expense; malpractice expense was added later). The fourth outcome is often referred to as "Standardization and redefining global services." Whereas the intent of RBRVS was to reduce the inequality between fees for cognitive services and payment for procedures, there still remains much discussion that challenges whether this goal was ever actually achieved. Some of the criticisms include the basic principles that define the RBRVS system. As an example, the "Conversion Factor" (which is discussed in more detail later), which translates resource-based relative value units (RVUs) into physician fees, is not the same for private carriers as it is for Medicare. Even more controversial are the differences, in allocation of practice expenses across services. The volume of diagnostic and imaging procedures has increased far more rapidly than the volume of office visits, which benefits specialists who perform those procedures. A simple review of the Documentation Guidelines confirms that the documentation requirements of complying with E/M regulations are much more complex and difficult than coding for a test or procedure. There is also no consistency in the ability of the current reimbursement system to capture differences in work between procedure-orientated specialties and physicians in "cognitive" specialties, such as most who see patients with refractory headaches of various types. To understand these issues better, let us take a closer look at how the RBRVS payment system is structured.

Physician services are reported using the Current Procedural Terminology (CPT) coding system. The E/M codes, as well as the rest of the CPT codes, are published in the annual edition of the AMA CPT codebook. The CPT codes are copyrighted by the AMA and are maintained by them through an annual evaluative process. RBRVS attaches a relative monetary value or Relative Value Unit (RVU) to each CPT code. A RVU is a numeric value that has been developed to represent three components of each medical service. The components of an RVU are:

1. Physician's Work: This is the physician's time, skill, mental effort, risk, and psychological stress of an adverse outcome. The physician's work takes into account the physician's expertise and time spent in preparation and follow-up documentation of each service performed. The physician's work component accounts for 52% of the total RVU for each service.
2. Practice Expense: This is the cost to operate a medical practice. Practice Expense includes the staff, salaries, the rent, office supplies, and office equipment. The physician's practice expense accounts for 44% of the total relative value for each service.

3. Medical Liability Insurance: The professional liability insurance expense is also an estimate of the relative risk of services. The malpractice costs are based on time and specialty specific national averages. This accounts for 4% of the total value for service.

Therefore, for every CPT code, each of the three components of physician work is assigned a RVU and the sum is the total RVU for that CPT code. The Total RVU = Work RVU + Practice Expense RVU + Medical Liability Insurance RVU. There are annual updates to physician work relative values. This is through the RVS Update Committee (RUC) which is an AMA/Specialty Society committee formed in 1991 to make recommendations to CMS on the RVU's to be assigned to new or revised codes in the Current Procedural Terminology (CPT) coding system. There is also a requirement that any RVU changes be budget neutral, which means that for every additional dollar allocated to a given service there is a dollar less for those who do not use a given code. Thus an increase in RVUs for one service can result in decreased reimbursements for other physician services. The RUC is an expert panel inclusive of all health care professionals. Non-MD/DOs (such as nurses, podiatrists, and physical therapists) have an advisory committee and one voting seat on the RUC. The RUC is involved in reviewing direct practice expense inputs. The RUC may submit recommendations to CMS but the latter is entirely responsible for all modifications to the RBRVS.

When periodically updating the physician system, CMS factors in a geographic adjustment factor known as the Geographical Practice Cost Index (GPCI). The GPCI adjusts the RVU for regional differences and is therefore based on practice location. The components of the GPCI include the disparity in the cost of living, the disparity in rent and wages, and the disparity in malpractice premiums. Using the three components of RVU (RVU work + RVU practice expense + RVU liability), one can calculate the total adjusted RVU as follows: Total adjusted RVU = RVUw × GPCIw + RVUpe × GPCIpe + RVUpe × GPCIpe.

As mentioned previously, under RBRVS the reimbursement for any given CPT code is based on the RVUs assigned to the CPT code multiplied by what is defined as a Conversion Factor (CF). The CF is what translates the RVU's into dollar amount or actual payment for the services provided. Any change in the CF impacts all CPT codes proportionally. The CF is updated annually by CMS. Therefore, using the CF, the calculation for physician reimbursement for any CPT code is: Payment = RVU × CF. The CF is a multiple of four components that all affect reimbursement. The four components are: (1) Estimated Medical Economic Index; (2) The Estimated updated Adjustment Factor, which is tied to what is known as the "Sustainable Growth Rate" (SGR); (3) Legislation change; and (4) Budget Neutrality, which indicates that any increase greater than $20 million must be accompanied by an equivalent reduction. The second component or SGR is essentially the expenditure target and is determined by different components and calculations. There has been criticism that the SGR formula does not keep pace with the cost of providing patient care or practice cost increases. The Medical Economic Index (MEI) has been suggested as an alternative to the SGR.[5] The MEI is a measure of inflation faced by physicians with respect to their practice costs and general wages. It measures input prices for resources needed to provide physician services, which could be a better indicator when estimating the increase in the total cost for the average physician to operate a medical practice. The MEI also measures year-to-year changes in prices for the various inputs to fund a physician practice. A change from the SGR formula to the MEI measure would affect the CF.

The use of RVUs as a measurement of physician productivity is also rapidly gaining popularity. As an example, an increasingly common application of using RVUs to determine physician compensation is seen for emergency room doctors. Productivity or work output of the emergency physician (EP) is frequently determined by how many RVUs that physician generated during his or her shift. The RVUs then translate into physician income. This method of determining physician compensation has its pros and cons, which are beyond the scope of this discussion. This practice has the potential to have a significant impact on physicians and other clinicians practicing headache medicine, particularly those working in group practices.

Evaluation and Management (E/M) services often make up more than 50% of total Medicare physician payments and a large part of private insurance expenditures. However, in most headache practices, especially when treating patients with refractory daily headaches, E/M constitutes the majority of patient care. As can be determined from the review of RBRVS in the preceding text, the direct role that complex policies of reimbursement have for consultancy and the ongoing care of chronic headache patients could produce additional economic obstacles for appropriate payment for services rendered. Understanding how to document the Key Components and Contributory Components of E/M CPT coding is crucial if the headache physician is to be properly reimbursed. It is not uncommon for headache physicians to perform level 4 or level 5 CPT services only to be down coded because of noncompliant documentation. To assist in proper documentation, CMS developed and published the 1995 and 1997 Documentation Guidelines for Evaluation and Management Services. The physician who is dedicated to treating the chronic refractory headache patient is generally a concerned individual who is focused on providing the best patient care possible. That same physician deserves to be appropriately compensated for his or her devotion to patient care.

Writing a review of CPT coding is akin to writing a novel in which the reader knows the ending before buying the book. In addition, although the plot seems to build in intensity, it does not lead to a final conclusion or resolution. On the contrary, reimbursement for physicians is a dynamic process, with periodic changes, which does not have a defined ending. William Osler, the Canadian who many consider the father of American medicine, is often quoted as saying, "Listen to the patient, he will tell you the diagnosis."

That teaching remains a central paradigm in medical schools today. However, in modern-day medical education, unlike in the times of Dr Osler, such concepts as RBRVS, RUVs, Conversion Factors, and the E/M documentation requirements of Medical Decision Making, are also important concepts for young physicians to learn. Historically, while the clinical portion of medical school education focuses upon history taking, physical examination, differential diagnosis, understanding disease entities, therapeutic interventions, medical procedures, and numerous other important topics including the physician–patient interaction, understanding medical economics is often relegated to on the job training after graduation. This plays an even more important role in "cognitive" medical specialties as headache medicine in which the history and physical examination remain the paradigm for diagnosis and treatment of patients. Because headache medicine is focused on E/M services, improper CPT coding and noncompliant E/M documentation translates into reimbursements that often do not correlate with the high level of care provided. Physicians should be paid for what they do, but are often down coded or compensated less than deserved because they do not understand the regulations that determine compensation. The RBRVS system identifies the rules; the *Documentation Guidelines* define how to be compliant with the rules; the physician is held responsible for knowing the rules of coding and compliant documentation.

By understanding better the coding rules, including the distinction between the CPT E/M coding guidelines and the CMS 1995 and 1997 *Documentation Guidelines*, the headache physician will have a more level playing field in meeting the demands of our changing and complex health care system. As stated previously, the CPT codes are published in the annual edition of the AMA codebook and are copyrighted by the AMA. These codes describe services and procedures and provide guidelines for E/M selection. The CPT codes incorporate the seven components of providing that care: History, Physical Examination, Medical Decision Making, Counseling, Coordination of Care, and Nature of the Presenting Problem and Time. These components are discussed in detail throughout this chapter. The CMS *Documentation Guidelines* are not published in any edition of the CPT codebook. These E/M *Documentation Guidelines* are developed and published by CMS and indicate how the services represented by the CPT code should be recorded according to CMS rules. It is important to recognize these distinctions because although the AMA was a key contributor in the development of the *Documentation Guidelines*, the AMA does not assume the role of dictating a payer's reimbursement policy and defers the decisions related to the adequacy of compliant documentation to the recognized CMS regulations. Therefore the rules for compliant documentation are found in the 1995 and 1997 CMS *Documentation Guidelines for Evaluation and Management Services* and not in the CPT codebook. It is the physician's challenge to meet these economic requirements of our health care system while still providing quality patient care under the time constraints of a busy practice. A working knowledge of the E/M methodology accomplishes the goal of quality care while conforming to the CPT E/M regulations.

The traditional approach to identifying the proper CPT code is documenting the physician's care, then trying to identify the code for that level of service. This type of retrospective analysis is based on the premise that in traditional medical training we are taught the history and examination skills and then instructed to document our findings into the medical record using guidelines that preceded the introduction of E/M coding and the *Documentation Guidelines.* This translates into identifying the appropriate CPT E/M code after the medical encounter and then secondarily attempting to calculate the proper level of care. In reality, this often does not work. Frequently the information necessary for E/M documentation had not been recorded or the time needed to perform the numerical calculations is not available. It becomes important for physicians to understand that a well documented medical record that is *prospectively* designed to meet compliance will facilitate efficiency and compliance. In addition, to help ensure more accurate coding and better reimbursements, there are some key points regarding the CPT coding system that are important to review.

When the AMA first developed and published the CPT nomenclature in 1966, a four digit system was used. The initial purpose of developing the CPT system was not centered toward reimbursement but was more focused to help standardizing terminology among physicians. It basically was designed to be a more efficient way to simplify medical records for physicians and medical record clerks.[6] By the time the second CPT edition was published in 1970, it was recognized that the codes needed to be more inclusive. The codes were expanded to five digits to designate diagnostic and therapeutic procedures. Since that time, all CPT codes are five-digit codes. Currently, the CPT coding system includes thousands of codes and definitions for medical services, procedures, and diagnostic tests. Every year, the AMA revises and updates the CPT codes and those changes become effective each January 1. The AMA's CPT Editorial Panel is responsible for maintaining the CPT nomenclature. The panel is made up of 17 members. The panel contains representatives not only from several of the larger medical specialties but also representation from Blue Cross and Blue Shield Association, the Health Insurance Association of America, CMS, the American Hospital Association, and two nonphysicians representing the Health Care Professionals Advisory Committee.[7] Hundreds of codes may be added, changed, or deleted annually and all are published in the updated CPT code books. It is therefore recommended that all health care professionals maintain current copies of the CPT code books.

There are three categories of CPT codes. The development of these categories are founded on the premise that CPT codes should be tiered to accommodate not only codes to report performance measures but also codes for emerging technology, services, and procedures. All of the E/M codes are included in Category 1 CPT codes. Category 1 codes describe a procedure or service performed. The Category 1 codes have a five-digit numeric value and descriptor nomenclature. They are based on the procedure being consistent with contemporary medical practice and being performed by many physicians in clinical practice in multiple locations. The Category 1 CPT codes are restricted to clinically recognized and generally accepted services, not emerging technologies, services, and procedures. Two additional CPT code categories debuted in 2002. Category 11 codes are a set of optional codes developed principally to support performance measurement. These codes are intended to facilitate data collection, do not have a relative value associated with them, and are not required for compliant E/M coding. These codes have been developed for following the care and good outcomes in certain clinical conditions. The Category 111 codes are temporary codes used for emerging technology, services, and procedures. These codes may have reimbursement potential with different carriers if the coverage is prearranged. Category 111 codes are not covered by Medicare.

The E/M codes used by most physicians, including those in headache medicine, to report a significant portion of their services, are 99201 through 99499. The E/M codes are divided into broad categories such as office visits, hospital visits, new patient encounters, and consultations. Some of these categories are further subdivided into two or more subcategories of E/M services. For example, office visits may be new patients or an established patient. Hospital visits may be an initial evaluation or subsequent visit. As indicated previously, E/M services are composed of seven recognized components: History, Physical Examination, Medical Decision Making (MDM), Nature of the Presenting Problem (NPP), Counseling, Coordination of Care, and Time. The first three components, History, Physical Examination, and Medical Decision Making, are recognized as the "Key Components" of E/M. The Nature of the Presenting Problem, Counseling, Coordination of Care, and Time are considered "Contributory Factors" in the majority of patient encounters. It is not required that the contributory services be provided at every or any patient encounter, although, as we will see later, *time* may be a significant factor if counseling and/or coordination of care constitute more than 50% of the physician-patient and/or family encounter. Time may then be considered the key or controlling factor in determining the level of E/M service.

The E/M system designates four categories for each of the Key Components. The History includes the traditional: CC, HPI, PFSH, and ROS. The four levels of the Physical Examination are: Problem Focused, Expanded Problem Focused, Detailed, and Comprehensive. The four elements of Medical Decision Making include: Straight Forward, Low Complexity, Moderate, and High Complexity. The Nature of the Presenting Problem(s) (NPP), although not listed as a key component, is also an E/M category of importance. It is another one of the nontraditional terms within the CPT coding system that becomes an important element in the basic format of the E/M coding system. The NPP has five categories: minimal, self-limited or minor, low severity, moderate severity, and high severity. The role of this contributory E/M component in coding is discussed later in this chapter.

In an attempt to simplify the basic format for E/M coding, one may subdivide each patient contact into five components: (1) Every patient encounter is assigned a specific CPT code that defines the level of service but also designates the place or type of service (e.g., office, or other outpatient setting or hospital). (2) The content of service is defined (e.g., using the four categories for each of the key components, history, physical and medical decision-making, as described previously). (3) Counseling and/or Coordination of care is described when that type of E/M service is provided (e.g., more than 50% of the encounter). (4) The Nature of the Presenting Problem(s) usually associated with the given level of care is described. (5) Time may be important (e.g., especially when counseling and/or coordination of care is the sole determining factor in E/M code selection).

To a large extent, physicians practicing headache medicine use about four or five different types of service codes for the majority of care they provide. The most frequently used CPT codes for outpatient and hospital visits are listed in Table 24.1. To understand E/M compliance better, it is important to define some of the coding rules. All medical services are characterized by face-to-face services for the purposes of classifying new and established patient encounters. A new patient is an individual who has not received any professional services from the attending physician, or another physician of the same specialty who is a member of the same group practice, within the past 3 years. An established patient is one who has received professional services from the physician, or another physician of the same specialty who belongs to the same group practice, within the past 3 years. The question of cross referral to a subspecialist within the same group frequently comes up. Unfortunately, the CPT definitions do not explicitly address this situation. If a general neurologist in a group refers a patient to a headache specialist within the same group, can that patient be considered a new patient evaluation for the headache specialist? The answer is probably yes. It does appear appropriate for cross referral within the same group so long as the consultative services are met. However, since the question of subspecialty reporting within a given specialty is not precisely defined by CPT, it would be best if the headache subspecialist had a separate tax identification number to avoid an auditor's subjective interpretation of the rules.

Table 24-1 E/M CPT Codes

Office or other Outpatient Services, *New Patient*	99201–99205
Office or other Outpatient Services, *Established Patient*	99211–99215
Hospital Inpatient Services, *Initial Hospital Care*	99221–99223
Hospital Inpatient Services, *Subsequent Hospital Care*	99231–99233
Office or Other Outpatient Consultations, *New or Established Patient*	99241–99245
Inpatient Consultations, *New or Established Patient*	99241–99255

Another important distinction to make is the difference between a new patient Consultation (99241–99245) and a New Patient Referral (99201–99295). For Medicare patients, the reimbursement for the former is greater than for the latter. For purposes of CPT, a Consultation is defined as a service provided by a physician whose expertise regarding evaluation and/or management of a specific patient problem is requested by another physician or other appropriate source. There is no request for transfer of care built into the rules defining a consultation. In most cases, a consultation is expected to be a one-time visit. However, if necessary, the consulting physician may initiate diagnostic or therapeutic services at the same visit or at subsequent visits. Even though treatment is initiated, the initial service is still considered a consultative service. When the consultant completes the consultation, depending on the situation, he or she may assume responsibility for management of all or a portion of the patient's care. The E/M services provided by the consulting physician after completion of the consultation should be reported with the appropriate level of office or other outpatient service code.[8]

Although traditionally, the terms *Consultation* and *Referral* have often been interchanged, a physician referral to another physician is not automatically a consultation. To be identified as a Consultation, there must be a request for consult from another physician or healthcare provider, the suspected or known diagnosis requires determination by the specialist who renders his or her opinion, the referring physician and consultant specifies a reason for the consultation, the treatment is undetermined or may be known, and a written report to the requesting physician or referring source is forwarded by the consultant. When the referring physician requests another doctor to assume the care of the patient, it is defined as transfer of care. This type of referral for evaluation and management of the patient cannot be considered a consultation and must be coded as a New Patient Referral. It should be emphasized that all of the above rules are related to Medicare patients. Currently, it appears that non-Medicare payers have not yet implemented these regulations.

For new patients, both Consultations and New Patient Referrals, all three of the key components, History, Physical Examination, and Medical Decision Making, must be reported. In addition, to qualify for a particular level of service, all three key components must be met or exceed. As seen in Table 24.2, for level 4 services the history and examination must be Comprehensive and MDM must be Moderate Complexity. To code a level 5 service the H&P must be Comprehensive and MDM of High Complexity. For an Established Patient encounter, only two of the three key components must be met or exceeded. For example, a level 4 service (99214) may have a Detailed H&P and the MDM may be Moderate Complexity. For a level 5 service (99215), the H&P may be Comprehensive and MDM High Complexity (Table 24.3).

Many of the terms used in the preceding paragraph are nontraditional medical concepts which nonetheless define how physician reimbursements are determined. The level of service, the complexity of the encounter, whether the visit is problem focused or expanded problem focused, and other terms as

Table 24-2 New Patient and Consultation office visit (3 out of 3)

Code	History	Exam	Medical Decision Making
99201 99241	Problem focused	Problem focused	Straightforward
99202 99242	Extended problem focused	Extended problem focused	Straightforward
99203 99243	Detailed	Detailed	Low Complexity
99204 99244	Comprehensive	Comprehensive	Moderate Complexity
99205 99245	Comprehensive	Comprehensive	High Complexity

Table 24-3 Established Patient – Office/OP (2 out of 3)

Code	History	Exam	Medical Decision Making
99211	Minimum services; physician not required		
99212	Problem focused	Problem focused	Straightforward
99213	Extended problem focused	Extended problem focused	Low Complexity
99214	Detailed	Detailed	Moderate Complexity
99215	Comprehensive	Comprehensive	High Complexity

medical decision making and nature of the presenting problem is an entirely new language that was introduced with the CPT E/M coding system. In addition to identifying a new paradigm for recording clinical findings, the physician is also responsible for "compliance" in regard to the rules set forth in the CPT codebook and *Documentation Guidelines.* To maintain consistency in reporting E/M services and appropriately report the codes that distinguish an individual patient encounter, it is crucial that the physician understands the terminology and learns the words and phrases used for E/M documentation. Irrespective of who does the coding for a physician's practice, it is the doctor who is ultimately responsible, economically and legally, for that determination. For Medicare, auditors have the authority to assess penalties for "fraud," up to $11,000 per visit, if the level of E/M codes is consistently up coded or not supported by the necessary documentation according to the guidelines.[9] Private insurers also have their own audits, which could be associated with frequent down coding and/or expulsion from their panel of doctors. Demands for the return of overpayments are also becoming more frequent. Repayments to insurers could result in a significant economic burden for a practice. As someone known to all of us once said: "The buck stops here".

The Levels of E/M Services are the coding categories that describe the amount of E/M care given at a patient encounter. The different levels of

E/M service "...encompass the wide variations in skill, effort, time, responsibility, and medical knowledge required for the prevention or diagnosis and treatment of illness or injury and the promotion of optimal health".[10] The CPT codebook identifies code descriptors for the levels of E/M services for the seven components. The descriptors for the key components, History, Examination and Medical Decision Making, may not be the same as for the contributory factors, Counseling, Coordination of Care. There are also differences in the rules delineating the key components. The 1995 and 1997 editions of the *Documentation Guidelines for Evaluation and Management Services* have introduced numerical values for the History and Physical Examination. As will be seen, for Medial Decision Making, while the physician is asked to quantify the "amount" of data and at the same time define the "complexity" of data, the guidelines do not provide specific direction to make these determinations. There are no quantifiable parameters to help meet compliance. Based on the information found in the guidelines, determination of the level of MDM is, to a large extent, a subjective assessment. Therefore, while determining the level of History and the level of the Physical Examination more closely follows the traditional medical record documentation model, the concept of Medical Decision Making presents an even greater challenge.

The E/M coding elements of the history is similar to the H&P taught for years in physical diagnoses classes in medical school. It consists of the chief complaint (CC); history of present illness (HPI); review of systems (ROS); and past, family, and social history (PFSH). All levels of the history must include the CC. The completeness of the other three components of the history is what determines whether the coding level is Problem Focused, Expanded Problem Focused, Detailed or Comprehensive. The medical record should describe the appropriate number of elements for each part of the history. (Table 24.4) Documentation of the CC and HPI must be a part of each patient visit. The PFSH and ROS are obtained at the initial patient encounter. The Documentation Guidelines state "A ROS and/or a PFSH obtained during

Table 24-4 Summary of Coding the Key Components of the History

Elements	Problem Focused	Expanded Problem Focused	Detailed	Comprehensive
HPI History of Present Illness	Brief (1-3 elements)	Brief (1-3 elements)	Extended (4 or more elements)	Extended (4 or more elements)
ROS Review of Systems	None	Problem specific	Extended	Complete
PFSH Past Medical, Family and Social History	None	None	Pertinent	Complete

an earlier encounter does not need to be re-recorded if there is evidence that the physician reviewed and updated the previous information".[11] It is also important to emphasize that the physician does not need to personally be the data entry person for this section of medical information. Another health care professional (such as a nurse, nurse practitioner, physician assistant, or medical assistant), can obtain this information from the patient or the PFSH and ROS can be completed by the patient and acknowledged, signed, and dated by the physician.

The Physical Examination also follows the traditional medical education model which teaches documentation of both the positive and negative findings for every organ system. The 1997 edition of the *Documentation Guidelines* defined 12 categories of Single System Examinations (SSE). The guidelines also require that any abnormal or relevant negative findings should be described in appropriate detail. This rule also applies to any abnormal or unexpected finding on examination of an asymptomatic body area or organ. Just saying "abnormal" is not sufficient. On the other hand, saying "normal" or "negative" is sufficient for an uninvolved part of the anatomy. The Single System Neurological examination consists of 25 elements or bullets. Most headache medicine physicians would use the Neurological SSE. The CPT descriptors for a Problem Focused examination, Expanded examination, Detailed examination, and Comprehensive examination can be found in Table 24.5. The examination templates built into the 1997 *Documentation Guidelines* (not found in the 1995 Guidelines) are easy to follow and ensure compliant documentation if used properly.

Because of the multiplicity of comorbid issues often associated with treating the refractory headache patient, a comprehensive history and physical examination, in most instances, is a part of the initial evaluation. For the same reasons, the average patient follow-up visit would also be a comprehensive evaluation and management service. Based on this premise, it would mean that the first two of the three E/M key components, History and Examination, would be at a level 4, and often level 5, category of service. Essentially, for CPT E/M coding, the headache physician treating the refractive headache patient starts out of the gate ahead of the pack. But it is important to remember that E/M levels are determined by documentation of three of three components for New Patients or Consultations and two of three components for Established Patients. In addition, if any of the three Key Components do not meet the documentation requirements for that particular service, then the lower level of service would need to be selected. It is the inadequate documentation of Medical Decision Making that is often the cause for down coding even if the visit justifies a higher code. It is not uncommon for physicians to record MDM according to the traditional documentation of *diagnosis, recommendations, and treatment plan.* This is not MDM as defined by the E/M guidelines. Unfortunately, Medical Decision Making is not part of the traditional H&P template and deals with components of the patient encounter, which could be an intellectual challenge for many physicians. It now becomes necessary to rate the *complexity* of the decision making, plus rate the *complexity* of the

Table 24-5 Single System Neurological Examination

Elements (Bullets)				
Constitutional • Measurement of any 3 or 7 vital signs • General appearance of the patient **Eyes** • Ophthalmoscopic examination **Cardiovascular** • Examination of the carotid arteries • Auscultation of the heart • Examination of the peripheral vascular system **Neurological** • Higher cortical functions • Cranial nerves • Sensation • Muscle strength • Muscle tone • Deep tendon reflexes • Coordination • Gait and station	▪ 1–5 Bullets	▪ At Least **6** Bullets	▪ At Least **12** Bullets	▪ Perform **All** Bullets
	Problem Focused	Expanded Problem Focused	Detailed	Comprehensive

diagnosis and therapeutic options. The *amount* and *number* of items is to be documented. There is also a need to address the *risk* associated with the diagnosis, necessary tests and management options selected. To be more specific, the fundamental principles of MDM are measured by the three following elements:

1. The number of possible diagnoses and/or the number of management options that must be considered
2. The amount and/or complexity of medical records, diagnostic tests, and/or other information that must be obtained, reviewed or analyzed
3. The risk of significant complications, morbidity, and/or mortality, as well as comorbidities, associated with the patient's presenting problem(s), the diagnostic procedures(s) and/or the possible management options

The guidelines recognize four levels for each of the three components listed in the preceding text. The level of MDM for a given visit depends on the highest two out of these three elements. There are instructions for calculating the MDM which can be found in the *AMA Current Procedural Terminology CPT Codebook.* These calculations are based on the MDM grid published in the CPT codebook. Unfortunately, for many physicians the whole mechanism of trying to calculate MDM is so complicated and time consuming that the directives cannot be effectively employed. In addition, the *CPT Codebook* and *Documentation Guidelines* do not provide the necessary quantifiable parameters for compliance. Nonetheless, the requirements for documentation of MDM must still be met for outpatient initial visits, outpatient consultations, and established patient visits.

To help document the quantitative values under Number of Diagnoses or Management Options and Amount and/or Complexity of Data to be Reviewed different scoring systems have been developed by experts in the field of CPT E/M coding. Although the various methods are not part of the CMS guidelines, the computation tables have been widely accepted as a way of transferring MDM data into a numerical value. Examples of representative point systems that are commonly found in the literature and on the Internet can be found in Tables 24.6 and 24.7. It must be emphasized that because the government coding guidelines do not define one specific scoring system that would guarantee that Medicare or individual insurance carriers would accept a particular computation table for MDM calculations, every physician must still do his or her best to record all the significant details of the visit as best as possible.

Another important part of MDM which is frequently misunderstood by physicians is the importance of documenting the subjective impressions about a relative problem, or *differential diagnosis.* All too often there has been a misconception that for reimbursements, a specific diagnosis must be recorded and that a differential diagnosis or "rule out" diagnosis would not be acceptable. The principle of recording a specific diagnosis primarily applies to International Classification of Diseases (ICD) coding, and even then, there

Table 24-6 Number of Diagnoses or Treatment Options

Diagnoses or Treatment Options	Number	Points	Result (Total)
Self-limited or minor (Stable, improved or worsening)	Max = 2	1	
Established problem (Stable, improved)		1	
Established problem (Worsening)		2	
New problem (No additional workup planned)	Max = 1	3	
New problem (Additional workup planned)		4	

Table 24-7 Amount/Complexity of Data Reviewed (more than 1 may apply)

Data Reviewed	Points (Total)
Order/review clinical lab tests	1
Order/review from radiology services	1
Order/review from medical services	1
Discussion of tests results with performing provider	1
Decision to obtain old records/history/discuss case with provider	2
Independent visualization of image, tracing or report	2

are different interpretations regarding a "definitive" diagnosis and a "working" diagnosis. While MDM requires recording the number of diagnosis to help identify the level of coding, listing a number of ICD diagnoses does not necessarily increase the potential for a higher level of care. Although it is often appropriate to record more ICD diagnoses when indicated, it is important to recognize that the ICD coding system is used to code signs, symptoms, injuries, diseases, and conditions. It is the CPT coding system that describes the medical procedure or services. Therefore, the ICD code describes the clinical condition of the patient to support the medical necessity of the CPT procedure or service. Choosing the proper CPT code defines the level or reimbursement. When documenting the CPT component of Medical Decision Making, quantifying the Number of Diagnoses or Management Options, including a differential diagnosis, is important. The rules defining this component of MDM are clearly stated in the E/M Documentation Guidelines: "... for a presenting problem without an established diagnosis, the assessment or clinical impression may be stated in the form of a differential diagnoses or as a 'possible', 'probable', or 'rule out' (R/O) diagnoses."[12] Basically, the guidelines ask the physician to describe the differential diagnosis including alternative diagnoses. This may include descriptive adjectives as 'severe," "refractory," and "daily headaches." Just using ICD-9 diagnoses does not permit any narrative related to the patient's clinical condition. Under MDM, the Number of Diagnoses or Management Options is really asking for qualitative information to help describe the nature of the patient's clinical state.

The third element of Medical Decision Making, the Risk of Complications and/or Morbidity or Mortality, is another nontraditional part of MDM. This component considers the level of risk to the patient within the decision-making process, or more specifically: "the risk of significant complications, morbidity and/or mortality, as well as comorbidities, associated with the patient's presenting problem(s), the diagnostic procedure(s), and/or the possible management options."[13] The assessment of risk of the presenting problem(s) is based on the risk between the present encounter and the next one. The assessment of risk of selecting diagnostic procedures and management options is based on the risk during and immediately following the procedure or treatment. The guidelines also state: "The highest level of risk in any one category (presenting problem(s), diagnostic procedure(s), or management options) determines the overall risk."[14]

The identification and documentation of the appropriate level of risk is based on explanations provided in the Table of Risk. The Table can be found in the 1997 *Documentation Guidelines* and provides common clinical examples, within the three categories or risk, which serve as a guideline to help measure the risk inherent in medical problems and procedures. If a physician were to use the Table of Risk to classify the complicated refractory headache patient, there are features in the high-risk category which frequently characterize these individuals. Also, although documentation of the risk for only one category meets compliance for determining the overall risk, there may be added benefit in documenting another category if the risk is also at the higher level.

The Guidelines state: "Because the determination of risk is complex and not readily quantifiable, the table includes common clinical examples rather than absolute measures of risk."[15] Therefore, the Table serves as a guideline to help measure the risk inherent in a medical problem or procedure. When physicians in headache medicine apply these definitions to the care given to the complicated refractory headache patient, it becomes apparent that this group of individuals often meets the CPT criteria for high-risk designation. This is especially true in the risk categories of "Management Options Selected" or number of treatment options and "Presenting Problem(s), or the level or risk of complications and/or morbidity or mortality (Table 24.8). Thus, if the physician treating complicated refractory headache patients becomes familiar with the Table of Risk and uses the common clinical scenarios described in the table, it is likely that most patients would meet the criteria for "Drug therapy requiring intensive monitoring for toxicity" and/or "One or more chronic illnesses with severe exacerbation, progression, or side effects of treatment." This indicates that this group of patients would often be at a risk level 4 or level 5. A summary for scoring all MDM can be found in Table 24.9.

While the Table of Risk includes "Presenting Problem(s)" as one of the three categories defining the level of risk, it is important that the physician understand what role this component of CPT coding plays in determining the overall level of E/M care. The Nature of Presenting Problem (NPP) has already been referenced earlier in this section as one of the seven components of

Table 24-8 Table of Risk Comparison: Elements Relevant to Headache Specialists Extracted from Table of Risk

	Number of Treatment Options	Risk of Complications
Minimum	Rest	One self-limited or minor problem
Low	Over the counter drugs	Stable chronic illness
Moderate	Prescription drug management	One or more chronic illnesses with mild exacerbation
High	Drug therapy requiring intensive monitoring for toxicity	One or more chronic illnesses with severe exacerbation

Table 24-9 Summary of MDM

	Straightforward	Low Complexity	Moderate Complexity	High Complexity
Diagnosis/Management Options	≤1	2	3	≥4
Amount/Complexity of Data	≤1	2	3	≥4
Risk	Minimal	Low	Moderate	High

E/M coding. Although it is not one of the key components and listed as a contributory component, the significance of the NPP not only helps define *risk* in Medical Decision Making but also plays a central role in the CPT coding system. The Nature of Presenting Problem is another nontraditional term that was introduced in the Current Procedural Terminology literature and found in the Evaluation and Management (E/M) Services Guidelines section of the CPT codebook. Basically, the NPP is an evaluation of what level of care the patient will need after obtaining the medical history. It is an estimate of the complexity of care, which should then serve as guideline when completing the other two key components of E/M; the Physical Examination and Medical Decision Making. The NPP is not synonymous with the patient's Chief Complaint. The assessment of severity and/or potential functional impairment can best be determined after completing all the E/M components of the History. The degree of severity is also measured by what outcome the patient may have if their individual medical condition were not treated. In other words, just as seen in the discussion of *risk*, the NPP includes any potential morbidity and mortality associated with the patient's condition. The Nature of Presenting Problem is a disease, condition, illness, injury, symptom, sign, finding, complaint, other reason for the encounter, with or without a diagnosis being established at the time of the encounter.

CPT E/M guidelines include documentation of the Nature of Presenting Problem in the patient's medical record. As indicated previously, the CPT manual describes five levels of the severity of the NPP:

Minimal: A problem that may not require the presence of the physician, but service is provided under the physician's supervision.

Self-limited or minor: A problem that runs a definite and prescribed course, is transient, and is not likely to permanently alter the health status or has a good prognosis with management/compliance

Low severity: A problem in which the risk of morbidity without treatment is low; there is little to no risk of mortality without treatment; full recovery without functional impairment is expected.

Moderate severity: A problem in which the risk of morbidity without treatment is moderate; there is moderate risk of mortality without treatment; uncertain prognosis or increased probability of prolonged functional impairment.

High severity: A problem in which the risk of morbidity without treatment is high to extreme; there is a moderate to high risk of mortality without treatment or high probability of severe, prolonged functional impairment.

Documentation of the NPP therefore records the medical necessity for the visit. It should also be emphasized that depending on the findings on Physical Examination and determination of Medical Decision Making, the NPP may be adjusted at any point during the patient encounter. After documenting the NPP following the History, there should be an integration of the level of care on completion of all the E/M key components at the end of the visit. Another extremely helpful tip for determining code selection are the Clinical Examples found in Appendix C in the CPT codebook. This is an important part of the CPT coding manual that most physicians do not even know exits. Appendix C includes clinical vignettes which provide a comprehensive and helpful guide for physicians to help define the level of services provided to their patients. In addition to all CPT types of services, these clinical examples illustrate how the NPP can be correlated to a specific code for a New Patient Evaluation and Established Patient visit. For example, one of the vignettes for a level 5 (99205) New Patient Evaluation defines an initial office visit for a 49-year-old female with a history of headaches and dependence on opioids. She reports weight loss, progressive headache, and depression. Another vignette for a level 4 (99214) Established Patient visit is that of a patient with frequent intermittent, moderate to severe headaches requiring beta blocker or tricyclic antidepressant prophylaxis, as well as four symptomatic treatments, but who is still experiencing headaches at a frequency of several times a month that are unresponsive to treatment. A level 5 (99215) Established Patient visit includes a patient who has acute migraine with new onset neurological symptoms and whose headaches are unresponsive to previous attempts at management with a combination of preventive and abortive medication. Clearly for physicians involved in Headache Medicine, it would be worthwhile to become familiar with the clinical examples in Appendix C of the CPT manual.

By now it should be apparent, that with proper documentation and based on the definitions of the five NPP levels and vignettes in Appendix C, CPT coding for the refractory headache patient New Patient or Established Patient visit, in most instances, may be at an E/M level 4 or 5. However, although some of the clinical examples found in the CPT code book, as in the case illustrated above, are similar to many of the patients seen by headache medicine physicians, it should be emphasized that the vignettes are only general examples. They are not meant to be absolute correlations or templates for defining the level of CPT coding. In essence, the vignettes are guidelines to help the physician determine the level of care. It still comes down to the key components of E/M. The three components of History, Examination, and Medical Decision Making must be met and documented in the medical record to report a particular level of service. Even though the CPT E/M prompts and various vignettes found in the *Documentation Guidelines* Table of Risk and CPT Appendix C may support a level 4 or level 5 code for this more complicated group of headache patients, if the medical record is not in compliance with the E/M guidelines, physician reimbursements will not be at the higher levels of care. It is not uncommon, however, for headache specialists to spend large amounts of time obtaining a history and reviewing the patient's clinical situation, plus discussing risks and benefits of treatment, in lieu of repeating the physical examination at each visit. How, then, does a physician in a cognitive specialty such as headache medicine receive appropriate compensation for spending 30 to 60 minutes, or longer, talking to a patient and/or family without meeting the three key components of E/M coding. Fortunately, there are circumstances when time, and not the key components of H&P and MDM, may become the determining factor in E/M coding.

When Counseling and Coordination of Care comprises more than 50% of the patient visit, *time* is permitted to become the single essential element in defining the level of E/M service. Although the commonly used CPT E/M codes do include time in the visit code description, when the three key E/M components are used, the time values are averages to assist physicians in selecting the most appropriate level of E/M services. The specific times associated with each code may be higher or lower depending on the clinical situation. Therefore, times associated with each CPT code are generally not meant to be used to select the level of E/M service when the key components are used to describe the patient encounter. However, when Counseling and Coordination of Care takes more than half of a visit, time is then permitted to become the single essential element in defining the level of E/M even if the physician did not do an examination or document Medical Decision Making. If Counseling and Coordination of Care dominates (>50%) the encounter, these contributory components may be used in place of the three key components of E/M. When time is defined as the controlling element of the visit, it is crucial that the extent of Counseling and/or Coordination of Care be properly documented in the medical record. In addition, specific details about the type and content of counseling need to be included in documentation.

If time is considered the key or controlling factor to qualify for a particular level of E/M out patient service, it must be *face to face* time that the physician spends with the patient and/or family. On the other hand, for physician hospital services, CPT defines unit/floor time. This is the time that the physician is present on the patient's hospital unit and the bedside rendering services for that patient. Unit/floor time may include the time in which the physician establishes and/or reviews the patient's chart, examines the patient, writes notes, and communicates with other professionals and the patient's family. Conversely, for office visits, such visit components as review of x-rays or laboratory tests, phone calls, and the medical record documentation of the visit are not reflected in the CPT stated time but are included in determining the work value of an E/M service. All further discussion of *time* will be focused on outpatient Consultation and/or Coordination of Care physician services.

The CPT nomenclature for E/M coding refers to Counseling as face to face discussions regarding diagnostic results, impressions and/or recommended diagnostic studies. Important components of the discussion including prognosis, risks and benefits of management options, instructions for treatment and/or follow-up visits, importance of compliance with chosen management options, risk factor reduction, and patient and/or family education must also be recorded. In the practice of headache medicine, especially when treating the more complex refractive headache patient, these contributory components often dominate the visit. If the physician elects to report the level of service based on Counseling, the content of the discussion must be completely documented in the patient's medical record. The physician must also document that more than 50% of the encounter was spent in these activities. If Coordination of Care is also defined as part of the visit, the physician must also document the time spent in arranging and organizing the patient's care with other physicians or providers or even agencies if applicable.

The importance of compliant documentation of the medical record cannot be overemphasized. If Counseling and *time* becomes the determining E/M factor of the patient encounter, specific CPT guidelines that must be followed. The medical record should be legible and include the date of the encounter. Relevant history and the reasons for the encounter must be clearly defined. As indicated previously, discussion of the assessment and clinical impression, or diagnosis, should include appropriate health risk factors and the current treatment plan. The patient's progress, or lack of progress, must be explained. Any changes in therapy and the rationale for additional diagnostic tests must be justified. The CPT and ICD codes should support one another. If Counseling and/or Coordination of Care did dominate the visit, the documentation within the medical record should be complete enough to substantiate the implied claim that the amount of time spent with the patient would give reason for the CPT code chosen. The time spent with the patient should have some proximity to the time values that are listed in the CPT codebook for each type of E/M service and level of care.

Conclusion

The historical development of providing health insurance for Americans has been associated with greater demands on physician reporting of services rendered. What began 80 years ago as a 50 cent a month insurance plan for Dallas teachers at Baylor University Medical Center grew to the 1992 Medicare Payment Reform program with implementation of the Resource Based Relative Value System. It has been 17 years since the initial publication of the Evaluation and Management coding system in the 1992 American Medical Association CPT codebook. The first edition of the Health Care Financing Administration (now CMS) *Documentation Guidelines for Evaluation and Management Services* was published 14 years ago. Medicare introduced their next version of the *Documentation Guidelines* in 1997, 12 years ago. Ever since the introduction of the E/M system, there has been physician concern regarding the complexity and administrative burden associated with documentation and the rules of compliance. Although there have been proposed revisions to the guidelines to reduce some of the physician burden, the proposals were never finalized. Compliant documentation and coding must still follow the rules defined in the initial E/M publications. Physicians may use either the 1995 or 1997 Guidelines. Both versions may be accessed at: www.cms.hhs.gov/medlearn/emdoc.asp.

The E/M CPT system still remains the methodology that determines how physician's get paid in our current health care environment. In addition, both physicians and administrators recognize the challenges created by the ongoing changes in the Medicare and insurer reimbursement policies. To maintain E/M compliance, there is a need to understand the Medicare rules and regulations, which are, themselves, often ambiguous and sometimes open to interpretation. In addition, it is also important for providers to understand the different guidelines and rules that may differ from Medicare but appear in contracts with private party payers. This is especially true in cognitive specialties as Headache Medicine, which focuses on E/M.

Because Headache Medicine is a relatively new area of specialization, payers often do not understand the disability and dysfunction that accompanies the complex patient population treated by headache specialists. This is especially true when treating the refractory headache patient. Before the 1970s, there were very few headache specialty clinics and those that existed were primarily affiliated with an academic institution or hospital. As early as 1988, only 21 years ago, the first *International Classification of Headache Disorders*, ICHD-I, was introduced and 16 years latter, 2004, the ICHD-II was published. The definition of Refractory Migraine and Refractory Chronic Migraine was first published in June 2008 by Schulman et al.[16] Because of the newness of Headache Medicine as a specialty service, multispecialty Neuroscience initiatives have only recently begun to include "Headache Centers" as a component of the Neuroscience program. In addition, reimbursement for headache care is also undergoing a period in which payers are just beginning to understand the importance of appropriate headache management. Insurance carriers have always recognized their direct economic burden associated with less than optimal care for complicated and/or refractory headache patients. They are now beginning to understand the positive societal, personal, and quality of life benefits that are concurrent with optimal patient care. Quality care for headache patients also translates into cost savings for insurers. In a healthcare environment, where the economic future even includes the possibility of universal health insurance, there are many uncertainties. One thing, however, is certain. A physician specializing in Headache Medicine who understands the current E/M CPT regulations, and who is compliant with the document guidelines, will have a better opportunity for a level 4 and level 5 reimbursement for New Patient and Established Patient care. Those with little or no knowledge who follow the old traditional paradigm of documentation and/or rely on others to do their coding without personal involvement run the risk of poor reimbursements, or, at worst, an audit, with potentially serious adverse financial impact.

References

1. Blue Cross and Blue Shield Company History: www.fundinguniverse.com/company.../Blue-Cross-and-Blue-Shield-Association-Company-History.html

2. President Franklin D. Roosevelt's Executive Order Providing for the Stabilization of The National Economy. October 3, 1942; White House News Release.
3. Narration regarding the signing of Medicare in 1965, including a sound clip of President Johnson enrolling former President Truman as the first Medicare beneficiary www.socialsecurity.gov/history/mpeg/videosound.html#9
4. Hsaio WC. The Resource-Based Relative Value Scale: toward the development of an alternative physician payment system. *JAMA*. 1987;258:799–802.
5. Joint Recommendations on Eliminating the SGR and Supporting Efforts to Promote Health Care Quality and Appropriateness. www.aace.com/advocacy/leg/pdfs/MedicareReformPrinciples.pdf
6. Principles of CPT Coding, 4th ed. Chicago: American Medical Association; 2005:3.
7. Principles of CPT Coding. 4th edi. Chicago: American Medical Association; 2005:4.
8. Revised Medicare Claims Processing Manuel, January 1, 06. Related CR no. 4215: Consultation Services Current Procedural Terminology (CPT) Codes 99241-99255. www.cms.hhs/MedlearnMattersArticles/downloads/MM4215.pdf.
9. CMS website on Fraud and Abuse. www.lamedicare.com/provider/medguide/safeguards1.pdf
10. American Medical Association. *Current Procedural Terminology CPT 2007.* Chicago: AMA Press;2007:3.
11. Health Care Financing Administration. *Documentation Guidelines for Evaluation and Management Services.* Chicago: American Medical Association;1997:6.
12. Health Care Financing Administration. *Documentation Guidelines for Evaluation and Management Services.* Chicago: American Medical Association;1997:45.
13. American Medical Association. *Current Procedural Terminology CPT 2007.* Chicago: AMA Press;2007:7.
14. Health Care Financing Administration. *Documentation Guidelines for Evaluation and Management Services.* Chicago: American Medical Association;1997. p 47.
15. Health Care Financing Administration. *Documentation Guidelines for Evaluation and Management Services.* Chicago: American Medical Association;1997:47.
16. Schulman EA, Lake AE, Goadsby PJ, et al. Defining refractory migraine (RM) and refractory chronic migraine (RCM): proposed criteria for the refractory headache special interest section of the American Headache Society. *Headache.* 2008; 48: 778–782.

Index

Note: Page references followed by "*f*" and "*t*" denote figures and tables, respectively.